EVOLVING A CULTURE OF MEDICAL EXCELLENCE

The First Sixty Years of the Hawaii Permanente Medical Group: The "Permanente" of Kaiser Permanente of Hawaii

ALBERT J. MARIANI, M.D.

ISBN: 978-1-7167-1909-7 (sc)
ISBN: 978-1-7167-1910-3 (hc)
ISBN: 978-1-7167-1907-3 (e)

Library of Congress Control Number: 2020913988

Lulu Publishing Services rev. date: 08/27/2020

CONTENTS

PREFACE

I t was more than twenty years ago. In a casual conversation with the Kaiser Permanente Hawaii regional corporate attorney, he mentioned that to open up storage space and eliminate even miniscule liability, all the old regional records, including the Hawaii Permanente Medical Group (HPMG) archives, were to be purged. No one seemed to care. I was appalled.

I had been a student of history since childhood. That, in turn, spurred an interest in leadership as a tool to make things better. This paralleled a fascination with science that eventually translated to a medical career. I joined the Hawaii Permanente Medical Group as a staff urologist in 1980 immediately after completing my five-year urology training at the Mayo Clinic. The Mayo Clinic was to me a model of principled medical excellence and efficiency. Historically, it had been an early clinical model for Kaiser Permanente. Kaiser Permanente had added the social reform dimension of providing state-of-the-art, affordable health care for as much of the population as possible. For someone who had matured in the 1960s and 1970s, it was a great fit.

Active in student leadership since high school, the resolution to stay out of politics to concentrate on clinical medicine at HPMG was a failed mission. Within six months of my arrival, I had been asked to chair the Cancer Committee and reorganize the Multiphasic Screening program. Within two years of that, I was appointed chief of surgical services. For the rest of my over twenty-nine-year career with HPMG, I was deeply involved at an executive, insider level with the decision-making of HPMG. Upon retirement, this involvement had represented more than half of the entire history of the Medical Group and almost half of my life.

In the course of these duties I had come to know and work closely with many of the leaders and founders of HPMG, those of my own generation, and for a very satisfying five years, the current generation. The older physicians told vivid stories of hardship and hard-won victories spiced by hard lessons, bitter controversy, treachery, and idealism, especially idealism. HPMG has a rich heritage. It would have been lost with the destruction of the archives. At the time of my retirement, the few survivors of the first generation were already into their nineties, while the second generation had mostly retired and were in their midsixties.

Certain historical records were saved, but when would someone again look longingly at the storage space and decide that it could be better used for something else? Outside-sourced accounts of the early years of HPMG were often inaccurate as to details. They had come predominantly from the oral histories of national Health Plan and Permanente leaders and the historical narratives from other regions—often decades after the actual events. In these, references to Hawaii were digressions from the main narrative and occasionally inaccurate. I decided that my postretirement project would be to write an accurate history of HPMG to be completed in time for the sixtieth anniversary in 2020. Graciously, the current HPMG administration assisted with these efforts.

This book is a narrative and not an academic treatise. I have vivid, bad memories of reading unreadable management and corporate history books that were inflicted upon me as a result of management peer pressure. I resolved to make this narrative as readable and accurate as possible. Nevertheless, incorporating sex, violence, treachery, and triumph of the human spirit, the staples of media, into a corporate history would be a good trick. This narrative likely failed in this regard. Given the vast range of human behavior—good and bad, especially when describing political events where the stakes were high, as were emotions, such a narrative could get emotionally quite raw. Efforts at political correctness, while made to avoid egregious offense, were modest in the interests of accuracy and clarity. This is not a public relations piece.

This narrative is unlikely to be a best seller. That wasn't the intention. The topic—the story of the slow, successful evolution of a culture of excellence in a medium-sized medical group in a small state—is too narrow for general audiences. The book may, however, be of interest to four groups.

The first group would be those who might have an interest of the story of the doctors who care for almost a fifth of Hawaii's population and the exclusive partnership with Kaiser Permanente that made it possible. In my opinion, more than anything else, the founding principles of Kaiser Permanente made it possible. For those curious about how those principles contributed to the success of the Hawaii region are encouraged to skip directly to the epilogue first.

The second group would be the past and present doctors of the Hawaii Permanente Medical Group who are curious as to why things are the way they are in HPMG. More broadly, it may be of interest to all those who were associated with the Kaiser Permanente Hawaii region and who dedicated their career to its success. Without them there would be no story.

The third target group for this book are those doctors who, having mastered clinical medicine, are willing to give back even more by trying their hand at leadership to carry on and enhance the HPMG culture of excellence. It is to them that the book is dedicated. An important component of the evolution of this culture of excellence has been the purposeful provision of increasing amounts of formal training for those willing to go that extra mile. To the extent that this book might assist these educational efforts would give me great personal satisfaction.

Finally, the fourth group might be those who might be interested in the unvarnished realities of delivering health care at the ground level from a physician's viewpoint and given these realities how one group of doctors established a durable, virtuous cycle of continuous improvement.

Al Mariani, MD
May 15, 2019

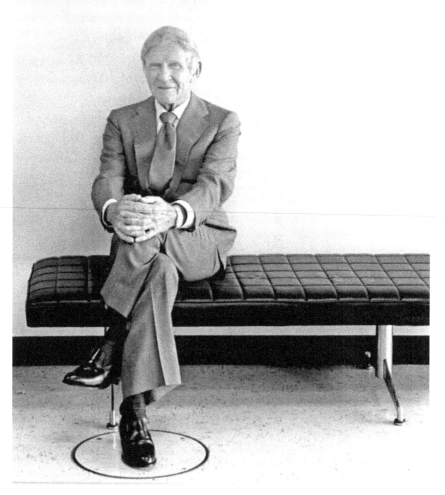

Sidney Garfield, MD, visionary cofounder of Kaiser Permanente.

CHAPTER 1

SIDNEY GARFIELD, MD: VISIONARY

Prepayment and Preventive Care: The Desert Experience

Perhaps it was the isolation and the harshness of the environment. The desert does focus the mind. It was during his desert experience that Sidney Garfield germinated a concept of a health care-delivery program that evolved into Kaiser Permanente—the largest civilian-managed care-delivery program in the United States.

It was 1933. The Great Depression was at its height, and almost a quarter of the US workforce was unemployed. Sidney R. Garfield, MD, was finishing his surgical training at the prestigious Los Angeles County General Hospital program. Employment prospects for a young general surgeon were bleak. One of the few opportunities for the unemployed in Southern California was the construction of the Colorado River Aqueduct (1933–9). It was a massive public works project designed to carry water from the Colorado River across the Mohave Desert to the population centers of Southern California. It employed up to ten thousand workers at a time. The work was dangerous. Being in the middle of the Mohave Desert, local fee-for-service medical care was nonexistent.

On the advice of a friend from residency, Garfield borrowed money from his family and constructed a twelve-bed hospital about six miles out of Desert Center—a gas stop/restaurant—in the Mojave Desert about halfway between the Colorado River and Los Angeles. While there was plenty of pathology to be treated, there was little reimbursement as insurance companies delayed or denied payment for services rendered.

Within a year, the hospital was facing bankruptcy as a result of payment denials. Ironically, it was the idea of two insurance executives, A. B. Ordway and Harold Hatch, employees of Industrial Insurance Exchange, that saved the hospital. Industrial Insurance Exchange was the largest insurer on the Colorado River project and was one-third owned by Kaiser Industries. It had the most to lose if Garfield's hospital closed. It would then have to ship every injury to Los Angeles.

Hatch proposed to Garfield a nickel-a-day premium (ninety-five cents in 2018 dollars) for the industrial injury care of the workers. Garfield accepted. Shortly after, Garfield proposed another nickel a day to the workers for comprehensive care of the workers and their families. Most workers signed up. With guaranteed payment, the financial situation immediately improved. Resources formerly spent on billing could now be devoted to medical care. With guaranteed prepayment, investments could confidently be made in staff and facilities to deliver better care. By the end of the project, the hospital had expanded to three hospitals and a string of clinics to serve work camps spaced over 150 miles.

More important, preventive care was now aligned with the economic interest of Garfield's medical care program. In a fee-for-service model, preventive care is at odds with the economic interest of a medical care program. Simply stated, in a fee-for-service model, if there is no treatment, there is no fee. The more treatment rendered, the more fees paid. In a prepaid program, the payment has already been received. The less treatment needed as a result of preventive care, the more resources are left over for other care—but only in a nonprofit model. There was now an economic incentive to prevent injury and disease. It now made sense to go to the work site where the nail puncture injuries were coming from, clean it up, and hammer down protruding nails, which was exactly what Garfield's caregivers did.

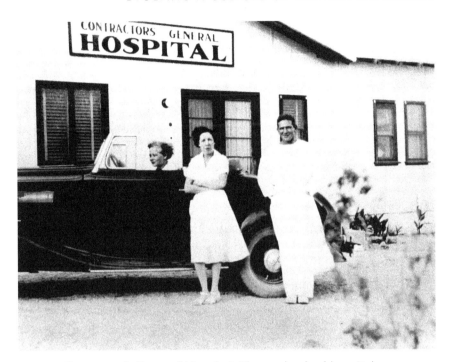

Contractor's General Hospital: The twelve-bed hospital on the middle of the Mohave Desert—prepayment saved it.

Group Practice and Integrated Facilities: The Grand Coulee Dam Experience

One thing that Garfield missed in the desert was the ability to practice his specialty in the collegiate atmosphere of subspecialty academic medicine. He had experienced this in his residency at Los Angeles County General Hospital. With subspecialized physicians, there was an improved level of care-delivery and efficiency. With salaried physicians, there was no economic competition among them and every incentive to cooperate.

In 1938, with the aqueduct project coming to an end, Garfield looked forward to establishing a private surgical practice in Los Angeles. Everything changed when he received a call from A. B. Ordway. He asked Garfield to meet with Edgar Kaiser to discuss health care for the fifteen thousand workers for the Grand Coulee Dam project. Edgar was the eldest son of Henry, whose company led a consortium of contractors who were to complete the work on Grand Coulee Dam in the semi desert of eastern Washington state. The relationship got off to a difficult start, but Garfield was convinced by the opportunity to provide prepaid, multispecialty care to a concentrated population with vertically integrated facilities. He was also impressed with the social consciousness of Edgar Kaiser, who felt that the contractors had an obligation to provide adequate health care in remote work sites—but not as a profit center.

Mason City had been built to serve the fifteen thousand dam workers. There was a preexisting, run-down, seventy-five-bed hospital that had served a dysfunctional two-tiered health care system that was unpopular with the workers. The Kaiser-led consortium promised a prepaid medical program that was eventually much preferred by the workers and their families.

With stable financing in place, Garfield upgraded and modernized the hospital. He understood the need for a high-quality, self-contained care program as essential to recruiting the high-quality medical group he envisioned. This was the first time that Henry Kaiser actually met Garfield. He grilled him about his vision of prepaid health care for almost a full day. He left Garfield with these words: "Young man, if your idea is half as good as you say it is, it is not only good for this project—it is good for the entire country."

Garfield set to work recruiting his medical group, many of whom he knew personally from his residency. They, in turn, helped recruit other young, recently trained physicians from the best training programs. The SR Garfield MD Associates Medical Group grew into an outstanding team of well-trained young physicians and surgeons. Many of them later figured prominently as Permanente first-generation founders and leaders.

At the isolated eastern Washington state dam site, the group became a socially tight, hardworking, professional unit. It was a precursor of the Permanente Medical Groups. Again, the effects of prepaid and affordable preventive care became apparent. Sidney Garfield said it best:

> Prior to this family plan, when walking through the corridors of our little hospital at Coulee, we would see very sick women and children. After the plan was in operation for three or four months, there was a noticeable change in

the severity level … The reason was simple: These people, with the barrier of cost for medical service removed, were coming to us early in their illness. Ruptured appendices changed to simple appendices, terminal pneumonias became early pneumonias. Certain conditions disappeared entirely, such as diphtheria [immunization] and mastoiditis [early treatment of ear infections].

By 1941, the Grand Coulee Dam was nearing completion. Preparations were being made to dismantle the Medical Group and the medical care plan for the dam workers. On December 7, Japan bombed Pearl Harbor—and the United States was in World War II. Within a few months, Garfield was faced with organizing what became the largest civilian wartime health care program in the US, which, in turn, became Kaiser Permanente.

Kaiser, a visionary in his own right, saw the potential of this model of health care-delivery for the whole country. The lessons learned at Grand Coulee about hospital construction, the integration of facilities, an exclusive partnership between the Health Plan financiers and the medical team through prepayment, group practice, and preventive care would serve Garfield well for his next great challenge. That challenge was to scale up the program by an order of magnitude, in the space of a few months, and under wartime emergency conditions.

World War II: Scaling Up

The loss of the Battle of the Atlantic—the submarine war—was the principle fear of Winston Churchill that would lose the war for Britain. He constantly worried that the Nazi U-Boat menace would cut Britain's lifeline to the United States. Kaiser Industries had been in the shipbuilding business since 1940 as a result of a contract with the British Admiralty. Thus, Kaiser Industries already had shipbuilding experience by the time the US entered the war. As such, Kaiser Industries was ready for the rapid expansion that was to come.

At its peak, the Kaiser shipbuilding effort employed ninety thousand workers in the vast complex of East Bay shipyards of Richmond, California, and another complex of shipyards in the Portland, Oregon and

Vancouver, Washington, area. These were soon supported by a large steel plant in Fontana in Southern California. By 1944, Kaiser's mass-production shipbuilding techniques were producing an average of one ship per day. During the war, 1,490 vessels were completed for a total tonnage of over fifteen million tons—27 percent of the total Maritime Commission construction by the United States. To put this into perspective, total allied losses to German U-Boats during World War II were 14.1 million tons. Kaiser Industries was soon building ships faster than the enemy could sink them.

Soon after Pearl Harbor, Sidney Garfield joined the US Army and was scheduled for duty in Burma with the Seventy-Third Surgical Evacuation Hospital Team. By then, he was well known to the Kaiser organization for his work first in the desert and then on the Grand Coulee Dam. About a month before he was to ship out, he was asked to consult on a health care program for the anticipated tens of thousands of shipyard and steel plant workers who would be flooding into the Kaiser industrial sites. It was immediately apparent to all that he could be of much greater service to the country organizing a health care program for Kaiser's war industry workers. Without Garfield's knowledge, the Kaiser organization, through A. B. Ordway, petitioned the maritime board to release Garfield from duty to organize health care at the shipyards. With a presidential order signed by Franklin D. Roosevelt, Garfield wasn't going to Burma.

The task was daunting. Initially, the men pouring into the work sites were old or classified 4F—not healthy enough for military duty. Eventually, the workforce was augmented by workers of all races and eventually women, celebrated by "Rosie the Riveter." There was inadequate housing, few available health care workers, too few hospital beds, and shortages of everything.

Garfield organized hospital design, and with Henry Kaiser's assistance, financing these hospitals. He organized on the fly, recruiting physicians and staff. Drugs and equipment were obtained in the face of strict rationing that was often controlled by physician boards that were hostile to the program.

Three important things emerged from the wartime experience. The Permanente Foundation was established as a nonprofit foundation funded by its own income—a new form of foundation. This formalized the nonprofit status of the program. The program had demonstrated clearly its ability to scale up to efficiently serve large populations even under adverse conditions. By the end of 1944, it covered 200,000 workers and dependents in four hospitals with a total of 790 beds by more than one hundred doctors. It was a model of cost efficiency. More important, it was a model of quality care.

Between 1943 and 1945, the Permanente Foundation Medical Bulletin published sixty-seven scientific papers documenting this care. This was in addition to the thirty other papers published in other medical journals. Among the topics addressed in these papers were pneumonia, appendicitis, hepatitis, trauma care, gunshot wounds, metal fume fever, ectopic pregnancy, and various infectious diseases. Based upon this scientific output, the quality of care was cited favorably by the prestigious *New England Journal of Medicine*. Prior to this, the superior clinical outcomes of affordable, prepaid, nonprofit, multispecialty care, delivered in integrated facilities, early in the course of disease had been only anecdotal observation. Now it was documented scientifically.

Near-Death Experience

As the end of the war approached in early 1945, the shipbuilding program was rapidly cut back. In a year, the medical program had gone from more than two hundred thousand members at its peak to only sixteen thousand. The Portland-Vancouver program, which eventually reached a nadir of 2,600 members and six doctors, avoided a successful dissolution vote only by a parliamentary maneuver that temporarily delayed the vote.

California went from one hundred doctors to a dozen. Fortunately, for the future of the program, the remaining doctors were a core group of true believers. Garfield and this group had begun the planning for the continuation of the program since 1944. With foresight, he had set aside from the operating margin a $1.5 million fund for this purpose.

When the shipyards closed, the former workers did not return "from whence they came." They liked California, and many decided to stay. The industrial growth of California and the West Coast, initially spurred by wartime production, became the foundation of an industrial peacetime boom that doubled the population of California in fifteen years. The success of the Kaiser Health Plan paralleled this West Coast demographic growth.

Many of the former shipyard workers, familiar with, and liking, the prepaid health care they experienced during the war, signed up for the Kaiser Health Plan when it became commercially available. It became the favored health care program for unions, civil service workers, and universities. Growth, especially in California, was rapid. By 1950, the program had grown to 120,000 in Northern California, 20,000 in Southern California, and 14,000 in the Northwest. The Kaiser Health Care Program was here to stay.

Organized Medicine Strikes Back

In 1934, the American Medical Association (AMA) modified its principles of medical ethics. It defined as unethical essentially anything other than unrestricted patient access to solo practitioners who were prohibited to advertise. Unethical practice, so defined, could then be used to deny AMA membership, board certification, and even threaten the medical licensure of a physician. This was clearly aimed at group practice and managed care.

From the 1930s to the 1970s, the American Medical Association and its affiliated local and specialty medical societies were much more powerful than today. AMA physicians dominated state licensing, specialty boards, and even military medical draft boards. A physician's standing with the AMA and affiliated state, county, and specialty medical societies could make or break a career. It was a professional act of bravery with this knowledge, or foolhardiness without it, for a doctor to join Kaiser Permanente well into the 1980s.

Garfield's desert clinic complex and later the Grand Coulee Dam health program were too obscure and remote to come to the attention of organized medicine. This changed with an established health plan that covered hundreds of thousands of members in major urban areas. During the war, the program had only been tolerated by organized medicine as a temporary war emergency program. With the end of the war, organized medicine's opposition to the program quickly ramped up.

Informally, new physicians were routinely advised by community physicians that joining KP would end their career as respectable members of the medical profession. Board certification often required letters of recommendation from the local medical and/or specialty society. These were hard to come by when program doctors were regularly banned from these societies for what organized medicine considered unethical practice.

Bill Dung, MD, the Hawaii Permanente Medical Group's (HPMG) second and longest-serving president (1970–1991), was asked by a community colleague upon joining HPMG in 1958 why he wanted to commit professional suicide. Dr. Yi Ching was an early HPMG pioneer and innovator and the long-serving chief of pediatrics who built one of the strongest departments in the Medical Group. He recalled a 1958 public health lecture in his senior year at Boston University Medical School. The professor stated that they would be leaving medical school shortly to pursue their careers in medicine. He wanted to warn them about joining a program on the West Coast that was both socialistic and unethical: the Kaiser Medical Care Program. Yi wrote the author, "So of course I did join."

PMG doctors, and even their families, were socially and professionally shunned by the medical community. This isolation from the medical community, while it made physician recruiting more difficult, had the unintended consequence of selecting for idealistic physicians willing to take personal risk because they believed in the principles of the program. Isolated from the medical community, the Medical Groups were forced to become self-sufficient. Without outside interference, they evolved a practice in their own clinics and hospitals that was radically different from fee-for-service practices. A new kind of practice would be required if the new prepaid, nonprofit practice was to be successful.

With the war's end, the AMA and its affiliated county medical societies wasted no time coming after the program. Formal harassment included a successful attempt to suspend Sidney Garfield's medical license in June 1946 over a hiring technicality, which was eventually overturned by the courts.

In 1948, formal charges of unethical practice were leveled against Garfield by the Alameda County (includes Oakland, California) Medical Association. They included charges of "advertising and solicitation of patients," putting "mass-production techniques" ahead of patient care, preventing free choice of physicians, rendering inadequate hospital service, diverting illegal profits into the Health Plan, and finally hiring unlicensed personnel. After an extensive investigation that took more than a year, in November 1949, he was cleared of all charges.

At the height of the Korean War, in 1952, the local medical society managed to manipulate the local draft board into inducting key KP physicians, including Sidney Garfield (then forty-four) and Morris Collen (then thirty-nine and whose asthma made him 4F during World War II). With the support of Henry Kaiser, Garfield successfully appealed the call-up by the local draft board, but it took a year to settle the issue after several key Medical Group physicians had already been inducted.

The greatest threat came with resolution 16, which was presented at the annual AMA meeting in 1954. The resolution defined any closed group medical plan, such as Kaiser, as an unethical practice. It was only the successful motion of Clifford Keene, MD, one of the founders of the program, to get resolution 16 referred to the AMA judicial committee. That parliamentary maneuver likely prevented a successful vote. There, the motion languished in committee for five years and then quietly died.

The root cause of the opposition was likely economic competition. Cecil Cutting, MD, the first TPMG president, was told on more than one occasion that if community physicians were allowed to treat program patients on a fee-for-service basis, the opposition would disappear. Cutting characterized this as a "shakedown." This, of course, would have ended the program. Kaiser Permanente Health Care is a program of salaried physicians. Salaried compensation isolates medical decision-making from direct personal gain. It is also a closed physician partnership that requires shared values, quality control, and teamwork.

These program victories were not entirely the inevitable outcome of sweet reason. The very considerable influence of Henry J. Kaiser weighed in firmly on the side of the program. In 1943, the Supreme Court had ruled in favor of the Group Health of Washington DC against the AMA. Group Health was a small government worker health plan that was being harassed by the AMA. It filed a restraint of trade suit against the AMA and won.

Based on this Supreme Court decision, at one point in 1948, "Mr. Kaiser" let it be known that if the California medical societies were to continue to harass "his" Kaiser Foundation Health Plan, this could be considered restraint of trade by the program—and the state of California would be required by law to dissolve the medical associations. He went on to say that he preferred a "spirit of peace." Neither Kaiser nor Garfield wanted to be "declaring war" on organized medicine. Fortunately, they favored the more rational, measured response.

Paul DeKruif, author of the classic *The Microbe Hunters* and a regular contributor to *Reader's Digest*, the largest circulation magazine in the US, was a powerful and effective advocate for the program in the mind of the public. He became enamored with the program during the war and continued his strong partisan support after. He presented the program as an innovative, futuristic program that could become the model for all medical care in the US.

While the positive public relations and powerful Henry Kaiser's "We're not going to hurt each other—are we?" position were undoubtedly helpful, this is not what turned back organized medicine. It was in the face of personal attacks against him, scurrilous gossip about poor quality, bad doctors, inadequate facilities and staff, diversion of funds, and accusations of communism that Sidney Garfield over many years patiently and persistently orchestrated the defense of the program.

Repeatedly, AMA physician representatives were invited to inspect the hospitals and clinics, interview the physicians, review the qualifications of the staff, and review the finances. To the chagrin of the AMA leadership, their own scientific studies of KP medical care-delivery clearly demonstrated that KP was at least the equal and usually superior to the non-KP care in any community studied, including Hawaii. It was the patient, rational, scientific demonstration of better-quality care, patient preference demonstrated by rapid growth, and financial success that guaranteed eventual victory. By 1960, with more than eight hundred thousand members and poised for rapid expansion, it became obvious that KP was here to stay—AMA or no AMA.

Growing Pains

By the early 1950s, what we now know as Kaiser Permanente was no longer a wartime experiment. It was a rapidly growing, high-profile, futuristic, health care alternative that was well equipped to defend itself from the coming onslaught of organized medicine. Garfield had functioned as the owner of SR Garfield Medical Associates—the ancestor of the Permanente Medical Groups. He was also chief medical officer of the Health Plan in partnership with Henry Kaiser and his executive team.

Kaiser personally was preoccupied with managing his extensive industrial empire. Principally, he provided financial backing, membership support through the unions associated with his industries, and the occasional high-profile defense of the program from its enemies—chiefly organized medicine. He left the day-to-day operations of the program to his Kaiser executives and Garfield and his physician leaders. There was an informal understanding that medical matters would be left to the doctors and that business matters would be left to the Kaiser executives.

Rapid growth—encompassing hundreds of thousands of members, hundreds of doctors and multiple hospitals and clinics geographically spread across the West Coast—eventually strained these informal understandings to the breaking point. Codifying these understandings was soon to be required or the very existence of the program would be at stake.

The cultures of medicine and business are vastly different. The stated mission of the medical culture is the health of the patient. Furthermore, most physicians see this as a moral imperative. There is no point to having a health care program without this mission except as a moneymaking scheme. The mission of the business culture is to increase productivity (providers and staff must work harder) and control costs (with fewer resources for care) and marketing (resources taken from medical care).

Without infinite resources, which is always the case, no margin eventually means no mission. This, in turn, means no mission, medical or business, for anyone. On the other hand, excessive resource restriction impacts medical care negatively. Excessive resourcing results in high medical cost with diminished medical outcomes. This, in turn, diverts resources from other societal needs. This is the essential dilemma of medical economics. Society ultimately decides what proportion of its resources will be devoted to medical care, and that is the "budget" for medical care. This "societal budget" for health care demands "rationing," which is something that no one, especially government officials, wants to talk about. Proper balance between the medical and business cultures to get the best medical care value for the "budget" provided by society determines the success or failure of a medical care program since all medical care plans are subject to the same societal "budget."

The coming crisis was brought to a head with the long illness and death of the beloved Bess Kaiser, Henry Kaiser's first wife. Garfield coordinated her long terminal care. He arranged for one of the best nurses in the Permanente Hospital—Alyce Chester—to provide live-in, nursing care for Mrs. Kaiser. Alyce was an attractive divorcee with a young son. She had been mentored in medical administration by Garfield himself and was part of his executive team. Bess Kaiser died on March 15, 1951. Three months later, Henry Kaiser controversially married the thirty-four-year-old Alyce Chester—reportedly with Bess's blessing. He was sixty-eight—twice her age. Garfield had become even closer to Kaiser during Bess's illness, but they were to become related soon. About a year after Kaiser married Alyce, with the encouragement of Henry and Alyce, Sidney fell in love with and married Alyce's sister Helen. Henry and Sidney were now brothers-in-law living next door to each other. Both couples were socially very close. This was to have fateful consequences for Garfield.

Henry Kaiser was a man of unshakable will with boundless confidence, energy, and international renown. His marriage to Alyce Chester increased his interest and involvement in the medical program. He paternalistically regarded "his doctors" as employees who had little or no role in business decision-making. Conversely, the physician leadership saw the Health Plan merely as a convenient financial instrument of their mission to provide medical care. They had no intention of being employees of Kaiser Industries. This was a time when the "Kaiser" physicians were actively defending themselves against charges by organized medicine of unethical medical practice as employees of Kaiser Industries. In 1952, the Health Plan and the hospitals had formally adopted the name Kaiser. When it was proposed that the Medical Groups also be named Kaiser, the Permanente Medical Group leadership refused. Mr. Kaiser was not pleased.

Henry Kaiser, frustrated by his inability to control the physicians, decided to give his capable young wife something to do. That something was the establishment of the Walnut Creek Hospital in an East Bay suburb of San Francisco, where she became effectively the hospital administrator. That hospital was organized independently from the rest of the Kaiser hospitals. The medical staff was recruited directly by Alyce. Scarce funds were diverted from the other hospital projects to build this showcase, luxury hospital. The staffing and budgeting were done with minimal involvement of the Permanente leadership. In September 1953, the Walnut Creek Hospital opened. It was resentfully called the "Country Club" by the non-Walnut Creek Permanente doctors. Kaiser's intention was to establish a Walnut Creek Independent Medical Group from the now-named Permanente Medical Group (Northern California region). The ultimate plan was to replace the unified Permanente Medical Group with many small, easier-to-control, independent medical groups. Worst of all, from the Permanente leadership standpoint, he planned to allow non-Permanente community doctors to practice in the hospital.

After a year of conflict and uncertainty, this plan was foiled when the Walnut Creek physicians refused to leave the Permanente Medical Group. The Permanente Medical Groups were now on a collision course with the formidable Henry J. Kaiser. Garfield had not opposed the Walnut Creek Hospital.

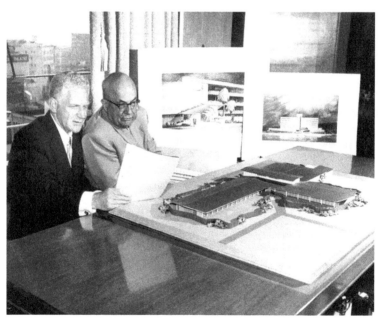

Dr. Sidney Garfield and Henry Kaiser review the plans of the controversial Walnut Creek Hospital in 1952.

It is amazing that the gentleman's agreements between the physicians and the Kaiser organization lasted as long as they did, but by 1954, the fault lines between them were wide enough to threaten the entire program. By early 1955, the program decision-making was paralyzed. The Permanente physician leadership called for a series of conferences with the Kaiser leadership to codify or dissolve the relationship. Garfield would be caught in the crossfire.

Garfield was a charismatic, high-energy visionary. From the program's beginning, he had solved problems—often brilliantly—on an ad hoc basis. In addition, he was peripatetically designing new hospitals and clinics, defending the program, and thinking through futuristic medical care-delivery. He was deeply respected for these efforts throughout his career and after. His strength, however, was not in disciplined day-to-day management and organization. Nor was he perceived to be the strong, partisan leader needed to confront the formidable Henry J. Kaiser to represent physician interests. It didn't help his standing with the physician leadership that Garfield playfully referred to Kaiser as "the boss," which Henry Kaiser loved.

The meetings that led to the "Tahoe Agreement" were held between April and July 1955. The final three-day meeting, which started in July 1955, was held at Fleur de Lac—the Kaiser compound on Lake Tahoe, which was later featured in *The Godfather II*. Kaiser's leadership style was very personal. He felt betrayed by Garfield's support of the doctors' positions. Prior to the start of this meeting, Kaiser told Garfield he wanted him out as program director. Garfield argued back, but then he said he would go if that was what the physicians wanted. To his surprise, the physicians backed Kaiser. Garfield was out of the power loop. From then on, his role was that of program visionary.

No minutes were taken of the last meeting, but participants recall rancorous partisan debate, posturing, demands, and counterdemands by both sides. It didn't hurt progress that Kaiser withdrew from the meeting after the first day, feigning illness when he saw that things weren't going his way. It was testimony to the dedication to the ideals of the program by the participants on both sides that the conference didn't fail.

By the end of the meeting, the blueprint for program governance was outlined. Kaiser Permanente would have a mutually exclusive group model partnership with the health plan rather than a staff employee model. The details would be defined by a periodically renewed medical services agreement contract. The Permanente Medical Groups would manage the health care-delivery and be paid by capitation—a fixed amount per patient served. Staffing, quality assurance, salaries and benefits, and outside services would be governed by the Medical Groups. Health Plan would control the hospitals, marketing, program financing, public relations, and government affairs.

The Tahoe Agreement led to the codification of the relationship between the Permanente Medical Groups and Health Plan, but it took three years to be implemented into the regional medical service agreements. The physicians through the Permanente Medical Groups would have a much larger say in the direction of Kaiser Permanente than they would have had if they were employees of Kaiser Industries—a staff model.

A relatively equal balance of power was now set up between the medical culture and the business culture for the program. It was now much less likely that the main mission of health care would be overwhelmed by business interests. This challenging, two-headed management model would force compromise and understanding between the disparate medical and business cultures. It required and still requires a dialogue, which is often difficult, between representatives of the medical culture and the business culture. Success of this model depends upon strong leaders of goodwill on both sides. They must have broad vision, energy, dedication, and a deep understanding of the mission of Kaiser Permanente. When the strength of such leaders is well-balanced on the Permanente and Health Plan sides, the program prospers mightily. When it isn't, the program falters and even fails.

The genetic code of Kaiser Permanente was now in place: (1) prepayment (2) capitation (3) nonprofit Health Plan, (4) salaried physicians (5) vertical integration through ownership of facilities (6) community rating, and a (7) mutually exclusive partnership between Permanente Medical Groups and Health Plan. This model led to a period of unprecedented program growth, prosperity, and influence until it became the largest vertically integrated HMO in the United States. Wherever and whenever it faltered or failed, it did so when it violated one or more components of the "genetic code."

Garfield was not a spiteful person. After Tahoe, he was left with the position of vice president of facilities and planning, which played to his visionary strengths. Despite his ouster from power, he remained a respected advisor of the Medical Groups and continued his close personal relationship with Henry Kaiser until Kaiser died. With day-to-day operational responsibilities no longer his concern, he was free to concentrate on the planning and design of facilities and to think deeply about the delivery of medical care. Decades before they became reality, he envisioned and promoted the electronic medical record, team models of care-delivery, and the preventive care of the well in addition to the care of the sick. He remained to his death a respected, often revered, advisor to the Medical Groups. He died in his sleep on December 29, 1984, at the age of seventy-eight.

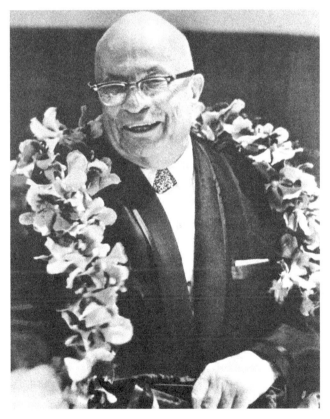

Henry J. Kaiser: Co-founder of Kaiser Permanente
on his 80th birthday celebration in Hawaii.

CHAPTER 2

HENRY J. KAISER: ENTREPRENEUR EXTRAORDINAIRE

H enry John Kaiser was born May 9, 1882, in Sprout Brook in upper New York state. Despite the legend that he promulgated, he
dropped out of school after eighth grade not because of poverty,
but because he was impatient to learn the business of business. He began as
a photography apprentice, and by age twenty, he was managing the studio.

With his savings, he moved to Washington state in 1906 and quickly
developed a reputation for competence and integrity. In 1914, he founded
a paving company that built roads, successfully pioneering the use of
heavy construction equipment. In 1927, the firm expanded with a large
contract to build roads in Cuba. By the 1930s, his firm was large enough
to participate as a major contractor in the western boom of dam building
including the Hoover Dam on the Colorado River and the Bonneville and
Grand Coulee Dams on the Columbia River. By the start of World War
II, his experience with large, complex construction projects had positioned
him for war production—most notably shipbuilding. Prior to his 1939
contract with the British Admiralty, he knew virtually nothing about
shipbuilding—a testament to his energy, self-confidence, and innovative
and entrepreneurial spirit.

Writing a hagiography of Henry Kaiser does the reader a disservice.

Henry Kaiser was a complex man. To understand the founding of the Hawaii region of Kaiser Permanente, it is helpful to understand him.

The root cause of Kaiser's success was that he was an action-oriented visionary. He saw large things in a large way. Problems were obstacles to be overcome—not reasons to avoid doing important things. When he succeeded, he succeeded spectacularly. The Hoover Dam, Grand Coulee Dam, wartime shipbuilding, and the postwar Kaiser Industries were groundbreaking successes. He had an equivocal attitude toward experts. On one occasion, he mused how he surrounded himself with people smarter than himself, and on another, he stated that sometimes the smartest move was to ignore the experts. He did both. When he had the right mix of listening to or ignoring his experts, he was fabulously successful. When he didn't, he failed. In his foray into car manufacturing in the early fifties, he lost $111 million—almost $2.9 billion in 2020 dollars. Much of the early history of the Hawaii region is about the recovery from his missteps establishing "his" health care program against the advice of most of his advisors. Overall, his visionary style succeeded far more often than it failed.

Kaiser had integrity. From early in his career, he was known for keeping his commitments. This was especially important in the construction industry where it is very difficult to provide accurate bids. He was known for coming in on budget and on time—even ahead of time. When he didn't, he would take a loss to cover his commitments. While he expected a fair profit, he was not a profiteer. Because of his reputation for integrity and performance, and successful public relations, he was awarded progressively larger, usually government, contracts. During World War II, war contract profiteering was a national scandal. It was Harry Truman's investigations into war profiteering that propelled him from obscurity to become Franklin Roosevelt's 1944 vice presidential running mate and then president. Despite efforts to prove otherwise, there was never any credible evidence of war profiteering by Kaiser.

Much of Kaiser's success can be traced back to the blood, sweat, and tears of his management "family." Kaiser had rare charisma. His managers were intensely loyal to him. For Kaiser, the separation of personal from business was not clear. His managers were his "boys." Two of them, Henry Jr. and Edgar, really were his children. Kaiser lived for the business—and that was his expectation of his managers.

Kaiser lived well and entertained lavishly. His seventeen-acre compound on Lake Tahoe, Fleur du Lac, was among other things, the setting for the legendary Tahoe conference as well as the wedding scene in *The Godfather II*. It was also the base for his terrifyingly fast speedboat rides—clearly remembered by many of the managers. To be in the Kaiser business "family" inner circle was to be part of this life.

Kaiser was constantly pushing his managers to higher and higher performance levels, which they usually met. He could be petulant when things didn't go his way. He was constantly talking and brimming with ideas—not all of them good. It was the difficult duty of his managers to turn him away from the bad ones. When they did, he often took it personally, and they risked permanently falling out of favor. Phil Chu, MD, the first HPMG medical director, characterized Henry Kaiser in a 1970 presentation: "He is like a happy elephant. He smiles and leans against you. After a while, you know that there is nothing to do except move in the direction that he is pushing."

Early on, Kaiser understood good labor relations would foster success. He took care of his workers, and his workers reciprocated. While health care for workers on remote work sites was legally required, it was not required for dependents. Nor were health care quality requirements well defined. His partnership with Sidney Garfield sensitized him to the health care issues that led him well beyond legal requirements to the concept of prepaid medicine and Kaiser Permanente. The concern for his workers led to a generally cordial relationship with organized labor. As verbalized by a later CEO of Kaiser Permanente David Lawrence: "If not for organized labor's active marketing support immediately following World War II, it is unlikely that Kaiser Permanente would exist today."

Kaiser was a diversity pioneer. Discrimination was not allowed. His success was summed up by longtime African American foreman and friend James "Totem" Shaw. To paraphrase Mr. Shaw: Mr. Kaiser mixes brains and money. I mix mud and money. Kaiser loved it. "Rosie the Riveter" was styled after the thousands of women employed in the Kaiser shipyards. The childcare provided at these factories was far ahead of its time.

Finally, he was a master of publicity, which he used effectively to obtain and carry out government contracts. His public relations skill was the envy of competitors. He was the subject of dozens of magazine articles touting his innovations and successes. An example is a hyperbolic quote from *Mechanics Illustrated* from 1942: Kaiser had "accomplished five times as much building in one lifetime as did the four pharaohs of Egypt ... he built three dams in a decade each one larger than the tomb of Cheops ..."

In 1944, Kaiser's popularity was such that he was briefly considered by President Roosevelt as a potential vice presidential candidate. If he had been selected, he would likely have succeeded FDR as president of the United States. In a 1945 Roper Poll, he was named the civilian who did the most to win the war. In the postwar years, this popularity would help him effectively defend "his" health care program against the attacks by organized medicine.

By 1956, when Kaiser "retired" to Honolulu, Kaiser Industries was listed as the 151st largest corporation of the Fortune 500. It was an international umbrella organization made up of more than one hundred companies covering often unrelated industries, including aluminum, steel, and cement production, mining, automobiles, international large-scale construction projects, broadcasting, banking, and real estate. Kaiser Industries had been pivotal in the industrialization of the West Coast. By 1959, Kaiser was gone entirely from the management of Kaiser Industries as he concentrated on his Hawaii ventures.

The next generation of Kaiser Industries' leadership lacked Kaiser's singular authority, vision, daring, and flexibility. The industrial empire began to crumble. Reasons offered have included the inability to coordinate the disparate industries, inability to diversify into newer industries, office politics, short-term management goals, and the overall decline of heavy industry in the US. With the value of the individual companies greater than the stock value of Kaiser Industries, the corporation began a voluntary breakup in 1977, which was 90 percent completed by 1980. The last of the shares of Kaiser Industries were liquidated in 1985.

On one hand, this could be taken as an object lesson in succession planning. On the other hand, it may be seen as proof what an extraordinary person Henry J. Kaiser was. Kaiser had rare vision, force of character, energy, and integrity. In 2006, in the *Forbes* magazine listing of the twenty most influential businessmen of all time, Henry Kaiser was voted ninth. For a given predicament, if you asked yourself, "What would Henry do?" your answer would not likely be far from the right one. Without Henry

J. Kaiser, in partnership with Dr. Sidney Garfield, it is unlikely that there would have been a Kaiser Permanente and certainly no KP Hawaii region.

Mister Kaiser "Retires" to Hawaii

Elsewhere on earth, at 21 degrees north latitude, the land is mostly desert. Hawaii is an exception. The prevailing northeastern trade winds cool the islands as they pass over the volcanic peaks rising abruptly out of the ocean. This condenses what water vapor there is into the abundant rainfall that waters the islands. This mountainous terrain creates microclimates. At sunny Waikiki Beach, the yearly rainfall is a semidesert twenty-two inches. Five miles away, in the cloud-covered Koolau Mountains, the yearly rainfall is 260 inches—enough to support a dense rain forest. The sharply vertical, cloud-covered, verdant peaks, the white coral beaches, the blue sunny skies, and the deep royal blue of the ocean provide some of the most stunning vistas on earth. The semitropical location, cooled by trade winds, results in air temperatures that rarely go below sixty-five in winter or above ninety degrees F in summer. Water temperatures in this part of the Pacific range from seventy-five to eighty-five degrees F.

What really makes Hawaii special is its people. The aloha spirit was built on a bedrock of such native Hawaiian values as harmony and cooperation (lokahi), justice and righteousness (pono), personal responsibility (kuleana), family (ohana), conciliation and forgiveness (ho'oponopono), and love and respect for the land (aloha aina). This culture was modified and enriched by the subsequent waves of American, European, Chinese, Japanese, Filipino, Korean, and Pacific Island immigrants who, in turn, absorbed many Hawaiian values. This rich cultural tapestry based upon aloha makes Hawaii one of the most interesting and tolerant societies on earth. More than half the marriages are interracial. Aloha is real. Even in traffic-choked Honolulu, it is unusual to hear a blaring horn, and if you do, that is likely to be done by a visitor to the islands.

It is not surprising that Hawaii, called "the Paradise of the Pacific," attracts more than ten million tourists per year. Hawaiian beaches and hotels routinely figure prominently in world top ten lists. The renewable resource of tourism directly or indirectly accounts for almost half of the economy of the state. It wasn't always that way.

When Henry Kaiser retired in Hawaii in 1956, it was a very different place. It was a US territory. Statehood wouldn't come until 1959. Political and economic control by an oligarchy of mostly Caucasian, many of them missionary descendants, was only beginning to break up. The population was 580,000 compared to 1,431,063 in 2015. Hawaii is one of the most isolated places on earth. The distance from Hawaii to the nearest continental landfall near San Francisco is similar to the distance from San Francisco to Washington DC. Travel to Hawaii was expensive, requiring a five-day ship cruise or a rough eight-to-eleven-hour one-way propeller plane ride. In 1956, there were 133,000 visitors to Hawaii compared to the almost ten million today—a seventy-five-fold increase. The economy then was dominated by agriculture and support services for the military rather than tourism.

Kaiser's ties to the islands went back to 1940's military construction contracts. Henry enjoyed the islands immensely and visited frequently first with Bess, and after her death, with Alyce. He tried retirement for six months and failed. During an earlier trip, he had difficulty finding accommodations in Waikiki and decided that Honolulu was underdeveloped.

As his retirement project, he set out to correct this. Soon he was up at five o'clock every morning, doubling the hotel bed capacity in Waikiki with the Kaiser Hawaiian Village Hotel (now the Hilton Hawaiian Village), the largest hotel in Hawaii. With the hotel came the beach and the lagoon that he constructed. KHVH-TV (now KITV channel 4) and KHVH radio 990 were established to advertise his Hawaiian enterprises. KHVH stands for Kaiser Hawaiian Village Hotel. Kaiser Cement broke the Dillingham cement monopoly by doubling the cement production of Hawaii. Kaiser Construction grew with the construction to include heavy equipment and dredges. His largest project—the Hawaii Kai subdivision—turned a swampy lagoon into a community that now houses thirty thousand people. He induced the state government to double the capacity of the Kalaniana'eole Highway to serve that community and then bid successfully for the contract to build it. There is a story about him visiting the Hawaii Kai site prior to a publicity event the next day. He noticed that there were no palm trees. It was Hawaii. Mr. Kaiser wanted palm trees. The next day, there were real palm trees in the publicity shots.

Kaiser Pink—a garish purplish pink—was his trademark color. The story given was that it was his wife's favorite color, but it was also a marketing tool. When the author started with HPMG in 1980, doctors were issued one pink and one blue smock as a sort of uniform. Kaiser pink construction equipment, catamarans, and jeep rentals were everywhere. Kaiser also publicized his Hawaii enterprises through his broadcasting network and by sponsoring the popular "Hawaiian Eye" ABC network program (1959–1963), the offices of which were set in his Kaiser Hawaiian Village Hawaii. While there were Hawaii setting shots, the program was actually shot on the Warner Brothers Lot in Los Angeles.

Kaiser's "retirement" transformed the state of Hawaii. From his arrival in 1956 to his death in 1968, the population increased by almost 25 percent—and the visitor count increased tenfold. Kaiser's enterprises in Hawaii are now gone—defunct or owned by others—but in any economic development history of Hawaii, Henry Kaiser must figure prominently.

While he was reengineering Hawaii, Kaiser decided that he was going to establish his own health care program there. Having been frustrated by the Walnut Creek Hospital adventure thwarted by the Permanente Medical Group, this time, he was going to do it without Permanente Medical Group's interference.

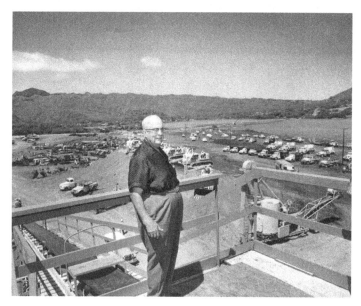

Henry Kaiser Reengineering Oahu

CHAPTER 3

MR. KAISER ESTABLISHES HIS HAWAII HEALTH PLAN

E mblazoned on the "Kaiser Pink" concrete mixer trucks of Kaiser Cement was Kaiser's motto: "Find a need and fill it." Kaiser's deviation from his own motto resulted in the difficult birth and near demise of the Hawaii program.

In early 1955, when it was apparent that Henry Kaiser was coming to Hawaii, representatives of the Hawaii Medical Association (HMA) asked Kaiser not to establish a health plan in Hawaii. He responded that if HMA would establish its own health plan with prepayment and group practice, he would support it. Not surprisingly, given the 1950s position of the AMA, he never heard back from them.

In 1956, the Stanford Research Institute published an eighty-seven-page monograph that concluded that Oahu's hospitals and the Hawaii Medical Services Administration (HMSA)—the Blue Cross Blue Shield affiliate in Hawaii—were adequately serving the needs of the population. Subsequently, Fred Pellegrin, MD, the chief of medicine at the Walnut Creek Kaiser Hospital, and trusted by Alyce and Henry Kaiser, was invited to live with them at Kaiser's Honolulu estate for six months. His assignment was to quietly research the Honolulu medical infrastructure to determine the feasibility of establishing a Hawaii Kaiser Health Plan. He worked full-time at this assignment and did a thorough job. Often he had to meet with community physicians at four or five o'clock in the morning in out-of-the-way places. They didn't want to be seen with him.

Curiously, in the evenings, Kaiser rarely spoke with Pellegrin about health care but about other unrelated subjects. At the end of the assignment, Pellegrin wrote a final report recommending that Kaiser not build a hospital because there were available beds in existing hospitals. He also recommended that Kaiser not establish a new medical group, but to affiliate with an existing group. This was not what Kaiser wanted to hear.

As Pellegrin stated in an oral history given decades later in 2011:

> Forty-eight hours later I was on a plane back to the Mainland. I never saw Mr. Kaiser again. I never heard from Mr. Kaiser again. That was the end of our relationship.

Up to that point, Dr. Pellegrin had been Henry Kaiser's on-call personal physician and had been close socially with Alyce and Henry. Pellegrin later learned that Kaiser had already been working with an architect planning his hospital.

The Kaiser Foundation Hospital

On a beautiful site overlooking the Honolulu waterfront and the Ala Moana Yacht Harbor in Waikiki, in early 1958, Kaiser began construction of his health plan's new hospital. The fact that there was no health plan, membership, or medical staff did not slow him down. It was a "build it, and they will come" venture. He personally supervised the fast-tracked construction. Concrete was being poured even before final approval was received from the city's building department. Kaiser visited the site as often as six times per day, urging faster construction to the consternation of his architects and engineers. A lava rock facing that he wanted had been completed on two floors of the hospital before city inspectors pointed out that this was not in compliance with the building code. Lava rock allowed tree rats to climb up the sides of buildings. Because he had excess concrete and steel, a tenth floor was added without prior approval. It wasn't discovered until years later when the hospital applied for a modification of the tenth floor, and the inspectors responded, "What tenth floor?"

Thus, the hospital was built in ten months and was ready to open by the end of November 1958. Haste did make waste. Designs that were innovative in California did not necessarily work in Hawaii. The outside access to patient rooms and open-air corridors, which could not be air-conditioned in often-humid Hawaii, were subject to flooding and blasts of wind during tropical storms. The elevators were too small to hold a gurney, and the kitchens were inadequate. The medical staff and patients had to, and did, adapt.

Most of the problems were fixed after the fact, but it took years. Despite all of this, the first Kaiser Medical Center served the program well for twenty-eight years. The view from the medical offices and the patient rooms was unsurpassed. It was a high-visibility fixture at the entrance to Waikiki. It was seen on the very popular *Hawaii 5-0* and referred to in one episode by character Chin Ho as "Kaiser's Hospital." Its demolition in October 1985 was used as the backdrop for a season-ending *Magnum PI* television show where Magnum is trapped in the building just as demolition charges were about to detonate. It was designed for seventy-five thousand members, but with modifications, it served 138,000 when hospital services ended in 1985. The hospital and the land cost only $4 million to build in 1958. The land alone sold for $28 million in 1985. The profit from the sale of the land went a long way in financing its successor: the award-winning Kaiser Moanalua Medical Center. The site of the old hospital is now occupied by the thirty-two-story luxury Hawaiian Prince Hotel. Gone but not forgotten, there remains to this day a well-known surf spot called "Kaiser Bowls." It was named for the Kaiser Hospital building that served as the landmark for this surf location for the twenty-seven years of its existence. "Bowls" refers to a surf spot where the wave energy suddenly impacts the shallow reef, causing a sudden increase in height and concavity up to the point of making a "tube."

Pacific Medical Associates

The Hawaii medical establishment was surprised and chagrined on May 22, 1958, when the *Honolulu Star Bulletin* reported the establishment of the Pacific Medical Associates. This was to be a group of five prominent community doctors. They were supposed to organize the Medical Group that would serve the members of the new Kaiser Health Plan. They included Samuel Yee, MD, a general surgeon who also did some general medicine. He was one of the first Asians from Hawaii to have graduated from Harvard Medical School and was former chief of staff at Queens Hospital and president of the Hawaii Medical Association for 1957–8. Dr. Richard Durant was a general surgeon and past president of the Honolulu Medical Society. Homer Izumi, MD, was a successful high-volume general practitioner and former HMA delegate to the American Medical Association. Dr. W.B. Herter was a respected pediatrician, and Dr. Richard S. Dodge was an orthopedic surgeon and the first medical director of the Rehabilitation Center of Hawaii.

A second newspaper article on the same day was entitled: "Kaiser Health Plan Announcement Is Greeted with Mixed Reactions." In it, an "influential voice" said he was "utterly shook." "Two of them [PMA partners] had never indicated any interest in such an affiliation and one doctor had repeatedly expressed disinterest in joining Kaiser." He went on to suggest that those doctors with positions in the medical society should resign those positions. The newly elected president of the HMA said while they were free to practice as they see fit, "They know the [negative] sentiment of the group [HMA]." The president of the Honolulu Medical Society surmised that they must be doing it for financial reasons. Given their previous stated positions about a Kaiser Health Plan and subsequent behavior, he was probably right.

Henry and Alyce Kaiser were at the center of the social whirl of Honolulu. Important people and movie stars were his frequent guests. They would be invited to his special table at the Kaiser Hawaiian Village Hotel to be entertained by such locally famous entertainers as Alfred Apaka. Kaiser understood that he was going to need physicians to lead his medical group, but he intended to control it. He wanted nothing to do with the Permanente Medical Group (TPMG). After the Walnut Creek conflict, TPMG wanted nothing to do with him or his Hawaiian adventure.

Being at the pinnacle of Honolulu society in his typical high-profile approach to things, Kaiser set about to recruit the most prestigious local physicians he could find. Dr. Durant, Herter, and Dodge were three prominent Caucasian physicians who were known to him socially. They were respected physicians and proven leaders of the state and county medical establishment. They shared office expenditures but were not partners. Kaiser managed to convince them to lead his health program. Kaiser's experienced Kaiser Industries manager Eugene Trefethen suggested to Kaiser that an all-Caucasian medical group might sharply limit the attractiveness of the program in multiethnic Hawaii. Samuel Yee, MD—of Chinese descent—and Homer Izumi, MD—of Japanese descent—were added to the founding group.

They were pure fee-for-service, establishment physicians who knew little or nothing about prepaid health care-delivery. Kaiser's overwhelming personality overcame any misgivings they may have had. After all, how could alignment with the fabulously rich tycoon who was transforming Hawaii be a bad financial move?

In the summer of 1958, Kaiser arranged for Scott Fleming, a prominent Kaiser Industries attorney and subsequent corporate counsel for Kaiser Permanente, and Clifford Keene, MD, effectively the Kaiser Health Plan CEO, to conduct a two-week intensive evening course for the partners on the principles of a prepaid medical care program. Kaiser attended many of the sessions and participated actively. His expansive approach tended to paper over the difficulties of what would be the ultimately unsuccessful effort to switch from fee-for-service to prepaid medical care-delivery by the partners.

Keene expected to stay on as possible medical director or at least as an advisor, but this was not to be. This was going to be Kaiser's show. After the sessions were completed, Fleming and Keene were flown back to the mainland. Keene was made to understand that he was to have nothing to do with the Kaiser Hawaii Health Plan and that he should stay out of Hawaii. He had a bad feeling that on some future day, the emergency call would come from Kaiser—and it did. Pacific Medical Associates would survive less than two catastrophic years before its contract was abruptly canceled. That is why the fiftieth anniversary of the Kaiser Health Plan was celebrated in 2008—while that of HPMG was celebrated two years later in 2010.

The seeds for the failure of the Pacific Medical Associates were sown from the start. Henry Kaiser allowed the five partners to continue their fee-for-service practice alongside the Kaiser prepaid practice. This would not

ALBERT J. MARIANI, M.D.

have been allowed in the traditional Permanente Medical Groups (PMGs). Prepayment and fee-for-service cannot comfortably coexist within the same medical group. The financial incentives for each are at cross-purposes. This was the first fatal flaw.

With prepayment, the budget is fixed but funds are immediately available because it is prepaid. The strategic goal is to provide the highest level of care with the lowest expenditure of resources. This conservation of medical resources allows for more care for the same cost, or similar care at lower cost than fee for service-based financing. The new Kaiser Health plan required a mix of both better benefits and low cost if it was going to be able to compete against the established HMSA. The quality of that care must be a given.

To conserve medical resources, preventive care, efficient care, and the avoidance of unnecessary or ineffective care are incentivized by prepaid financing. The prepaid fixed and immediately available budget allows for a preplanned organization of care to accomplish these goals. For prepaid medical care to work, physician salaries must be uncoupled from fee for service.

While physician compensation is less than one-fifth of the total health care budget, physician actions leverage nearly all of it. For health care costs as a whole, the cost of services generated by physicians is leveraged by five times more than the cost of physician salaries by the physician-driven cost of those services. This leveraging includes the cost of other consultations, laboratory, diagnostic imaging, drugs, surgery, and the need for office space and hospital services.

In traditional Permanente Medical Groups, the salaries are fixed, based only upon the market value of a given specialty. This is necessary only so that a high-quality medical group can be recruited and retained. The physicians are expected to earn their salaries by practicing preventive, high-quality, efficient medical care and taking responsibility for the avoidance of evidence-based, unnecessary, or ineffective care. Because they are salaried, their income is uncoupled from individual medical decisions. There is no incentive to provide unnecessary or ineffective care. It would just mean more work for the same salary. This is an actual disincentive to provide unnecessary care.

Conversely, in pure fee-for-service, the more services delivered, the more compensation. Compensation is directly linked to medical decision-making. Payment is largely determined by the number of services delivered—a form of piecework. In fee-for-service compensation, there is an actual financial disincentive to provide preventive care since it could reduce the need for future fee-for-service paid services.

In 1959, preventive services usually weren't a covered benefit anyway. Unnecessary care and even ineffective care were financially incentivized as long as it was covered by insurance. Fortunately, the high ethical standards and professionalism of physicians would usually guide them to protect their patients. To their credit, the worst abuses were avoided despite the temptation of these perverse financial incentives. It is not surprising, however, that physicians and patients equated more services, useful or not, with better care. People tend to do what they are paid to do. Doctors are people. Most physicians felt that it was up to the insurers to determine which services were worthwhile and would be compensated. These doctors felt that defining medical practice based upon preventive care—elimination of inefficient, duplicative, or ineffective care—was not their job but that of the insurers. Medical care-delivery would be defined and incentivized by what was covered or not covered.

At that time, medical cost containment by indemnity (fee-for-service) health plans was in its infancy. As a result, there were huge health care cost inefficiencies that could be eliminated by a well-run, prepaid, non-profit Kaiser Permanente-type program. Nonprofit KP had the potential to translate these efficiency-based savings into better care, more care, and less expensive care. This margin gave KP a huge value advantage in its early years, which was the key to its success. This was true, however, only if the potential advantages of prepaid medical care were effectively implemented. The efficiencies of KP medical care were not effectively implemented by the Pacific Medical Associates group. This led to the financial failure that caused its downfall.

The establishment of a two-class medical group by the partners was a second fatal flaw. In a traditional PMG, all doctors are salaried, and any coexisting fee-for-service is prohibited or at least narrowly defined and frowned upon. All qualified physicians are eligible to become partners after relatively short (two or three year) trial periods. While salaries are fixed and based on specialty-based market value because of necessity, any budget surplus as a result of care-delivery efficiencies is equally divided among all the partners. This financially fair system has gone a long way to keep the doctors in Permanente Medical Groups together during periods of crisis.

Henry Kaiser gave a free hand to the original five partners to form whatever kind of medical group they wished to build to service the Health Plan members. The partners hired additional physicians to care for the growing Health Plan membership under contract to them. At the time when the contract was terminated in August 1960, in addition to the five original partners, there were eventually thirty-three additional "hired hands." They were hired physicians and salaried by the partners at approximately one-quarter of the partners' base compensation. There was no provision for future partnership. Unlike the partners, they were not allowed a fee-for-service practice within the partnership. This two-class structure guaranteed conflict from the start.

Health Plan enrollment was slower than expected. There were only five thousand members when the hospital opened. To open the program on a sound financial basis, a minimum of fifteen thousand members were required. There were many obstacles. The union population, a traditional source of membership, was not as numerous in Honolulu as on the West Coast. As noted, there really wasn't a perceived need for a new Health Plan or hospital in Hawaii by a population that was already tightly bonded to their personal physicians—often on an ethnic basis.

HMSA had no interest in Kaiser's success. Very low rates were set by HMSA to financially starve the Kaiser program into submission before it established a beachhead. HMSA almost succeeded. The Kaiser program was required to respond with better coverage and lower rates. This forced a level of austerity, which made the early years very difficult. Nevertheless, the program slowly grew. By the summer of 1960, there were forty thousand members, but that still wasn't sufficient to fund an inefficient care-delivery program that was operating at a $2 million loss.

When a physician has two sources of income—one fixed and guaranteed (the salary) and the other variable based upon production (fee for service)—disproportionate effort will go into the fee-for-service component. This is exactly what happened. It is not entirely surprising. The partners had an excellent understanding of the financial incentives associated with fee for service. At the same time, they had little understanding of, no experience with, and little motivation to enact the financial incentives that make prepaid care successful. The definition of productivity did not go much beyond pushing the hired physicians to see more patients for their $1,000–1,100 per month salary.

Patient complaints to management began almost immediately. Fee-for-service, non-Kaiser patients were getting red carpet treatment such as personalized care, priority appointments, and free parking. Simultaneously and in the same Kaiser Health Plan-funded clinic, Kaiser Health Plan patients were subject to long waits and thin service. The non-partner physicians were clearly understaffed with doctor-to-patient ratios that were less than half of that of the community. The partners saw no problem in canceling their Kaiser Health Plan clinics on short notice to attend to other interests while pushing the hired doctors to work more hours and to see more patients.

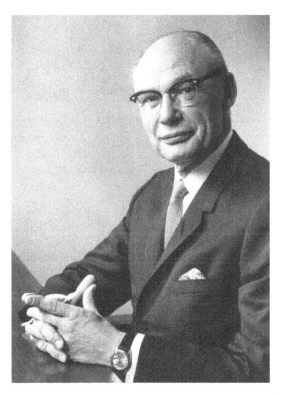

Clifford Keene, MD, Was willing to put his career on the line for Kaiser Permanente in Hawaii. He was later CEO of Kaiser Foundation Health Plan and Hospitals (1960–1970)

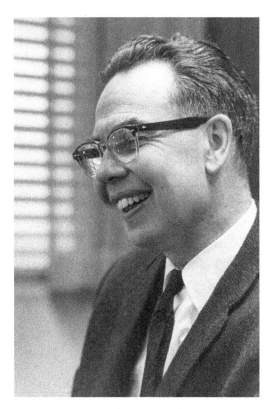

Ernest Saward, MD, medical director of Northwest Permanente from 1945–1970. He worked closely with Dr. Keene to establish the Hawaii Permanente Medical Group in 1960 and again in 1970 during the Philip Chu, MD, succession crisis.

Two Kaiser Permanente pioneers should be recognized as heroes of the Hawaii Permanente Medical Group (HPMG). One of these was Clifford "Cliff" Keene, MD, the de facto CEO (1956–1968) and later first CEO (1968–1975) of the Kaiser Foundation Health Plan. Dr. Keene was an experienced and well-trained board-certified general surgeon. He served four years in an administrative role in the US Army during World War II, achieving the rank of lieutenant colonel. He was a world-recognized authority on prepaid health care-delivery. His role in the Pacific Medical Associates crisis of 1960 and again in the presidential succession crisis of 1970 helped save the Medical Group. It is clear from his oral history that managing the Hawaii crisis of 1960 was one of the most difficult yet successful tasks of his career. He died on February 7, 2000.

The second HPMG hero was Earnest "Ernie" Saward, MD. Dr. Saward was the founder and medical director of the successful Northwest region centered in Portland, Oregon. He was a true founder of Kaiser Permanente and HPMG. After serving as medical director of the Northwest region for twenty-five years (1945–1970), he resigned for the altruistic reason that a new generation of leaders for the Northwest region needed to develop. He spent the remainder of his career in academic medicine, promoting the principles of Kaiser Permanente. He died in 1989. During the Hawaii region leadership crises of 1960 and 1970, he was the operational partner of Cliff Keene.

While Dr. Keene provided the bold strategic decision-making needed at the highest levels of KP, Dr. Saward, in a complementary fashion, provided tactical, day-to-day, on-the-ground management support for the fledgling HPMG leadership. He served as advisor to Dr. Keene and the new HPMG leaders, and part-time "auxiliary" medical director.

Out of the blue, the dreaded, but not unexpected, call from Kaiser came to Dr. Keene in the autumn of 1958, and Henry Kaiser demanded an immediate list of things to equip the hospital. Of course, no such list existed. Keene had been kept out of the loop on purpose by Kaiser. Thus began Keene's reinvolvement with Hawaii. A list was frantically cobbled together. He became involved with the hospital construction, and the hospital did open on time. He then turned his attention to the operation of the new Health Plan. Soon he had to address the problems of poor patient service, poor financial performance, and the quickly deteriorating situation between Pacific Medical Associates doctor partners and the Health Plan. This was in addition to his other worldwide responsibilities.

By March 1960, things were very bad and getting worse. Eugene Trefethen, at the suggestion of Dr. Keene, asked Dr. Saward to investigate the situation. Trefethen was a highly placed and successful manager of Kaiser Industries. He appears many times in the history of Kaiser Permanente as a positive force smoothing the stormy interface between Kaiser and his medical program.

Arrangements were made for Dr. Saward to practice in Hawaii during the month of April 1958. He said he was there to observe how such a practice worked. He was really there to figure out what was going wrong. He concluded that the partners were exploiting the "hired hand" physicians.

The hired physicians figured out the purpose of his visit and were not reluctant to tell him of the abuses that they felt that were being perpetrated. He made judgments about the quality of the medical talent and the leadership potential of the non-partner physicians. He concluded that the prepaid KP style of medical care was not being delivered by the partners and that the partners were favoring their own fee-for-service patients over the plan patients. Furthermore, the partners were exploiting the hired physicians, and the hired physicians didn't like it. This presented a possible opportunity. He shared his findings with Dr. Keene. When the crisis came to a head three months later, his inside knowledge of these operational details was essential to the successful establishment of HPMG.

The partners increasingly blamed Kaiser and what they characterized as his ill-considered health care program when the financial bonanza that they expected didn't materialize. They did not accept any operational responsibility for the financial shortfall. They expected Kaiser to simply bail out what they considered an underfunded program and blamed him when he didn't. The partners had a five-year contract with the Kaiser Health Plan, but there were escape clauses that could be activated at any time by either side. By the summer of 1960, the relationship between PMA and the Health Plan had completely broken down. That and the shunning of the Pacific Medical Associates physician partners and their families by the rest of the medical community was just too much for them.

On Saturday, July 20, 1960, the PMA partners submitted what they characterized as their final offer of a yearly salary of $60,000 per partner to Health Plan representatives. According to a statement issued by Kaiser, reported in the *Honolulu Advertiser:* "Dr. Richard Durant, medical director of PMA, pounded the table and replied 'By God, this is our final offer and you will meet it or else.'"

On Friday evening, August 19, a month later, Clifford Keene, MD, informed the partners that Health Plan would not be meeting their $60,000/year demand. On that same day, Durant informed the non-partner physicians that since Health Plan did not meet their "or else" demands, they regarded their contract with Health Plan repudiated. He also said that the partnership would no longer be responsible for paying the non-partners. This, of course, unsettled the non-partner physicians who were caring for the bulk of the 39,000 Health Plan patients, including those currently in the hospital. It was time to act.

Keene and the other program leaders had sadly watched the deterioration of the Hawaii situation. He and others had concluded that if the contract with PMA continued, the Hawaii program would die. Keene cleared his next move with Edgar Kaiser, now CEO of Kaiser Industries, Eugene Trefethen, Scott Fleming, and finally Henry Kaiser. They agreed to back what was to become the boldest decision in the history of the Kaiser Foundation Health Plan of Hawaii. It was the decision that saved the Hawaii program. It required personal courage on the part of Keene because it was made clear to him that the responsibility for the outcome was going to be entirely his. Kaiser told him, "Clifford, you're all on your own. If you come a cropper on this, you are just out the back door. You'll lose everything." In other words, he would be fired. Keene was staking his career on the outcome. As Keene said in his oral history, it was time to "roll the dice".

A meeting was called by Keene, the next day, at noon on Saturday, August 20, 1960. At this meeting, the partners and their hired doctors were told that the Health Plan regarded the recent actions of PMA as repudiation of the contract. Therefore, the contract was terminated, and the doctors were to vacate their offices. As the physicians got up to go, he asked the non-partners to stay. He invited them to form a new medical group. That group was to become the Hawaii Permanente Medical Group. A statement that Scott Fleming proudly characterized as a masterpiece of legal brevity was presented to them. Thirty-one out of thirty-three non partners signed it that day. Thus, HPMG was born.

For the partners, playing chicken with Henry Kaiser and his experienced management team was a very bad idea. The decision to take him on in the newspapers and the courts was an even worse idea.

The Pacific Medical Associates Take on Henry Kaiser

By declaring the contract with the five Pacific Medical Associates partners ended, Dr. Keene essentially rebooted the health program. He and Dr. Saward had correctly assumed that the partners were unpopular with the "hired hand" doctors because of their perceived exploitation while under contract to them. Keene and Saward knew that the Permanente Medical Group model was a proven concept and that the partnership would be seen as a much fairer program by the non-partner physicians. The non-partner physicians were also reluctant to abruptly abandon the Kaiser Health Plan patients. Dr. Keene called them on this. It was not surprising that most of them signed on to organize the Hawaii Permanente Medical Group on the afternoon that the contract with the PMA was ended. Dr. Saward, while still medical director of the Northwest Permanente Group, would work closely with the new medical director, Philip Chu, MD, on a part-time basis to establish the new Permanente group—the first new Permanente Medical Group since the founding of the program.

It is possible that, suddenly leaving forty thousand patients without medical care, that the partners expected Kaiser to knuckle under. That would have been their best bargaining chip. By immediately organizing the non-partner physicians into HPMG, Keene had boldly neutralized the continuing-care issue. This left the partners out in the cold, facing an eviction notice. At this point, they probably had little interest in continuing their affiliation with Kaiser in any case.

The partners had plenty of warning of Keene's plan to end the contract. Well before the August 20 confrontation, they had contracted Kenneth Young, a local attorney, to represent their interests. Their apparent plan was to delay their immediate expulsion from their medical offices in the Kaiser Hospital and to obtain a financial settlement with Kaiser. They embarked on a legal and public relations campaign to achieve just that.

The basis of their public relations campaign was sixfold. (1) They would claim that the program had exploited their reputations to establish the plan. (2) That the health plan, unwilling to pay their salaries, was discharging them without warning, thus breaking the contract. (3) They had carried out their duties in good faith and that the program was failing because it had been poorly managed by "suitcase executives from the mainland" who were trying to run the hospital and health care program like they would run a "cement plant." (4) They reiterated the old, discredited AMA accusations of ethical violations, of understaffing, and the hiring of unlicensed doctors. (5) They represented Kaiser's Health Plan as an out-of-touch, mainland juggernaut, disrupting the local Hawaii medical establishment. (6) Finally, they presented themselves as innocent, duped victims remaining above the fray while their attorney acted as their spokesperson.

By this time, Kaiser was deeply disappointed that his second attempt to establish a health care program managed directly by him had again been foiled by physicians. At the same time, he was heavily involved in a vast network of enterprises that was transforming Hawaii. He could have washed his hands of the whole mess. It would have had a negligible impact on his other Hawaii ventures. It was to his credit that he personally organized the response to the partners to defend "his" Kaiser Health Plan—even if he had to do it "partnering" with another Permanente Medical Group.

Anyone who knew Kaiser should not have been surprised by this. He really did believe that the health care program that he pioneered with Sidney Garfield was needed and would transform medical care in Hawaii and America—if not the world. He was also someone who was not going to back away from a legitimate fight. He did have some significant advantages. He had been successfully dealing with world-class controversies for more than fifty years. His public relations skills were the envy of his competitors. He owned popular local radio and television stations that had pioneered local news in Hawaii. Naturally, they would tilt toward his side of the story.

Finally, he was not seen as a disruptive outsider by the people of Hawaii. It was obvious that he truly loved Hawaii and was devoting his considerable energies to making it a better place. He had a reputation for integrity with the state government and the people and was credited for helping to break up the financial and industrial monopoly of the "Big Five" local corporations that had dominated the Hawaii economy—often with monopoly pricing. Facing a direct, high-profile, righteous challenge, it was "game on" for Mr. Kaiser.

In 1960, there were two large-circulation newspapers in Honolulu. There was the morning *Honolulu Advertiser* and the evening *Honolulu Star Bulletin*. On Monday evening, August 22, 1960, two days after the termination of PMA contract, in the *Star Bulletin* there was an article making vague references to "medical staff changes" and rumors of doctors being discharged.

The Kaiser spokesperson was less than forthcoming, saying that doctors had not been fired at the Kaiser Hospital:

> "Firing is not the word," he said. "If doctors do leave the Foundation they would do so by 'resignations due to disagreement.'"

On Tuesday, the *Star Bulletin* reported that the five partners were going to leave the hospital over salaries. On Wednesday morning, the partners got in the first punch. In the *Advertiser*, they were presented as among the most prominent physicians in the community who had lent their prestige to the establishment of the Kaiser Health program. This had been done in the face of heavy criticism by their colleagues and that they were lending their name to a "mass-production medical center" that was "basically a form of socialized medicine."

The Kaiser Health Plan local corporate response was lame. The *Advertiser* reported"

> The Kaiser spokesman was asked for a statement on comments that the Kaiser Foundation Hospital, after successfully using the talents of the five prominent Honolulu physicians for twenty months, now no longer felt it needed their talents, services, and reputations at the price being paid. The Kaiser spokesman would make no comment on this.

On Wednesday evening, the *Star Bulletin* reported that the five partners would be leaving Kaiser for salary reasons. An anonymous community physician who reportedly had previously worked for the Southern California Permanente Medical Group was quoted as saying: "Abrupt hiring and firing has been a traditional pattern at Kaiser hospital operations. It's just this simple. The doctors are hired help and as such are subject to being replaced." Of course, the five partners, being above the fray, had no comment. By Wednesday evening, August 24, Kaiser Health Plan was badly losing the publicity battle.

The tide turned with the personal entry of Henry Kaiser into the fray.

In a Thursday evening interview with the *Advertiser*, he punched back. As quoted by the Friday morning edition, he stated:

> The implications in the previous *Advertiser* stories are so completely contrary to the history of the Kaiser Foundation Hospitals and Health Plan that I owe a duty to state certain facts. The 40,000 Health Plan members here as well as the public, need to be protected from baseless fears and misinformation being manufactured currently by the local "rumor factory." In Honolulu, the Kaiser Foundation organizations would not suddenly reverse the principles and practices followed since the beginnings of the present medical care program twenty-seven years ago.

By the Friday-evening edition of the *Star Bulletin,* it was open warfare. In forty-five-point type, the headline read: "KAISER, DOCTORS BARE HOSPITAL ROW." The entirety of page 13 was dedicated to competing statements. Kaiser led off by effectively refuting the anonymous doctor who said that doctors were hired help. Interestingly, he fell back upon describing a standard Permanente Medical Group model. He pointed out that doctors partnering with the Health Plan were in independent medical groups now consisting of more than four hundred partners. Many had been with the program for decades, the turnover was less than 3 percent, and it was rare to be discharged for cause after passing the probationary period. He pointed out that no Northwest PMG physician had left program in the past five years. Finally, he pointed out that none of these partnering independent medical groups had ever repudiated a contract with the health plan—and that this was a first. He stopped there, having effectively rebutted the "doctors as hired hands of the Kaiser Health Plan" argument.

Instead of focusing on one issue, the PMA statement issued by their attorney was a litany of incautiously worded complaints. It was full of erroneous statements that were now in print and could be systematically refuted. Over the next few days, Kaiser took apart each one of these inaccurate statements, which seriously undermined the credibility of the partners.

They characterized "Mr. Keene" (Clifford Keene, MD) as "a suitcase executive from the mainland." They maintained that he had suddenly canceled their five-year contract not for cause but because he didn't like their "attitude." It stated that the non-partner physicians were hired directly by the Kaiser Health Plan. He went on to say, "Dr. Saward, a doctor not licensed in the state of Hawaii who had just arrived from the mainland would become director of professional services under the Kaiser Health Plan." They stated that Saward was directly employing the non-partner physicians as Kaiser Health Plan employees. They went on to say that these changes had affected morale badly, that PMA hired doctors had resigned, and the program was now understaffed. They concluded by saying, "In brief, the doctors in the Pacific Medical Associates are tired of being pushed around by a myth of gigantism. They have not and will not permit a hospital under their medical control and supervision be operated as some might operate a cement factory."

In the Saturday-morning edition of the *Advertiser,* it was the front-page lead story: "'UNETHICAL' SAY FIVE; 'NOT SO' SAYS HENRY J." A full-page article had the doctors' statement on the left-half side of the page, and "Kaiser's Reply" was on the right half. The doctor's statement was almost a verbatim copy of the doctor's statement covered in the Friday-evening *Honolulu Star Bulletin* piece. In contrast, Kaiser came out blazing. This time, he focused on their contention that they had faithfully performed their duties and then were suddenly fired without cause. Kaiser replied, "The five doctors' repudiation and termination of their contract to manage and supply medical care for Health Plan members culminated more than nine months of fruitless efforts to get them to live up to their obligations."

He then attacked their income demands:

> On June 18 the partners had received net personal incomes in 1959 of totaling approximately $45,000 each and in the first seven months of 1960 at a rate that would extrapolate to a $50,000 yearly income for each partner. Their new demands [$60,000] would have raised the professional medical care costs a fantastic amount that could not under any circumstances, be passed on through higher dues to the 40,000 Health Plan members. Consequently, Kaiser Foundation Health Plan officials replied that these

demands were "utterly and fantastically ridiculous and impossible."

It should be noted that in 1960 the US Census Bureau reported that the average family income in the United States was $5,600—and that the top 1 percentile was at just under $25,000. Kaiser went on to say that the partners, not the health plan, had repudiated the contract because the Health Plan would not meet their demands for $60,000 to continue to provide services to the members. Thus, Kaiser positioned himself and the program administrators as the protectors of the Health Plan members from the greedy doctors. That became the headline in the morning *Advertiser*: "'I WON'T PAY DOCTORS $60,000 EACH ANGRY KAISER DECLARES.'

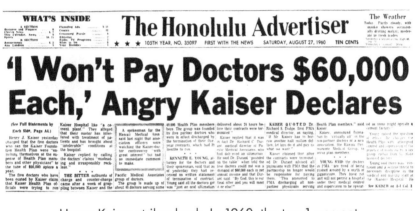

Henry Kaiser strikes back. In 1960, the top 1 percent income bracket was about $25,000.

Kaiser went on to point out that virtually all of the non-partner physicians had immediately and voluntarily reorganized as the Hawaii Permanente Medical Group. He pointed out that the partners had refused to hire sufficient numbers of physicians and that any short staffing was due to that. He also noted that the partners had not equitably shared the dollars received by the partnership with the non-partners. Thus, any low morale by the non-partners was due to the actions of the partners and not the Health Plan. Finally, he placed the financial problems of the program squarely on the partners' shoulders due to a "failure of leadership" and failure to provide "efficient medical management in the interest of assuring comprehensive medical services to the members at reasonable cost."

On that busy Saturday, August 27, a sidebar to the main article, "Lee to Look Into Hospital," stated that Dr. Lee, the Hawaii director of health, would have one of his staff check out the allegation that unlicensed physicians (Drs. Saward and T. K. Lin) were practicing medicine in the Kaiser Hospital. The response by the program was published the following Wednesday, August 31, in the evening *Star Bulletin* and in the morning *Advertiser* on September 1 that Drs. Lin and Saward were not practicing but were performing administrative duties. This was legal, and that was the end of it. In another sidebar, a spokesperson for the Oahu County Medical Association stated that the society would not be investigating the Kaiser Hospital because that duty was held by the American Hospital Association. He dismissively went on to say, "This hospital [Kaiser Hospital] as far as we know has never been accredited by the AHA. It may have been so accredited, but we do not know it."

In the same edition, an article, "New Group of Doctors Claims Kaiser Plan Care," described the establishment of the Hawaii Permanente Medical Group and the fact that it would assume the care of the Kaiser Health Plan patients. It pointed out that the chairman of the board of HPMG was Philip Chu, MD, and that Ernest Saward, MD, was a consultant. An image of the "Declaration of Associateship" with the signatures of the thirty-one founding doctors was published with the article. This positive article reassured Kaiser Health Plan members that there would be continuity of care.

The press war reached its climax in the *Advertiser* on Sunday, August 28, 1960 with a 1 3/8-inch red capitalized headlines: COURT BLOCKS KAISER FROM FIRING DOCTORS." There was an accompanying front-page editorial cartoon of Henry Kaiser with a big smile on his face, fencing with scalpels with five scowling doctors, one of whom was down and out.

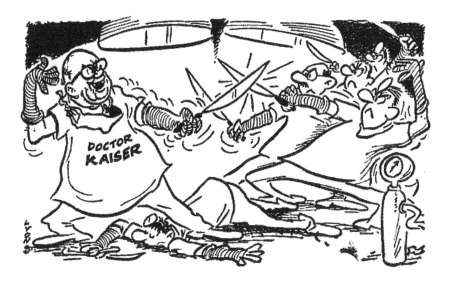

Scalpel fight between Henry Kaiser and Pacific
Medical Associates doctors.

The headline was somewhat inaccurate. It referred to a ten-day temporary restraining order obtained at six thirty on Saturday evening to prevent Kaiser Health Plan administrators from evicting the five partners from the hospital until a case could be heard in the courts on September 6. The Circuit Court judge, William Fairbanks, had agreed to the restraining order to give the partners time to make the transition out.

In side-by-side front-page statements, Kaiser and the partners exchanged charges again. The partners claimed that they were making a salary of only $24,000 a year. This was in response to Kaiser statements, who on the previous day, had given the newspapers a copy of the certified public accountant's statement of the partner's total 1959 income statements showing that they made $45,333.88 each from their Health Plan affiliation. The $24,000 was salary for plan patients, and the rest was from their fee-for-service practice with the billing and overhead covered by the Kaiser Health Plan. The fine distinction between salary and fee-for-service income was likely lost on the reading public who would have focused on the doubled "1-percenter" income. The rest of the statement was a summary of a list of grievances that later would be the basis of a lawsuit that was filed a week later.

By Sunday, Henry Kaiser's publicity offensive must have been hitting home. The partners complained that "Pacific Medical Associates are astounded at the burst of propaganda emanating from the Kaiser pressroom." Kaiser led off with a two-paragraph detailed description of the impressive medical qualifications of Dr. Keene who the partners had previously referred to as "Mr. Keene ... the suitcase executive from the mainland." He presented this as the first of many "falsehoods" found in the partners' press releases. He attacked the partners for their "reckless accusations" that were causing anxiety in plan patients. As for charges of confusion and poor morale in the hospital, he responded, "Patient care is proceeding efficiently and the only 'hospital confusion' has been created only because the five partners are not cooperating in an orderly transfer of their responsibilities to the new association."

He characterized the five doctors' plan to use the attorney as their spokesperson as a form of cowardice: "I have heretofore said to the press that there is nothing secret about the operation of the Kaiser Foundation Hospital and Health Plan and the recent statements given to the press have been given by me personally. It comes as a surprise to me that the 'five doctors' have hidden behind this attorney." He then went on to attack the attorney for ethical violations.

The restraining order was also the headline in the Sunday evening *Star Bulletin*: "Court Halts Kaiser Hospital Firings. Judge Signs Restraining Order." There was a shorter summary of the back-and-forth arguments. There was another political cartoon featuring Henry Kaiser with a stern look on his face listening to the chest of a doctor labeled Pacific Medical Associates with a stethoscope. The doctor with an angry scowl on his face was, in turn, listening to his. Both are saying, "YOU'RE SICK! SICK! SICK!"

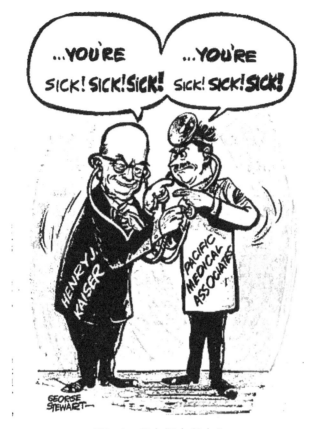

"You're Sick Sick Sick."

On Monday morning, August 29, the *Advertiser* had a prominent story on page A6: "Kaiser Plans Fight Against Restrainer." The restraining order challenge would be heard on August 31. Neither Kaiser nor PMA spokespersons would comment on what now would be a court case.

On Monday, August 29, in response to accusations that Kaiser Health Plan patients would be without doctors, the newspaper printed the founding document of the Hawaii Permanente Medical Group to demonstrate that medical care would be assumed without interruption by the HPMG doctors.

A declaration of association as the Permanente Medical group by remaining doctors at the Kaiser Medical Center.

The Hawaii Permanente Medical Group Founding Document.

Mysteriously, the *Advertiser* got its hands on the Kaiser affidavit. On Tuesday, in a full-page article, it liberally quoted from Kaiser's twenty-point defense—actually more of a counterattack against the PMA. This gave Kaiser the last punch. That evening, the *Honolulu Star Bulletin* also summarized the case to be heard on the following day. By this time, both sides were in active negotiation and close to a settlement, so the hearing was delayed. The *Star Bulletin* headline read: "Kaiser Hospital Hearing Delayed 'Peace' Rumored." It pointed out that two of the partners had either already moved out or were moving out of the hospital.

The headline in the Thursday morning September 1 *Advertiser*, "Kaiser Victor in Medical Dispute," described the agreement reached between the PMA partners and Health Plan. The agreement stated that the partners had until September 20 to vacate their offices. Until that time, they could care for their non-plan private patients in the Kaiser Hospital. They could no longer care for Kaiser Health Plan patients and must turn over the care of such patients to the Hawaii Permanente Medical Group. Both parties agreed to cooperate and "eliminate any friction" during the transition.

The evening *Star Bulletin* article, "5 fired Doctors to Stay Partners Outside Hospital," said, "The five doctors of the Pacific Medical Associates, who lost the first round yesterday in their heated fight with the Kaiser Foundation Health Plan, announced today the continuance of their partnership outside the Kaiser Hospital."

On Friday, another *Advertiser* article, "Kaiser Winner in Hospital Row," restated the agreement.

So, in ten days, it was over. What had happened according to the oral history of Kaiser attorney Scott Fleming was that he had received a call over the weekend from Kenneth Young, the attorney for the partners, proposing an end to the press war that was now going very badly for them. Mr. Fleming's response was in essence: Sure—since the press war was your idea to begin with. The controversy suddenly disappeared from the newspapers, but not before both the *Honolulu Advertiser* and the *Honolulu Star Bulletin* had declared Henry Kaiser the winner.

The dispute sputtered on in the form of lawsuits. On December 30, 1960, there was a small article in the *Star Bulletin* in which the PMA partners were suing Kaiser Health Plan for $1.7 million. They claimed $750,000 for breach of contract, $750,000 for interference with their medical practice, and $200,000 for punitive damages. There was a similar article in the *Advertiser* the following day.

On Saturday March 4, 1961, the *Star Bulletin*'s "Kaiser Plan Makes Counterclaim For $620,962 from five Doctors" claimed $400,000 in damages and $220,962 in alleged overpayments. The story was repeated by the *Advertiser* the next day. On March 20, 1961, the *Star Bulletin* reported that the partners sued the Kaiser Hospital for an additional $3,011,723. The next day's *Advertiser* totaled the claims against Kaiser in an article entitled "Doctors Ask $4,711,723 From Kaiser Health Plan." Scott Fleming saw this as a potentially serious case and organized a mainland team of legal heavy hitters. The partners' legal team, possibly feeling overmatched, settled the suit for a token $80,000. This approximated their legal costs. A small article in the *Honolulu Star Bulletin* article on April 25, 1961, noted that the Pacific Medical Associates had amicably dissolved their partnership.

CHAPTER 4

THE GENETIC CODE AND THE KAISER PERMANENTE GOLDEN AGE

T he Tahoe conferences provided only the blueprint for a power-sharing agreement between the Kaiser Foundation Health Plan (KFHP) and the Permanente Medical Groups (PMG). This blueprint was tested for a full six years before a stable understanding was achieved. Both entities vied for dominance during this interval. The insider jargon for this set of operational and power sharing understandings was the Kaiser Permanente "genetic code." For more than thirty years, these understandings provided the basis for the phenomenal growth and an increasing national and international influence of Kaiser Permanente.

Important factions in Health Plan, including Henry Kaiser, did not feel that doctors should have any role in management, but they should function as highly skilled employees. Similarly, factions within the Medical Groups felt that they did not need the services of Health Plan. These ideas had been tested in 1960 in Hawaii. Health Plan had fired the original medical group (Pacific Medical Associates) personally recruited by Henry Kaiser but was forced to fall back on the Permanente Medical Group model to survive. To preserve the KP program in Hawaii, Henry Kaiser, to his credit, did not resist the establishment of a PMG model and strenuously and successfully defended the reorganized program from the subsequent negative publicity onslaught of the Pacific Medical Associates.

In 1961, it was the turn of the Northern California Permanente Medical Group (TPMG) leadership to return the favor. Since 1960 had been a good year for TPMG, it began 1961 with a significant financial surplus, a stable medical group, and a rapidly growing membership. A faction of the TPMG leadership thought it was time to prove that they did not need Health Plan to manage the business side of a health care program. They identified an opportunity in San Diego. At that time, there was no KP or other prepaid health care program in this rapidly growing city separated from Los Angeles only by the Marine Corps training base, Camp Pendleton, to the north. The TPMG leadership was authorized by a strong majority of the associates to purchase for $475,000 the forty-six-bed Murray Hospital and to initiate there "a medical care program under the ownership, control, and operation of the Permanente Medical Group." The new program was to be called Pan-Medical Inc.

Morris Collen, MD, was to be the leader of this effort. Dr. Collen was a militant defender of the physician's role in any health care program and an important program founder. By choosing Dr. Collen to lead the effort, TPMG was demonstrating the seriousness of the initiative. He had been the first chief of medicine of the first Kaiser Health Plan for the shipyard workers. He had gone on to lead the research effort to prove that the Kaiser care was equal to and often superior to conventional medical care. He had been a lead negotiator for the Medical Groups in the Tahoe negotiations. He was to go on to a long list of lifetime program achievements, but this was not going to be one of them. He died at the age of 100 in 2014, still working part-time promoting Kaiser Permanente health care.

Initially, Health Plan management and the Southern California Permanente Medical Group (SCPMG) were cautiously supportive. As soon as Henry Kaiser found out about it, however, he was furious. He correctly saw this as an effort by TPMG to establish a competing Health Plan to weaken or even kill the mutual exclusivity understanding of the medical service agreement between Health Plan and the Medical Groups.

Mr. Kaiser's reaction spread to the Health Plan leadership and negotiations with TPMG stalled. The rapidly growing Southern California Permanente Medical Group (SCPMG) leadership also began to realize that this initiative, of which they were to have no part, would seriously impede any future expansion plans they might have into the adjacent, rapidly growing, and potentially lucrative San Diego market. Things were getting complicated. The potential of the Health Plan to terminate the medical services agreement with TPMG, just as had been done in Hawaii a year earlier, loomed over everything. This would have destroyed the program.

A critical meeting was called between Henry Kaiser and Cecil Cutting, MD, the president of TPMG. The meeting was well described by Dr. Smillie in his TPMG history. Both were program founders, both had fought many battles together to defend the program, and Dr. Cutting had actually lived with Kaiser for ten months during Bess Kaiser's terminal illness ten years earlier.

Kaiser met with Cutting on the top floor of the Kaiser building in Oakland. Looking out over Lake Merritt, Kaiser rebuffed Dr. Cutting's approach and remained silent. Finally, Cutting broke the ice and said, "Mr. Kaiser, would you really destroy this plan because of San Diego?"

Kaiser replied that he would.

Cutting responded, "In that case, Mr. Kaiser, I will assure you that the Medical Group will not go through with its plans."

At that, Kaiser turned to face his old friend and said, "Can you do that, Cecil?"

Cutting said he could, and he would—and he did.

On September 18, the TPMG partnership voted to sell the hospital, which it did for a tidy profit. That was the end of Pan Medical Inc. If Henry Kaiser and Cecil Cutting had not been founding fathers of Kaiser Permanente and personally invested in the success of the program, would they have compromised their egos and backed away from their entrenched positions? It is an interesting question, especially for today's program leadership.

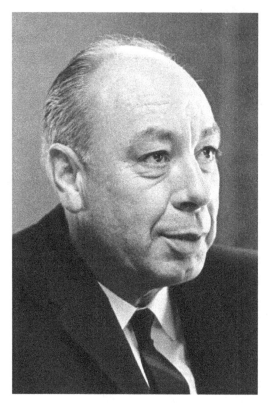

Cecil Cutting, MD, was one of the founding fathers of Kaiser Permanente. He was the first medical director of the Permanente Medical Group of Northern California.

As a participant in the 1987 Kaiser Permanente Stanford Executive Training Program, a highlight of the program for the author was the presentation by Dr. Cutting. Since his retirement as medical director of TPMG in 1977, he saw as his continuing mission the need to communicate the founders' vision of Kaiser Permanente to the new generations of leadership. That vision had evolved into the genetic code of Kaiser Permanente.

The genetic code espoused the principles of (1.) prepayment for comprehensive medical care to incentivize preventive care and the early treatment of disease through stable financing, (2.) cost-effective care through broad community rating so that the care is affordable by as much of the population as possible, (3.) vertical integration of facilities to control costs and provide a cultural environment in which preventive, cost-effective, scientifically based care can be safely delivered by the medical staff, (4.)

dual option to avoid forcing patients into the program, which by necessity had a closed panel of doctors, and finally and most important, (5.) the exclusive Health Plan-Medical Group partnership to balance interests of economics and medical care. It is worthwhile to spend some time on each of these elements of the genetic code.

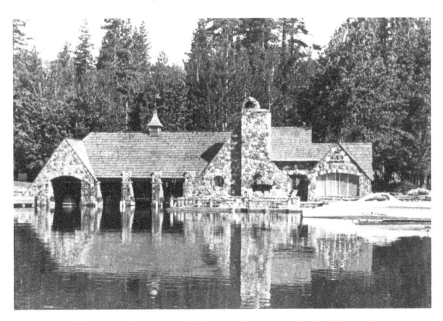

Fleur de Lac—the Henry Kaiser residence on Lake Tahoe. Some of the Tahoe agreement meetings were held here. These meetings established the fundamentals of the Kaiser Health Plan and Hospitals and Permanente Medical Group relationship.

Prepayment for Comprehensive Care

As noted in chapter 1, Sidney Garfield's desert clinic was on the verge of bankruptcy until A. B. Ordway and Harold Hatch of Industrial Insurance Exchange proposed prepayment based upon the number of patients served (capitation) rather than fee for service. That changed everything.

With guaranteed prepayment, the financial situation immediately improved. Resources formerly spent on billing and fighting insurance companies for denied or delayed fees could now be devoted to medical care. With guaranteed payment, planned investments could confidently be made in the staff and facilities to deliver better care. More important, preventive care and the early treatment of disease now aligned with the economic interest of the care program. In a fee-for-service model, preventive care is at odds with the economic interest of a fee-for-service care program. If there is no treatment, there is no fee. The more treatment rendered—worthwhile or not—the more fees paid. In a prepaid program, the payment has already been received. The less treatment needed, the more resources are left over for more care, more coverage, or lower, more affordable premiums. It only works this way in a nonprofit setting. In a for-profit setting, the temptation would be to divert any cost savings from decreased care to profits, which would be used to fuel stock dividends, stock options, and high salaries for executives.

Cost Effective Care and Broad-Based Community Rating

While often excellent—but not always—expensive health care outside of the reach of most of the population is not very useful to society. A goal of Kaiser Permanente was and is to provide excellent health care that would be affordable to the average working person. It was an article of faith that this could be achieved by a combination of efficient, evidence-based care, and economies of scale. Prepayment would avoid the perverse economic incentives of the medical industrial complex and fee-for-service payment mechanisms.

The purpose of health insurance is to cover the cost of catastrophic illness by spreading that cost over a large population and time. Thus, for a modest cost, the insured would have the peace of mind of knowing that the cost of a catastrophic illness would be covered. Catastrophic illness is bad enough. To compound it with financial ruin is often overwhelming. It actually impedes the healing process.

A broad-based community rating would provide the large population necessary to spread the financial risk over time and numbers. The goal would be to sign up as many community members as possible. The Health Plan would then determine the necessary budget to care for this population and set a per-member, per-month charge (capitation). As long as the members represent the average health of the community population, a broad-based community rating works well.

The flaw in community rating is narrow rather than broad-based community rating. The 50 percent of the population that uses only 10 percent of health care resources pays for the 5 percent that use 50 percent of the health care resources, including the 1 percent that use an astounding 28 percent of the resources. Figure out how to exclude that 5 percent of the population through marketing only to young, healthy populations, limiting coverage, and product design, and there is a lot of money to be made by for-profit health plans.

In an environment of legal cherry picking, for the health plans that don't cherry pick, they are left with the more expensive sicker patients. This leads to a health plan "death spiral." Since these plans have to charge more for the sick patients, premiums must be much higher. Only high-risk, sick patients are willing to pay the high premiums, while the healthy patients migrate to the cheaper plans. As premiums go higher and higher to accommodate the increasing disease burden, eventually the premiums are so high that no one can afford them—and the expensive health plans simply go out of business. The end result would be prohibitively expensive or nonexistent health insurance for those who need it and inexpensive health noninsurance for those who don't. This form of pseudo-health insurance negates the whole social mission of health insurance.

From the sixties through the early nineties, broad-based capitation worked well for Kaiser Permanente. Membership rates were affordable because of the large, representative, capitated populations that were being served. This and the medical benefits and cost efficiency of comprehensive care were a formula for success. Things would change in the early 1990s, which would threaten the financial health of, and more so, the soul of Kaiser Permanente.

Vertical Integration of Facilities

With prepayment came the capital to build the program's own hospitals, clinics, and pharmacies. By building facilities based upon clinical need rather than investing in new facilities to increase market share that may never occur, costs were better controlled. Owning its own facilities allowed the program to internalize care. Better quality and cost control of internalized care was now possible. Internalized care protected KP from outside local monopoly providers. Thus, it avoided monopoly-based subsidies to the competition, which would need to be passed on to members with either increased premiums, fewer covered services, or both.

More important, ownership of its own facilities provided a professionally safe environment to evolve and exercise evidence-based, rational, cost-effective medicine. It could be uncontaminated by the perverse incentives of the medical-industrial complex and fee-for-service medicine often delivered by a hostile outside medical community.

The "big money" to be saved in medical care is not made by fancy financing, complicated product design, marginally better contracts, or buying medical care at below cost because of market oversupply (which is always temporary. The big money is saved by medical care being delivered scientifically, systematically, and rationally to a representative segment of the population. This was and is a core strength of Kaiser Permanente. It happens best when the care is internalized.

Voluntary Membership: The Dual Choice

In the early years, a persistent criticism of the Kaiser Permanente program was that patients were being forced into a "socialistic" health care program with a limited choice of doctors who were "owned" by the Kaiser Industries. The Permanente Medical Groups were eventually able to neutralize the false Kaiser Industries "ownership" argument by emphasizing their independence from the Kaiser Foundation Health Plan.

The argument that patients were being forced into a "socialist health care system" with a limited choice of doctors was disposed of by the "dual choice" policy. Dual choice meant that a patient offered Kaiser would, wherever possible, have the choice of a non-Kaiser plan. This "dual option" had a twofold advantage for the program. First, patients who would not be happy with KP didn't have to join. This siphoned off those who were already skeptical of the plan and therefore would be hard if not impossible to please. The second advantage was that it forced Kaiser Permanente to compete with non-Kaiser programs on cost, service, and quality. Dual option became less important as Kaiser Permanente established itself as a model program for US health care. Nevertheless, it served its purpose, and even today, most Kaiser Permanente patients have the option not to join the program when health care decisions must be made.

Exclusive Partnership of Kaiser Foundation Health Plan and the Permanente Medical Groups:

Arguably the most difficult and the most important component of the code is the exclusive partnership between Health Plan and the Permanente Medical Groups. The partnership had been sorely tested by the Walnut Creek, Hawaii, and San Diego ventures. By 1961, a sort of detente between the Health Plan and the Medical Groups had been reached. Because of his Hawaii work, Clifford Keene, MD, was now widely respected and accepted as effectively the CEO of the Kaiser Foundation Health Plan. The Medical Group and Health Plan leadership of the existing four regions—Northern California, Southern California, Northwest, and Hawaii—were established and stable. The partnership was poised to bear fruit.

The partnership was, and is, by no means easy. The disparate cultures of business and medicine are difficult to reconcile, but it is precisely that reconciliation that makes the program successful. It required skill, patience, understanding, and forbearance. Regions with well-balanced, competent Health Plan and Medical Group leadership prospered mightily. Those that didn't stagnated—sometimes for years. Some regions failed. The successful regions have been an argument for the genetic code, especially the partnership. The same is true for the failed regions that ignored the genetic code. There is a huge difference between a partner relationship and a vendor relationship. When working optimally, the partnership is more of a covenant than a contract.

Between 1960 and 1970, during Dr. Clifford Keene's time at the helm of Kaiser Foundation Health Plan, Kaiser Permanente grew from 800,000 to 2,200,000 members and had spread from three to six regions.

James (Jim) Vohs led the program from 1970 until 1992. He began his career with Kaiser Industries as a mailroom clerk after graduating from high school. After obtaining his degree at the University of California at Berkeley in 1952, he joined the labor relations department of Kaiser Industries. In 1954, he transferred to the Northern California Kaiser medical program because, as he said, he wanted the opportunity to do something "for the public good." He rose rapidly in the Health Plan. By 1957, he was the employee relations manager in Southern California region, and six months later, he was offered the Health Plan manager position. By 1970 he was effectively the CEO of Health Plan.

Vohs was a courtly, principled, other-centered gentleman who believed deeply in the founding principles of the program, including prepaid group practice, the Medical Group-Health Plan partnership, and a decentralized organizational structure. In other words, he believed in, and managed by, the Kaiser Permanente genetic code. He had a special interest in promoting quality assurance. For his efforts promoting quality assurance, the yearly Kaiser Permanente James A. Vohs Quality Award was named after him. Under his leadership, the program grew from 2.2 million members to 6.6 million members and from six regions to twelve regions.

Both Keene and Vohs believed in the code and managed by its principles. It was a golden age for Kaiser. Membership increased more than eightfold, and Kaiser Permanente had evolved from being a peculiar West Coast health care entity to a nationwide, rapidly growing organization that was being studied as a model for health care both nationally and internationally. In his typical self-effacing way, when Jim Vohs retired, he stated that he was leaving the organization in good hands—hands that would take it to the next level of performance. That was not to be, but that's another story for later.

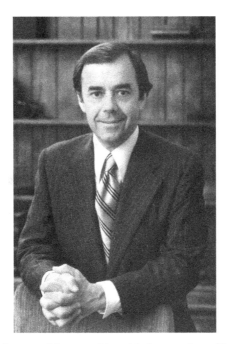

James A. Vohs: president and/or chief executive officer of Kaiser
Foundation Health Plan and Hospitals from 1970 to 1992.

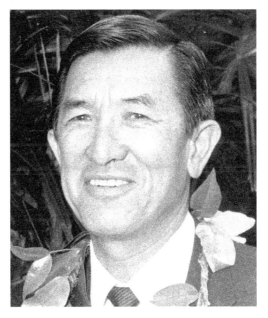

Dr. Phil Chu: the founding medical director of the
Hawaii Permanente Medical Group.

CHAPTER 5

PHILIP CHU, MD: THE FIRST PRESIDENT OF THE HPMG

n his oral history, Dr. Keene described how he chose Dr. Chu to lead the first Permanente Medical Group outside of the original California and Oregon regions. At the end of one long day, as he was leaving the hospital, he ran into Dr. Chu as he was waiting outside for a ride from his wife, Phoebe. Since both were surgeons, they had something in common. As they spoke, Dr. Keene was so impressed with Chu's charisma and leadership potential that he decided on the spot that if he got the opportunity to promote one physician from the group to be its leader, it would be Dr. Chu. Who was this Dr. Chu who was to be the founding president of the Hawaii Permanente Medical Group?

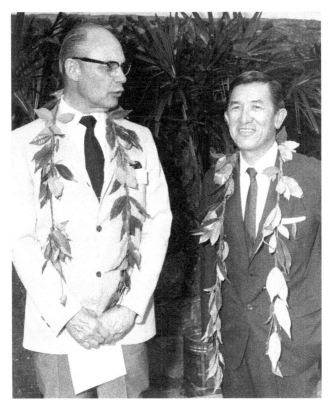

Drs. Clifford Keene and Philip Chu.

Philip Chong Chu was born in Honolulu on September 3, 1918. He received his BS degree at the University of Hawaii in 1940. He obtained his MD from the Pennsylvania Medical School of St. John's University in Shanghai, China, in 1944, which was at the time an affiliate of the University of Pennsylvania. He went on to his internship at St. Luke's Hospital in Shanghai from 1944–5 during the difficult and dangerous Japanese occupation of the city.

After the Japanese surrender, from 1945 to 1947, he was the regional medical officer for the China Division of the United Nations Relief and Rehabilitation Administration. He returned to the United States in 1947 to continue his medical studies in pathology at Jefferson Medical College (1947–52) and then in general surgery at the State University of New York in Syracuse (1952–6) where he completed his general surgery residency. He obtained his board certification in general surgery. After his residency, he served as a surgeon and medical officer in charge of the US Public Health Service Indian Hospital at Sacaton, Arizona (1957–8) and then as senior surgeon and deputy chief surgeon at the US Public Health Service Hospital in Detroit (1958–9).

He then returned to Honolulu. The timing was fortuitous. Pacific Medical Associates would soon break up, and someone would be needed to lead what would become the new Hawaii Permanente Medical Group (HPMG). That a physician with such clinical and administrative experience was available and willing to join the program was a stroke of extraordinary good fortune for the future of HPMG.

The first general staff meeting of HPMG was held five days after Dr. Keene dissolved the Pacific Medical Associates and reformed what was to be HPMG from the PMA-hired doctors. Dr. Saward presided over the first meeting as chief of professional services on that Tuesday evening at five o'clock on August 22, 1960. Dr. Saward stated that he was acting in a temporary advisory role. He announced that individual fee-for-service payments, which had been a major source of discontent within PMA, would no longer be allowed. Any fee-for-service income by the members would be placed into the HPMG general fund to fund HPMG medical services. He announced, in consultation with Dr. Keene, a temporary HPMG governing committee that would consist of the acting chiefs of the major services: Philip Chu, MD, surgery and chairman of the board, T. K. Lin, MD, medicine, Alma Chun, MD, pediatrics, Arthur Zacks, MD, hospital services, James Bennett pathology, and Willis Butler, MD, outlying clinics. While Hawaii would be the first new region, he recommended that it follow the model of the established Permanente Medical Groups in California and Oregon.

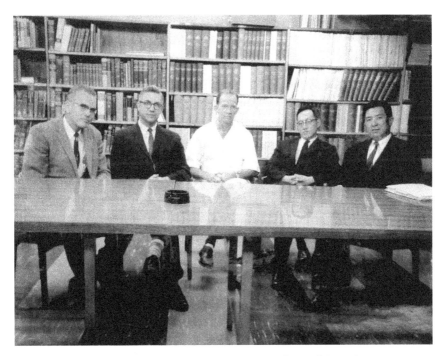

The first HPMG executive committee (L to R) Drs. Jim
Bennett, J. Dempsey Hewitt, Willis Butler, T. K. Lin, Phil
Chu. Drs. Alma Chun and Arthur Zacks were absent.

Dr. Chu presided over subsequent general staff meetings. During the next
three weekly meetings, basic operational policies were established. The
name Hawaii Permanente Medical Group was formally adopted. Clinic
hours were to be 9:30 a.m. to noon and then 1:30–5:30 during weekdays
and 9:00–1:00 on Saturdays. All physicians were expected to work five and
a half days. The roles of Health Plan and HPMG were clarified relative to
the hospital. Laboratory and diagnostic imaging were to be administered
by HPMG.

Dr. Chu then went on a two-week tour of the California and Oregon
regions. He was personally tutored by Kaiser Permanente founders Ray
Kay, MD, Southern California medical director, Cecil Cutting, MD,
Northern California medical director, Cliff Keene, MD, acting CEO of
Kaiser Permanente, Scott Fleming Kaiser Permanente corporate counsel,
Eugene Trefethen of the Kaiser Permanente board, and Ernest Saward,

MD, Northwest medical director. These legendary program founders believed deeply in its principles.

Despite the Hawaii region's inauspicious beginnings, they wanted to be sure that the medical director of the first expansion region was going to be successful and that he understood the underlying principles of Kaiser Permanente. They had made many personal sacrifices on behalf of a program that they felt should be the model of health care in America if not the world. This missionary spirit was to last almost forty years until it reached a peak of twelve regions spread over the US by the late 1990s. This was paralleled by an active Kaiser Permanente International effort that was intended to spread the concept of the KP model internationally.

Phil Chu was a good student. Upon his return to Hawaii at the September 30, 1960, staff meeting, he articulated the Kaiser Permanente founding principles that would be the strategic and operational hallmarks for the new HPMG: a nonprofit Health Plan, an HPMG Medical Group-Health Plan exclusive partnership with mutual accountabilities, salaried physicians under Medical Group management, financing predominantly by prepaid membership dues, vertical integration of services, an emphasis on preventive care, and the voluntary enrollment (dual option) of members. He emphasized that while the program was nonprofit, it was not a charitable program. Patients were to be treated as private, not charity, patients. Arguably, these Kaiser Permanente founding principles remain to this day best preserved in the Hawaii region and have been the reason for its steady progress.

The Pacific Medical Associates partners had failed because they were unable to make the transition from the economic imperatives of fee-for-service to the almost opposite economic imperatives of prepaid medical care. While KP on the mainland had been delivering large-scale prepaid care for almost two decades, there were no models for the very different Hawaii health care environment. While the HPMG leadership was well mentored in the theoretical advantages of the KP model, translating that model to the day-to-day care of tens of thousands of patient interactions required much ad hoc ingenuity and experimentation.

During the decade of Dr. Chu's leadership, almost every decision was setting a Hawaii region care-delivery precedent. All this was being done in the face of very tight finances and a hostile local medical environment. The leadership needed to deal with rapid membership and geographic growth. In some years, the membership grew more than 10 percent. Between 1960 and 1970, the program went from one clinic integrated with the hospital to five clinics geographically dispersed on Oahu and two on Maui.

Many operational challenges needed to be overcome. The well-documented minutes of the general staff meetings described these problems and their ad hoc solutions, often in vivid detail. One of the most difficult problems was recruiting physicians in the face of low salaries. This was due to very low pricing by the dominant carrier HMSA. To be competitive clinical resources within the KP Hawaii region were very tight. This was further complicated by a hostile medical community.

Rapid internalization of specialty care was critical to the survival of HPMG. Internalization required a population base that was large enough to support a given type of specialist both financially and clinically. If a specialist did not have enough clinical material, clinical skills would be rapidly lost. Because the Medical Group started with only thirty-one physicians, many specialists needed to be recruited by physicians not in that specialty—a difficult task. Once recruited, these one-person specialty departments faced twenty-four-hour, seven-day-a-week call for tens of thousands of patients. There was little willingness by community physicians to provide coverage or support. There was one incident in which the pioneering, lone HPMG orthopedic surgeon Grant Howard, MD, was promised coverage by a community orthopedic surgeon so that he could take a vacation after a long stretch of solo coverage. Due to medical community pressure, the covering physician went back on his commitment, forcing a last-minute cancellation of the leave. Low salaries, onerous call, and medical community hostility increased physician turnover, further complicating recruiting.

Underperforming Physicians

With rapid growth and low salaries, the inadvertent recruitment of underperforming physicians was inevitable. At that time, there was little in the way of comparative objective data to validate physician performance. Due process procedures were primitive compared to those of today. There was always the risk of legal disputes. Fortunately, the Medical Group, which at the time was governed as a committee of the whole, was vigilant and careful.

Firmly guided by Dr. Chu and a strong executive committee, disruptive, unproductive, or clinically unskilled physicians were identified and discharged in a timely fashion. The temptation to turn a blind eye to poor performance must have been great given the recruiting difficulties. Nevertheless, the minutes of the general staff meetings document that poorly performing physicians were regularly removed from the Medical Group for cause, and there were no reports of wrongful discharge suits. In later years, as the labor legal environment became more complex, HPMG was to develop a sophisticated physician evaluation program with specific due process and remedial opportunities for underperforming or impaired physicians.

Medical Establishment Hostility

The Honolulu County Medical Society, a subsidiary of the Hawaii Medical Association, was hostile to Kaiser Permanente from its inception. In January 1964, two qualified HPMG physicians applied for membership and were rejected. The total was now five rejections in the previous six months without explanation. This was serious because rejection by the county medical society implied that the HPMG physicians were unqualified. This was an idea that was subtly and sometimes not so subtly promoted by the Hawaii Medical Association since the program's founding. Board certification essentially required membership in good standing in the county medical society. HPMG decided to take on the medical society.

During a long discussion on January 6, 1964, at the general staff meeting, options were considered, ranging from lawsuits to a more passive approach. Henry Kaiser was still alive and at the pinnacle of his power and influence in Hawaii. There had already been a Supreme Court legal precedent for a successful restraint of trade suit against the AMA by Group Health of Washington DC.

Mr. Kaiser had in the past threatened similar legal action against the Alameda County Medical Society when it was harassing the Northern

California program, which caused the medical society to back off. During the HPMG medical staff meeting, cooler heads prevailed. It was decided that the five rejected physicians should send a letter of inquiry requesting specific reasons for the rejection of their application for membership. They would then reapply after six months. By then, the leadership of the Honolulu County Medical Society would have changed. This patient, persistent, strategy was reminiscent of Sidney Garfield's approach to organized medicine from the previous decade, and it was successful.

From then on, HPMG members were no longer arbitrarily barred from membership in the local medical society, but that was a long way from acceptance. HPMG members rarely achieved officer status in the county society, and membership in the affiliated specialty societies was a long time coming. For example, urologists were not allowed into the Hawaii Urologic Society until the late 1970s. HPMG ophthalmologists, after initially being admitted to their specialty society, were suddenly expelled in the mid-1980s. They were eventually invited back, but by then, there was little interest in rejoining.

In the early 1970s, the Honolulu County Medical Society, a component of the Hawaii Medical Society, proposed a medical society-controlled health plan that would directly compete with Kaiser Permanente. It didn't materialize, but that was only after HPMG members, who now made up a significant portion of the HMA membership, threatened to withhold dues and the Kaiser Health Plan legal department threatened the county society with legal action. As in the California and the Northwest Permanente Medical Groups, the medical establishment's scorn and isolation of Hawaii Permanente Medical Group had the unintended consequence of strengthening and unifying the Medical Group during the critical early years.

Reputation

From the beginning, there were young, energetic, and skilled doctors in HPMG. Many were proud idealists who saw the program as the future of medicine. They did not like the derision of the medical establishment. They were determined to prove the critics wrong by actions that belied the criticism.

Peer-reviewed, published, medical research papers by HPMG physicians would be concrete documented proof of state-of-the-art practice. Would-be HPMG physician researchers had the benefit of a large, growing, and relatively stable patient population as well as centralized medical records.

Carol Tom, RN, previously from the Mayo Clinic, had organized the KP Tumor Registry, which summarized the care of every cancer patient treated in the program since its founding in 1958. This included care delivered outside of the program. At that time, while there was extensive medical research on specific disease therapy from academic medicine, there was little research about the practical application of these therapies to large populations to guide physician practice. This aspect of medical research was wide-open to KP physician investigators, and they took advantage of it.

While not mandatory, clinical research was encouraged and incentivized. In time, HPMG physicians could apply for an extra one-week, all-expenses-paid educational package per year to cover the costs of attending a national or international meeting where an HPMG paper was being presented. Eventually, HPMG physicians, who represented only about 5 percent of the state physician population, were producing a disproportionate amount of the clinical research coming from Hawaii.

From 1963 on, HPMG sponsored an annual research symposium organized by Dr. Clifford Streahley. One of the presentation requirements was that the HPMG presenter had to invite a prominent community physician to critique the paper. Hawaii is a small state. Many of these studies were eventually published. Through this program and the HPMG clinical research featured in the peer-reviewed international specialty literature, the word got out to the medical community. It became increasingly difficult for local doctors to describe HPMG medical care and its doctors as substandard. It became especially difficult when a 1969 published study of health care in Hawaii sponsored by the Hawaii Medical Association and the University of Michigan demonstrated that KP Hawaii health care was superior to private health care for most of the HMA predefined prospective measurement parameters. The principle reason was thought to be due to the low barriers to specialty care for patients in the KP program.

From the beginning, physician continuing medical education was also incentivized. Within two years of its founding in 1962, extra compensation and later educational leave were made HPMG benefits on a use-it-or-lose-it basis. This was a powerful incentive for the HPMG doctors to keep up to date. Since almost all HPMG physicians participated and then attended Saturday Grand Rounds, the collective knowledge base of the Medical Group increased. For the community private practice physicians, there was a strong economic disincentive to travel to continuing education programs. Lost time from practice and the travel and tuition to attend educational meetings were a major expense and not a reward. It was to their credit that they attended when they did.

As HPMG grew with the KP membership, it specialized to internalize as much patient care as possible. Internalization resulted in care that was more integrated, subject to internal quality assurance and service measures, and much lower cost. As specialty departments grew, individuals could subspecialize within the specialty, enabling them to increase their skill level to international state-of-the-art levels as their subspecialty caseload grew. This was possible because, within a department, there was no economic competition for cases. Indeed, sub-specialization fostered intradepartmental interdependence and cooperation, which was strongly encouraged by HPMG leadership. This growing skill level became increasingly apparent to local physicians through HPMG physician participation in the local specialty societies in addition to their scientific output.

In time, growth in membership and resources, standardized policies and procedures, standardized recruiting, an eventual requirement for specialty board certification, improved compensation, quality assurance, and quality of service had an effect. As organized medicine in Hawaii gradually declining in political influence, the size and clinical capability of HPMG grew. By the early 1990s, HPMG was by far the largest medical group in Hawaii. It was a stable, growing, skilled, and unified medical group encompassing nearly a fifth of the practicing doctors in Hawaii. The deliberate HPMG multipronged response to its critics had, by the late 1990s, converted the scorn of the Hawaii medical establishment to grudging respect if not envy.

Membership Growth

By 1965, membership stood at fifty-three thousand, and the program was on solid footing. For HPMG to grow in numbers and clinical talent, proportionate Kaiser Health Plan membership growth was required. Much of this growth from the late 1960s to the 1980s came as a result of an agricultural health care revolution in Hawaii. Labor-intensive, large-scale agriculture—dominated by sugar and pineapples—was the main source of population growth in Hawaii from the mid-nineteenth to the mid-twentieth century. Hundreds of thousands of contract agricultural workers were brought to Hawaii first from China, then Japan and Portugal, and finally the Philippines. Most stayed. Agribusiness in Hawaii organized itself around paternalistically managed, self-sufficient plantations that dotted the islands. Typically, there would be a large plantation served by a small, self-contained company town—complete with housing, schools, stores, community centers, and either a clinic or small hospital. These facilities were served by physicians and other medical staff contracted by the plantation companies. While the care was basic and variable, it could boast some impressive public health care achievements relative to rural health care elsewhere in the US. Best of all, the care was nearly free.

The plantation health care system reached its peak in the 1930s and 1940s. In the July edition of *Plantation Health*, which was sponsored by the Hawaii Sugar Planters' Association (HSPA), it was reported that there were twenty-nine doctors, eighteen plantation hospitals, seven smaller receiving hospitals, and three government facilities caring for the plantation workers. The relationship between the agricultural companies and the workers represented by their aggressive labor unions was spirited and sometimes even violent. This resulted in conditions that were typically better than for agricultural workers elsewhere in the country. By the 1960s, the agricultural companies were looking to get out of the medical business, and the unionized workers wanted access to the more sophisticated private medical infrastructure that was available to the rest of the population of Hawaii.

On May 27, 1970—less than two months before his sudden death—Phil Chu was the plenary speaker of the 1970 Group Health Institute, which was holding its convention in Honolulu. His speech, "Development of the Kaiser Medical Care Program in Hawaii," described the first ten years of the development KP Hawaii—the first Kaiser Permanente program outside of the founding regions in California and Oregon. He described the important role that KP Hawaii played in the transition from plantation to private medical care.

> Our involvement in the sugar industry began in the spring of 1967 when we were invited by Mits Fukuda vice president and Industrial Relations, Castle and Cooke, Inc. and Mr. Ed Bryan vice president and General Manager of the Ewa Plantation to provide medical services to Ewa Plantation's 2,300 employees and dependents. This was our first invitation from a "Big 5" organization, Ewa plantation at the time being a Castle and Cooke subsidiary.

A contract was signed on July 1, 1967, and KP proceeded with the difficult task of absorbing these patients. Dr. Chu noted:

> If we are to take full advantage of the membership potential offered by the sugar industry, we must find an answer to this basic question: "Can we work out the methodology of providing quality medical care to a rural population from what is essentially an urban-based program?"

With a lot of work, this effort proved successful because by mid-1968, a second industrial medicine contract was signed with the Lahaina Maui Pioneer Mill, which was owned by AMFAC. The 2,400 employees and dependents were to be cared for out of the old agriculture research and quality control building, which was converted to the Lahaina Clinic. This was the first KP clinic outside of Oahu.

This successful Maui KP endeavor led to the opening of the much larger Wailuku clinic by the summer of 1970. KP was no longer an urban, Oahu-only program. This successful neighbor island expansion was eventually to lead to a KP statewide presence with clinics on all of the major Hawaiian Islands.

At the time of his presentation, Dr. Chu projected that a successful conversion of plantation medicine to KP could be worth seventy thousand members at a time when the total KP membership was only eighty thousand. Most of this potential was realized and provided substantial increases in membership at critical times between the late 1960s and the mid-1980s as plantation after plantation converted to KP membership.

The success of the neighbor island program proved that the program was flexible enough to provide the KP standard of care to the thinly populated, predominantly rural, neighbor islands. Because of the need to organize a medical infrastructure to provide medical care to these populations, it gave KP a serious advantage over its chief competitor: HMSA.

As an indemnity insurance program organized to pay for medical services on a fee-for-service basis, HMSA accepted little responsibility for, or control over, the organization of a medical infrastructure of these rural areas, which was left to underfunded, free market and state subsidized economic mechanisms. In these same rural areas, KP established local clinics to provide primary and locally available basic specialty care.

Where the local membership would not support a full-time specialist, traveling Oahu-based medical center specialists provided the remaining specialty care. Efficient and medically covered transfer of patients to the Kaiser Medical Center in Honolulu was provided for patients requiring major surgery and other tertiary specialty care not readily available locally.

Neighbor island expansion forced KP to figure out how to deliver a Honolulu level of care to the neighbor islands. By 2015, KP had been on Maui for forty-five years. Almost 40 percent of the Maui population was KP, which gave KP an important advantage when it successfully competed for the Maui Memorial Hospital management contract that year.

By 1960, pineapple production had peaked. Hawaii growers were supplying 80 percent of the world's canned pineapple. After 1966, pineapple production in Hawaii began a steady decline, and by 2000, large-scale pineapple production in Hawaii was finished. Production was limited to fresh pineapple for local consumption. Similarly, the sugar industry reached peak production in 1966; then, it too went into steady decline. By 2009, there was just one remaining sugar mill in Hawaii, which closed in 2016.

While the sugar and pineapple Hawaii plantation economy is gone because of lower-cost foreign production, the contract workers and their descendants were an important source of growth for KP at a critical time in its history. The operational efforts required to accommodate the rural population of the neighbor islands led to a robust KP statewide presence. These efforts proved that the program was flexible enough to successfully provide an urban level of medical care to thinly populated rural communities separated by ocean.

Medicaid

Medicaid, a program to provide health care to the poor, was passed into law in 1965. Unlike Medicare, which is a federal program, Medicaid, although backed by federal funding, is administrated by the individual states. In his May 1970 address to the Group Health Association, Dr. Chu proudly presented KP Hawaii's imminent signing of a contract with the Hawaii Department of Social Services. This contract was to care for an initial pilot project of 2000 Medicaid patients. This was to be the first Medicaid KP contract in the country. Unlike most KP regions, the Hawaii region through most of its history treated a Medicaid population that was proportional to the Medicaid population of the state, but Medicaid participation is controversial.

Medicaid patients tend to have unmet health needs. Therefore, they are often sicker and more expensive to care for than non-Medicaid patients. Medicaid also tends to reimburse poorly—sometimes below the cost of delivering that care. When costs don't cover reimbursements, the program ends up subsidizing Medicaid. The reality is that the program is just a pass-through. It isn't the program subsidizing Medicaid, but the other non-Medicaid members who are paying higher KP monthly dues to offset the KP Medicaid subsidy—a hidden tax for KP members. Is the program thus violating its fiduciary duty to the non-Medicaid members? The program initially took the high-minded stance that as the second largest health care provider in Hawaii, this was its social contribution to the state. Later, as the cost discrepancy has widened, it was more practically justified as an important defense of the KP nonprofit tax status.

Throughout the Hawaii region's relationship with Medicaid, no care distinction was made between Medicaid and non-Medicaid patients. The same resources were available to Medicaid patients as to all other patients.

They were not treated as charity patients. This is a long-standing policy for which the program is justifiably proud. When other health plans to cut their costs to lower their bids, offered lower levels of service for Medicaid patients, KP—led by HPMG—refused this option to lower the KP bid. Some Medicaid members were thus lost to low-bid, low-service programs. Nevertheless, as of this time, KP Hawaii regularly remains in the top five Medicaid-quality providers nationally while still caring for twenty-nine thousand (2015) Medicaid patients, which is about 9 percent of the eligible Hawaii Medicaid population. Medicaid patients are among those with the greatest need for quality health care. Providing quality health care for as many as financially possible has, after all, been the KP mission from the beginning.

HPMG and Free Speech

Willis Butler, MD, was one of the most interesting personalities in HPMG history. He was born in New Orleans in 1918 and graduated from Tulane Medical School. He came to Hawaii in 1952 to work as a general practitioner plantation doctor on Molokai where he delivered babies, performed surgery, and tended to the other medical needs of the plantation workers. As a vociferous advocate for the workers and an associate of Jack Hall, Hawaii's leader of the International Longshore Warehouseman's Union (ILWU), he came into conflict with plantation management and eventually set up his own practice in Mauna Loa, Molokai. In April 1959, he joined the fledgling Kaiser Health Care program as a Pacific Medical Associates (PMA) contract physician. He was a charter member of HPMG after the dissolution of PMA in August 1960, and he was appointed one of the permanent members of the original HPMG executive committee.

Dr. Butler engaged in a lifetime of political activism. He had been active in the civil rights movement, and in 1965, he was a founding member of the Hawaii Committee to End the War in Vietnam at the height of that war's popularity. At that time, polls showed three-to-one support for sending troops to Vietnam. Opposition to the war did not equal and then surpass support for the war until after the Tet Offensive in February 1968. Dr. Butler's outspoken, high-profile anti-war activities were frequently reported in the local press. With a large resident military population, feelings ran high for and against the war in Hawaii. At their height, in 1970, the University of Hawaii ROTC offices were occupied, and in 1971, they were set afire.

The Vietnam crisis came before HPMG, in 1966, as a result of Dr. Butler's activism. According to court documents, on October 17, 1966, President Lyndon Johnson was to deliver an outdoor foreign policy speech at the East West Center at the University of Hawaii. Prior to his scheduled speech, a crowd of pro- and anti-Vietnam War protestors gathered. Among the most prominent of the protest displays was an apparatus that suspended a life-sized cowboy effigy of Lyndon Johnson and another figure labeled "Pentagon" both hanging by the neck with a sign: "Nuremburg Justice for War Criminals." Pro-war protesters began jostling the anti-war protesters to push them away from the stage.

As one pro-war protester began to tear down an anti-war sign, a police officer threated that person with arrest. He stopped. Things were getting unruly. A police officer approached Dr. Butler and asked him to remove the effigies. Dr. Butler refused and grabbed one of the supporting poles. On the third request, the officer said that the effigies were causing a disturbance and that if he did not remove them, he would be arrested.

Dr. Butler replied, "Go ahead and arrest me. What are you going to arrest me for?"

When the policeman told him he would be arrested for disorderly conduct, Dr. Butler turned to the crowd, gestured to them, and said, "I am not disorderly—the police are." At that point, he was arrested. The disorderly conduct charge later went to jury trial, and Dr. Butler was convicted. At the next HPMG general staff meeting on December 12, 1966, the issue was raised.

The debate was passionate but nuanced and tightly reasoned. It was recorded in great detail by Sumi Croydon. Ms. Croydon had been the HPMG executive secretary since its founding; therefore, she knew all of the personalities very well. Sumi was an important figure in the early history of HPMG. She believed deeply in the program and was a motherly mentor for many young physicians learning their way around HPMG, including the author. It is of interest that in the first fifty-two years of the program, there were only two executive secretaries of HPMG: Sumi Croydon (1960–1989) and her protégé Shelly Young (1989–2012). During that era, they were responsible for audio recording-based detailed and accurate general staff, board, and executive committee minutes. Those minutes are a historian's dream.

The last item on the agenda of December 12, 1966, was the consideration of a motion of no confidence for Dr. Butler's continuation on the permanent executive committee of HPMG. As quoted from the minutes:

> Dr. Huitt reiterated that he found Dr. Butler's demonstration personally offensive and that Dr. Butler should not continue to serve as a long-term [permanent] member of the executive committee. Dr. Huitt felt that the issue was not war or peace or political.

He went on to say, "Dr. Butler's actions bring potential jeopardy and discredit to the Hawaii Permanente Medical Group. He can accept Dr. Butler as an associate and a friend, but he cannot accept him in the position of leadership in the group." Dr. Huitt was a founding member and influential in HPMG. He then turned the floor over to Dr. Butler.

Dr. Butler began by stating that he "felt no guilt, that he was not there with a sense of obligation to defend himself or expiate himself for his performance." He challenged his accusers to produce evidence of harm to the group. He then went into a detailed condemnation of the Vietnam War, citing facts to reinforce his anti-war position. "At this point Dr. Baugh called for a point of order. He stated that the Vietnam War was not the issue," but Dr. Butler's "behavior" was.

Dr. Dizon next asked the question: "What is the difference between a member of the group's conduct and a member of the executive committee's conduct? If any removal is contemplated, should he be removed totally from the group?"

Dr. Huitt answered "that he had no basic quarrel with Dr. Butler being in the group or his being a friend but that he had a quarrel with his continuing in his position of leadership."

Dr. Straehley read a prepared statement where he expressed his own opinion of the Vietnam War as being "ill-advised" and that "the importance

that the right of the citizen to thoughtful and responsible dissent be preserved. I stress the words *thoughtful* and *responsible*."

> I do not feel that Dr. Butler's recent actions can be char-
> acterized in this way. His highly emotional behavior has
> tended to offend most of us, whether or not we agree with
> his opinions.
>
> We are engaged in the practice of medicine and are
> intimately involved with our patients in a relationship de-
> manding not only professional competence but also faith,
> sound judgment, confidence, and respect. It is evident
> that Dr. Butler's flagrant manner tends to undermine his
> professional image and by virtue of his association with
> the Hawaii Permanente Medical Group, it is felt to be
> damaging to the confidence which the community has
> reposed in all of us. Dr. Butler has an obligation to temper
> his public actions and expressions with that thoughtful
> restraint which one rightly expects of a physician. He
> has brought the focus of public attention sharply upon
> himself; therefore continued membership on the executive
> committee will inevitably be construed by the public to
> mean that we as a group approve the method that he has
> chosen for protest.

Additional opinions were solicited. Issues of censorship, freedom of speech,
freedom of conscience, and the failure to resolve this on a colleague-to-col-
league basis were raised. Clearly, there was discomfort about making this
a public HPMG action. A motion to table the motion indefinitely was
made by Dr. Mehta, an internist. The motion passed by a show of hands
with eighteen affirmative votes, ten negative votes, and five abstentions.
Dr. Butler continued his high-profile anti-war activities.

The issue would not go away. It was again raised at the August 28,
1967, general staff meeting. By then, Dr. Butler had been convicted in
the lower courts for disorderly conduct. The issue was again carefully
defined not as political but behavioral and not as an individual doctor
but as a leader of HPMG. Speakers stated as a leader of HPMG his highly

publicized actions reflected on the Medical Group. Dr. Straehley questioned whether the time spent on external political activities detracted from Dr. Butler's service on the executive committee. The members of the executive committee all stated that it did not.

Dr. Brown one of the operational leaders of the Medical Group stated:

> That he had been pushed into the position at times of having to defend Dr. Butler's actions to members of the press and others and that he had done so reluctantly. He felt that in a group situation any member of this Group owes a prime obligation to all the other members of the Group. It is his personal feeling that Dr. Butler's behavior and political actions have definitely reflected upon our group in a derogatory way.

As quoted in the minutes:

> Dr. Hewitt stated that he has been in the group eight years and knows of no controversy which has arisen in this group that has divided the group and caused more dissention and more turmoil than simply Dr. Butler's conduct. He pointed out that he felt that this was not the kind of leader he would commit his entire professional life to and especially when we are on the edge of such rapid professional growth.

The minutes continue:

> Dr. Butler replied that if no one has even shaken up the group as he has, it was because there had never been a Vietnam War before.

Dr. Straehley then restated his motion as follows:

> A vote of no confidence in the continued service of Dr. Willis Butler as a permanent member of the executive committee of the Hawaii Permanente Medical Group.

The final vote was twenty-seven expressing no confidence in Dr. Butler, eight expressing confidence in Dr. Butler, three abstentions, and two absent.

HPMG had been careful to separate freedom of speech from his role as an executive committee member of HPMG. As defined in the debate, this was a nonbinding motion advising Dr. Butler to resign if he felt that the moral imperative of his high-profile political activities took precedence over his leadership role of the Medical Group. At no time was his status as a clinician in HPMG ever threatened. Despite the lopsided vote, Dr. Butler did not resign from the executive committee.

High-profile statements, often exaggerated, by Dr. Butler's non-HPMG supporters implied that the Medical Group was persecuting him for his beliefs followed in the press and on television. He did little to correct this misinformation. Dr. Butler's leadership role in HPMG had now become a public issue.

Prior to the next HPMG general staff meeting, a petition was circulated:

> We the undersigned, move to un-table the motion of December 12, 1966, and that the question with regard to Dr. Willis Butler's continued service on the executive committee of the Hawaii Permanente Medical Group be put to a vote.

It was signed by thirty of the forty-six associates. Thus, Dr. Chu had no choice but to present the issue before the general staff meeting on December 18, 1967. Dr. Butler led off by requesting that he be allowed to make an audiotape of the meeting. This was granted in a separate motion unanimously as long as the audiotape was kept in the permanent possession of the secretary of HPMG. He then went into a carefully reasoned and detailed defense of his actions.

> I think that I don't agree with those who say, "You've got the right to your political views, but we object to your methods." I reject this. I claim you cannot distinguish expression of political views and their content from the manner in which they are expressed. This is a false assumption.

Because the very manner of expression becomes part of content: and if you deny a man the choice of the manner in which he expresses himself you are inevitably limiting the content of his message. I think this has been reiterated and corroborated many times in court decisions. It is basic in our First Amendment. Behavior is a mode of expression—doing something to a flag, doing something to an effigy, marching, demonstration—whatever. The manner of expression becomes part of the content and it is protected by the First Amendment.

He later went on to say, "Nobody has the right to tell me how I am going to express my political views, and nobody has the right to tell me what these views are going to be."

Later in the debate, Dr. Straehley countered:

As members of a group, we do have the right to have confidence in the leadership of those who are in positions to guide our destinies; and furthermore, there is no constitutional or inalienable right anywhere in the United States Bill of Rights or Constitution which guarantees a citizen has the right to serve on the executive committee of [the] Hawaii Permanente Medical Group. This issue has been a leadership issue pure and simple.

The question was called. Of the thirty-eight associates present, the vote was twenty-seven to remove Dr. Butler from the executive committee and eleven votes for Dr. Butler to remain on the executive committee. There were no abstentions. Dr. Butler was removed from the executive committee of HPMG.

Dr. Butler was eventually vindicated in the courts when the case was appealed to the Hawaii Supreme Court. On May 22, 1969, the conviction was overturned on the basis of the right to free speech and that the state had not demonstrated an imminent threat of public disorder.

Dr. Butler continued to practice as a HPMG physician for another year and a half until he resigned effective July 1, 1970.

Dr. Chu, ten days before he died, reported in the July 6, 1970 board minutes:

> He had long discussions with Dr. Butler concerning his resignation. Dr. Butler felt at this point in time and at his age being in general medicine he would like to look for some other challenges. He leaves the Medical Group with great memories of the early beginnings of the Medical Group and with kind thoughts and wishes for the continued success of our program.

Fortunately that wasn't the end of Dr. Butler's involvement with HPMG. He was welcomed back to the Medical Group in April 1978 and retired with full benefits in June 1982.

Dr. Butler remained an activist to the end. As quoted from his obituary in the *Honolulu Star Bulletin* of February 9, 2008:

> Butler was later prominent in opposition to American involvement in Central American politics, he was a member of Physicians For Social Responsibility, a national opponent of developing nuclear weapons. In recent years his letters to editors made clear he did not like the invasion of Iraq and the influence of industrialists on the government.

He died at the age of eighty-nine on June 14, 2008, at the St. Francis Hospice.

The Death of Dr. Chu

One of the most important but quiet successes of American medicine has been a two-thirds reduction in coronary artery disease mortality since the late 1960s when it was at its height. This was accomplished by cumulative advances in cardiology, cardiac surgery, drugs, diet, and lifestyle changes. In September 1968, Dr. Chu was hospitalized for his second myocardial infarction. He had been and continued to be on then state-of-the-art preventive care under the direction of Dr. T. K. Lin, the well-respected

HPMG staff cardiologist in consultation with Dr. Kuo from the University of Pennsylvania cardiology department. After his recovery, he remained without symptoms.

On July 16, 1970 he flew to Maui to oversee operational details of the recently opened Wailuku Clinic—the second on Maui. Like other HPMG physicians providing Maui coverage from Oahu, he would overnight in one of the tourist hotels on beautiful Ka'anapali Beach near Lahaina. On Friday morning, July 17, 1970 at 6:50 a.m., Dr. Chu called down to the hotel front desk to tell them that he was short of breath and to call for help. By 7:45 a.m., the ambulance had arrived, but he had already died. His body was flown back to Honolulu by HPMG on a chartered flight.

An emergency general staff meeting was called on July 20. Dr. Keene rearranged his schedule to fly to Hawaii to address the HPMG physicians. He recommended that the next president be chosen from within HPMG and that the board take its time choosing Dr. Chu's successor. He provided words of encouragement and offered the advisory support of the recently retired medical director of Southern California, Ray Kay, MD, and the familiar Ernest Saward, MD, medical director of Northwest.

Dr. Chu's sudden and unexpected death was a tremendous shock to the Medical Group and the Hawaii region as a whole. Dr. Chu was respected at Kaiser Permanente corporate headquarters in Oakland, was a natural leader, and had been the only president that HPMG had known. During the decade of his leadership, HPMG had survived and prospered against long odds. It had grown from thirty-one doctors to fifty-six. With eighty thousand members, Kaiser Health Plan now had sufficient membership to support the internalization of all the major specialties. More important, this membership was diversified. It was no longer dominated by Kaiser Industry employees and unions—but also state and federal employees, Medicaid recipients, agricultural and industrial workers, and the university. The program had gone from an experimental money-losing Henry Kaiser (now deceased) adventure limited to urban Honolulu to a successful, well-financed, established—even model—program serving all of Oahu and Maui. There was an annual research symposium, staff publications, a surgery residency affiliation with Stanford Medical School, and a University of Michigan study demonstrating equivalent or superior outcomes compared to the competition affirmed its clinical capabilities.

Myriad operational problems had been overcome under the firm leadership of Dr. Chu to achieve these successes. Now he was gone with no obvious successor.

By necessity, Dr. Chu was a strong, decisive leader. In the 1960s, the standard workweek was five and a half days with the half day being on Saturday. The story is told that a physician made an appointment to inform Dr. Chu that he was no longer going to work on Saturdays. Dr. Chu responded that not only did he not have to work Saturdays—he did not have to work for HPMG at all. In a prophetic, heartfelt, handwritten letter to Conrad Bohuslav, his Health Plan counterpart, on December 7, 1969, seven months before he died, Dr. Chu reflected upon the need to make group governance more democratic. This had been prompted by the defeat of Robert Boyd, MD, to a vacant executive committee position.

Bob Boyd, MD, was the very capable, sole staff urologist for HPMG. He had been taking on increasing administrative responsibilities as assigned by Dr. Chu. He had an obvious talent for it, and in the minds of many, he was the obvious successor to Dr. Chu. With the strong support of Dr. Chu, he ran for a newly vacant position on the HPMG executive committee. He was defeated in the December 1, 1969, general staff meeting by a populist candidate twenty-eight to twenty-one. This disturbed Dr. Chu, but he correctly interpreted this as a referendum against his centralized leadership style. Prophetically, he realized that if something happened to him, the present centralized governance structure was not giving enough experience and training opportunities for physicians to develop the management skills necessary to provide a smooth succession. He stated that correcting this would be his next priority. He did not live long enough to carry out that goal. He was right about the succession.

After his death, HPMG would require five months of administrative drift and divisive, faction-driven political conflict before it could elect Dr. Chu's successor. William Dung, MD, inherited a group riven by factions that had been held together only by Dr. Chu's strong leadership. It would take Dr. Dung five years to suppress the factionalism and establish his own administration. It would be up to Dr. Dung to establish the wide-based, democratic, check-and-balance-based governance structure that survives to this day. It would be a long and very difficult road.

Phil Chu, MD, husband, father, experienced and successful clinician and administrator, humanitarian, educator, and amateur pilot left quite a legacy in his tragically shortened fifty-one years. HPMG was fortunate to have had him as its first president.

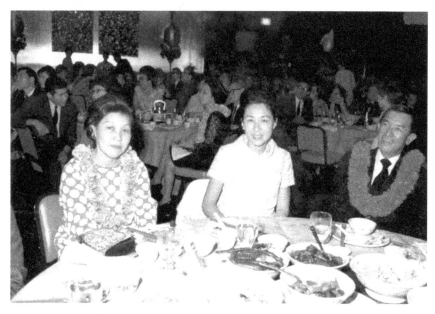

(L to R) Sumi Croydon, Phoebe Chu, and Dr. Phil Chu.
Sumi was the executive secretary to the president
and HPMG Archivist from 1960 until 1991.

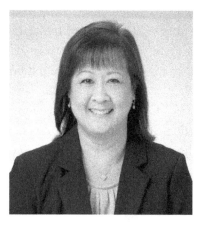

Shelly Young was Sumi Croydon's protégé and
successor from 1991 until 2012. There were only two
HPMG executive secretaries in fifty-two years.

CHAPTER 6

ARE PHYSICIANS GOVERNABLE?

I n the 1932 classic *Brave New World*, Aldous Huxley envisioned a futuristic, post-apocalyptic society that had eliminated suffering and civil discord. This was achieved by Soma, the anti-anxiety pleasure drug and by biologically engineering all human beings into five classes, ranging from the tall, attractive, hyper-intelligent alphas to the short, ugly, moronic epsilons. The alphas were predestined and trained to be in charge. They were, and they pitied those in the lower castes. Conversely, the epsilons were trained to do the dirty work of society, and to the extent that they could think about it at all, they were happy not to have to have the responsibilities of the alphas.

The nonconformist protagonist questions the justice of such a social order. A historical experiment was revealed to him by the lead alpha male: the "controller." In that experiment, twenty-two thousand alphas were "hatched," trained, gathered up, and then settled on the depopulated island of Cyprus and left to govern themselves. After six years of extreme civil discord and civil war, the remaining three thousand survivors begged for outside governance. Is this the inevitable fate of a medical group containing hundreds of doctors?

Unquestionably, physicians are among the alphas of society. While difficult to study, one of the best contemporary (1998) studies of intelligence quotients (IQ) by profession was done by the University of Wisconsin in which physicians scored highest (average 120). *Doctors are smart.* While IQ and EQ (emotional quotient) can assort independently, it is difficult for a doctor to succeed without being able to interact smoothly with others, such as patients and colleagues. In May 2014, the United States Department of Labor National Occupational Employment and Wage Estimates reported that the physician groups had the highest average pay by occupation. The Gallup poll has consistently rated doctors among the best of the professions in terms of reputation, and interestingly, the trend is up since the 1970s. In summary, physicians are typically very intelligent, articulate, independent, and confident. Deficiency of self-esteem is rarely a problem. They represent positions where there is a lot at stake: patient health and even lives. The governance of such a group is a real challenge.

How can a large group of doctors with a divergent complex of individual and group self-interests not result in a toxic brew of constant conflict? The dynamic range of human behavior from extreme other-centeredness and saintly self-sacrifice to totally self-interested, evil, sociopathic conduct never ceases to amaze. Fortunately, the process of becoming a physician filters out most of the sociopaths, but there aren't enough "saints" to staff a medical group large enough to provide health care for a significant portion of the population. While the average physician is likely to have a service orientation that is higher than that of the general population, the average physician is not a saint.

Almost from the beginning of its existence, factions began to form within HPMG from the natural grouping of physicians. Dr. Dung referred to these factions in one of his last presidential newsletters. Among them were primary care versus specialty care, hospital versus clinics, Oahu versus neighbor islands, and inter and intradepartmental conflicts over work responsibilities and compensation.

Within a few years of the founding of the HPMG, these factions had become sharply defined enough to cause serious conflict. Efforts spent fighting each other had the potential to seriously disrupt the health care-delivery mission of HPMG—and it did. It has been the ongoing mission of every HPMG president to prevent the centripetal forces of factionalism from tearing the Medical Group apart. Whatever governance structure emerged needed to align the self-interest of the average physician and the group in which they reside with the health care-delivery mission of the program. This is how HPMG has done it so far.

The Evolution of the HPMG Governance Structure

When HPMG was founded that Saturday afternoon in August 1960, under crisis conditions, it had a lot of help. Clifford Keene, MD, effectively the chief operating officer and chief executive officer of KP, had chosen Ernie Saward, MD, in early 1960 as his operational partner to save HPMG. Dr. Saward was the founder and medical director of Northwest PMG. He chose Dr. Saward because of his long experience and belief in a strong chief system for management. Together, they had been monitoring the Hawaii situation closely and in person since early 1960. They had a good sense of the capabilities of the remaining thirty-one "hired hand" physicians when the contract with the original five founders was canceled.

Clifford Keene recognized Phil Chu, MD, as a leader with tremendous potential, and he named him HPMG executive chairman and chief of surgery. Chu only accepted the position after Henry Kaiser, with his own funds, paid off the $2.5 million deficit (worth $21.6 million in 2020) accumulated by Pacific Medical Associates. HPMG was still a high-risk venture. Chu later noted that the program did not break even until 1961 and did not generate enough reserves to be self-sustaining until 1964. Four other doctors made up the first HPMG executive committee. This ad hoc arrangement was good enough for the thirty to thirty-five doctors in that crisis environment, and it lasted until 1963.

By the summer of 1963, the program was on a much firmer footing with forty-eight thousand members and growing rapidly. There were now sixty HPMG physicians. The Medical Group had outgrown the ad hoc four-person executive committee. For organizational and legal reasons, the need for a more formal governance structure was recognized.

Discussions ran through the summer and fall by the full membership at the general staff meetings. Proposals ranged from an overly strong permanent executive committee to an overly weak structure of frequently elected officers and chiefs of service. Consensus formed around a middle ground. At the November 27, 1963, general staff meeting, a new structure was ratified. There would be a president of HPMG nominated by the executive committee and then ratified by two-thirds of the associates for a six-year term. The executive committee would be formed by three elected permanent members who would serve for as long as they remained in HPMG and could perform their duties and four elected members who would be elected at four-, three-, two-, and one-year terms. This structure served its purpose for the remainder of the decade.

In July 1970, Phil Chu, president of HPMG since its founding, died suddenly and unexpectedly. There was a period of turmoil and instability until Bill Dung assumed the presidency the following December. By the beginning of 1971, there were ninety physicians in the Medical Group with five of them on Maui. Making policy using the entire Medical Group as a committee of the whole during general staff meetings was getting unwieldly. Dr. Dung proposed a re-organization and streamlining of the governance structure, which remains largely intact to this day. This was ratified by the general staff in November 1971.

The permanent members of the executive committee would become the HPMG advisory board of directors. It consisted of the vice presidents who today would be called associate medical directors. Also included were clinical chiefs of service and the clinic physicians in charge (PICs). Chiefs of service had primary responsibility for recruiting, quality assurance monitoring, and quality of service of their departments. They also served as PICs of their departments within the medical center. They were expected to work cooperatively with the PICs of the outlying clinics on quality of service and disciplinary issues. PICs were primarily responsible for care-delivery support for their clinics. The advisory board was to be responsible for day-to-day operational issues. Service chiefs, physicians in charge, and vice presidents would be appointed by the HPMG president subject to ratification—and then re-ratification every three years by the elected board of directors.

The elected board of directors would serve up to two consecutive three-year terms. This elected board was to be the board of directors for the legal corporation. They would be responsible for general policy, including staffing, ratification of associates, and compensation issues. The definition and separation of day-to-day operational policy from general policy was to prove to be very important to the success of HPMG. Bill Dung insisted that the elected board (policy) and the advisory board (operations) always meet together so that one could check and balance the other. He regarded this separation of powers as the most important accomplishment of his twenty-one-year term as medical director.

Checks and Balances

When the founding fathers set out to establish a democratic government for the thirteen former British colonies, they were aware that the few historical experiments with democracy had eventually failed. Typically, they degenerated into mob rule, and then to control the mob, dictatorships arose. Perceived British tyranny was the reason that the eight-year Revolutionary War had been fought to begin with. On the other hand, during the turbulent five-year postwar period under the weak Articles of Confederation, the country was on the verge of breaking apart. Shortsighted economic exploitation was being met by mob rule in individual states, and there was little that the weak national government could do about it. The European powers, especially England, watched with interest. They were standing by to pick up the pieces of the former United States of America.

The founding fathers understood that they needed to balance tyranny against mob rule. Whatever governance structure that was proposed needed to provide democratic outlets for dissent to protect against government tyranny. On the other hand, there needed to be government and policy stability, and protections under the law, to offset the tyranny of the mob. The result was the Constitution of the United States—the oldest functioning, and arguably, most successful, constitution in the world.

They concluded that the best way to protect against the tyranny of an easily incited, passionate, fickle mob was to slow down the process of government by having three branches of government that would "check and balance" each other. Major policy changes needed to pass two houses of Congress and then get the approval of the president who had the power of veto. A supermajority would then be required to override a veto. Passed legislation could then be reviewed by the courts for adherence to the constitution, which was difficult to amend. Any branch could check any other branch. Presidents would be elected every four years, congressmen every two years for direct accountability to the people, but senators would serve for six years on a staggered basis as a bulwark against political fashion. Supreme Court justices could serve for life. Major policy changes could take years or even decades to pass. By then, mob passions would have cooled.

HPMG leadership, no doubt based upon the subliminal grade-school civics lessons of American education at the time, on a much smaller scale, also evolved a government of checks and balances. Physicians are subject to human nature. The potential for mob rule or tyranny is at least as great. Physicians are smart and articulate, they are quick to see when their interests are threatened, and they are typically decisive and action oriented.

The chief instrument to balance government tyranny against mob tyranny in HPMG is the elected board of directors. Established in 1971, and little changed since then, every year, there is an election in which one-third of the board of directors is elected. All associates (partners) can vote, and any associate can run for the board of directors. Terms are limited to two three-year terms after which an associate must wait for one year to run again. By staggering the elections so that only one-third of the voting board can be elected in one year, takeover of the board by one faction is made much more difficult. To do so, such a faction would have to win all the board positions at least two years in a row. This slows down the adoption of some sudden political craze, thus preventing the instability of lurching from one policy extreme to another.

Attempts over the years to allocate board positions to specific factions such as neighbor island and primary or specialty care have been repeatedly defeated. The feeling always has been that board members need to represent the interests of the Medical Group as a whole—and not a specific faction. It was recognized that factionalism had and would sap the competitive energy of the Medical Group, thus threatening its survivability.

As time went on, an understanding evolved that the directly elected board of directors should represent the collective will of the associates. As such, it was responsible for general policies that would guide the actions of the executive branch of the Medical Group—the president and chiefs. Decisions about partnership, staffing, and compensation were within the purview of the elected board. The elected board also ratified the election of a president (executive medical director—EMD), the ratification after a six-year term and all presidentially (EMD) appointed associate medical directors (AMDs), department chiefs, and physicians in charge (PICs) initially and again every three years. Chiefs have failed to be ratified or re-ratified by the elected board in past years. While infrequently exercised, it has been an effective check against chiefs and other executive appointees who are perceived as underperforming or abusing power.

The two most important roles for the board are as a political pressure relief valve and as a recruitment mechanism for future leaders of HPMG. Any associate can run for the board of directors. They run for a number of reasons, which include dissatisfaction with existing policy or policies, an interest in leadership, and even simple curiosity. Sadly, baser motives such as financial self-interest, protection from disciplinary action, reduction of workload, escaping clinical responsibilities, or even revenge against a leader or the existing leadership can also be motives for candidacy.

The elections often filter out the candidates of negativism, self-interest, and revenge. Most HPMG physicians are people of goodwill who usually can see through these motives. To those who have run for reasons of self-interest and have lost an election, a powerful message has been sent. When they win, they are seldom successful in the long run as their motives are recognized through direct observation by their fellow elected colleagues who are continuously judging their behavior. Once the self-interest is recognized, they are usually outvoted and eventually ignored. Nevertheless, their voice, even if it is a negative one, has been heard. They then must accept the Medical Group for what it is, or less commonly, they leave it. When that happens, both parties are usually happier.

Most run for board positions to improve the Medical Group, to right legitimate grievances, to learn how "things work," and to test their interest in leadership. As such, this is a valuable HPMG resource.

Administrative reputations are often made by high-profile initiatives that more often than not increase the workload of those affected. To paraphrase some of Winston Churchill's leading military advisors: "Winston has many innovative ideas—a few of them are actually good ones." An important elected board role is to decide which initiatives improve the survivability of HPMG—and to push back when they don't. It is an important check on the executive branch of HPMG.

Beyond the board's political pressure-release valve role, for those who have experienced a term on the elected board, most will see that policy making in a large medical group (more than six hundred doctors in 2019) is a complex business and is almost always done properly and fairly. When a critical mass of current and former elected voting board members have had this experience, it is a bulwark against conspiracy theories, which are the fodder of demagogues. Once satisfied that things are complex and done properly, some elected board members may decide that they do not want to divert their energy from the practice of medicine, and they choose not to run again. From then on, they are typically quietly supportive of the HPMG leadership and their quality initiatives.

Arguably, the most important function of the board is the recruitment of future leaders. Many of the best leaders in HPMG history got their start on the elected board. Board experience allows a potential leader to see the work that a chief needs to do. It also shows them the potential for professional satisfaction that good leadership can provide. For those who have the interest and the personality for it, board experience demonstrates that the personal – non financial - rewards of leadership can be great. While a physician might positively affect ten or twenty thousand patient lives in a purely clinical career, an effective physician leader can positively affect the lives of hundreds of thousands or more—in addition to what they do as a clinician.

The Importance of Leadership

The Hawaii region was founded in 1958. Of the 1958 *Fortune* 100 list of the hundred most successful companies, only fourteen remained in the top 100 by 2019. An additional nineteen continued to survive but well down in the Fortune 500 listing. Most of the rest are gone. The ability to adapt to rapid change is essential for survival in a free market.

Medical group checks and balances, the requirement of a Health Plan-Medical Group partnership rather than a unified authority and large size all resist adaptation to change. At least one PMG leader referred to this as "bureau-sclerosis." The antidote to this "bureau-sclerosis" is principled, innovative, energetic, persistent, and technically skilled leadership. This has been recognized since the founding of the program.

Initially, future leaders were selected by the then current leaders on the basis of their observed performance. Mentoring was personal but of variable quality. By the 1960s, regional Health Plan presidents, medical directors, and high-level Health Plan administrators were being sent to the Harvard Advanced Executive Training Program, which was a three-month program of intensive study. It was a sort of a mini-MBA.

By the 1980s, mid-level administrators were being sent to the Kaiser Permanente Executive Training Program (KPEP) at Stanford University. This was a six-week course spread out over three two-week sessions. This course was Kaiser specific with considerable time spent on Kaiser history, principles (the genetic code), and culture. It was a valuable education and networking experience for those who took advantage of it. Many graduates went on to high-level executive positions. This program continued in various iterations but with progressively less Kaiser Permanente history and philosophy. It moved from Stanford to the University of North Carolina and is now at Harvard.

In the 1990s, "Medicine and Management" started as a combined effort of the Colorado, Hawaii, and Northwest regions. It reached even further down in the hierarchy to new and future leaders and has been a great success. Any KP leader who has gone through Medicine and Management, then the Kaiser Executive Training Program has a solid, albeit brief, education in management. This investment in leadership by the program has been one of its most successful endeavors.

However, leadership is more than executive training. Character is far more important. Indeed, executive training should be withheld from someone without character. It would just make them more dangerous. There is a difference between being a character and having it. In the leadership sense, character refers to individuals with integrity defined as honesty, sincerity, living by a high moral code of values, and taking responsibility for one's actions. As leadership responsibility increases, integrity becomes more and more important.

Citizen Chiefs

In the mid-1980s HPMG leadership passed three policies to establish "citizen chiefs" rather than "paid professional" chiefs. The first policy established modest administrative compensation (maximum ~10 percent of salary) so that physicians wouldn't seek leadership positions primarily for money. The second policy was payment for only one administrative position—even if multiple positions were held. This removed the incentive to collect many positions. It had the effect of spreading out the leadership and prevented individuals from becoming financially dependent upon piggybacked administrative salaries. The third policy was to restrict administrative time to no more than 30 percent with rare and usually temporary exceptions. This meant that virtually all chiefs had a full clinical practice. Thus, they would be among the first to recognize their own bad policies, if they had no other reason than they personally had to practice medicine under their own policies.

Characteristics of Successful Clinical Chiefs

As Dr. Chaffin, the third president of HPMG, would say, "Clinical respect is table stakes for leadership." Physicians must respect their leaders to follow their lead. Poorly performing physicians are not respected by their colleagues. Hence, they cannot lead effectively. Historically, poorly performing clinicians or clinicians aspiring to leadership positions to escape clinical responsibility have not succeeded as leaders.

While the subset of outstanding clinicians is the pool from which successful leaders should be drawn, not all outstanding clinicians will make good leaders. Some have no interest in leadership for the very valid reason that they don't want to do anything that might distract them from patient care. Others are extraordinarily sensitive. It would be simply too painful for them to discipline other doctors or to "fight" for certain policies that they believe in. This should not be seen as a criticism. Such sensitivity may well make these individuals better physicians and human beings.

Most potential HPMG leaders begin as very popular figures because of their clinical accomplishments and/or pleasant personalities. For those who would find loss of popularity too painful, leadership is not for them. Human nature is such that people want what they want, and they want it now. The leader who stands in the way of what they want becomes instantly unpopular to that person—at least temporarily.

A successful HPMG leader must walk a political tightrope. Successful leaders must represent their constituency to higher leadership but also higher leadership to their constituency. On one hand, there is the department chief who only represents department interests at the expense of Medical Group interests to build popularity with department members. Higher leadership, which has the difficult role of allocating limited resources, will brand this chief a "shop steward." Eventually, that chief loses credibility with the higher leadership, and the ability of that chief to obtain even necessary department resources declines. The department members begin to see that chief as ineffective, and popularity is eventually lost anyway. Now seen as ineffective with leadership and the department members, that chief fails.

The opposite situation is the chief, who trying to curry favor with higher leadership, commits the department to work projects that are not resourced. This chief will quickly be branded as a "sell-out" by the department members. Passive resistance to un-resourced, unpopular work almost guarantees the failure of these projects. The inability of that chief to lead the department will be quickly seen by leadership. Now unpopular with the department and seen as unable to lead the department by program leadership, that chief fails.

Either way, a successful chief will have to "spend" some popularity to do the job. The fair, hardworking chief who successfully negotiates this political tightrope will retain the popularity of those of goodwill and earn the respect of almost everyone. Popularity is fickle, but respect is much less so. In HPMG history, successful chiefs have been seen as a valuable resource and have served for decades. Those successful leaders who painfully sacrifice popularity but gain respect should be consoled by the words of one of history's most respected leaders. Winston Churchill said, "You have enemies? Good. That means you stood up for something in your life."

Strong Versus Weak Chief Program

"American democracy will survive until the people figure out how to bribe themselves." This statement is apocryphally attributed to Alexis de Tocqueville (1805–1859), an observer of early American democracy. What is to prevent a popularly elected HPMG board of directors from bribing HPMG with overstaffing, overpayment, and permitting low productivity, quality, and service? Ultimately, the answer to that is the free market—and that answer is a harsh one.

If HPMG is significantly less productive than its community competition, the program will be too expensive to market successfully by Health Plan. Kaiser Foundation Health Plan of Hawaii would then go out of business—and HPMG with it. This is not a desirable outcome, but try running for popular office on a platform of austerity.

For HPMG to survive, some entity has to be the interface between the raw, popular will and the realities of limited resources. That entity in HPMG has been the executive branch: the medical director, associate medical directors, chiefs, and clinic PICs. The difficult job of successful government is to fairly balance the near-infinite desires of the population with the finite resources available.

A legislative body, such as the elected board of directors, designed as it is to represent popular will and to slow down executive function, is a poor instrument to initiate and carry out policy. This is especially true if those policies require accommodation to unpopular limited resource realities. That is the role of the executive. The executive has the responsibility to initiate and carry out policies that will promote the survival of HPMG. *With this responsibility must come authority.* Checking excessive executive zeal has been the real role of the board of directors—not initiating day-to-day operational policy.

In a "weak chief program," the members of the executive are subject to frequent elections, chiefs are elected by their departments or rotated, and the elected board involves itself in day-to-day policy. The advantage of such a system is that individual doctors within the Medical Group are unlikely to be oppressed by their own leadership. The disadvantage is that they could be even more oppressed by rapidly changing policies governed by waves of popular enthusiasm or by indecision in the face of change. Both are disruptive to a clinical program.

The executive in a weak chief system is less likely to initiate programs to accommodate limited resource realities as these would usually be unpopular. If the executive proceeds anyway, it would likely be voted out in the next, soon to happen, election. Frequently elected department chiefs would be expected to promote "shop steward" behavior, and there would be no strong executive to expect better. The Medical Group's relationship and creditability—and therefore its bargaining position with Health Plan—would be critically weakened if it could not carry out its responsibility to effectively control staffing, pay, and quality. Worst of all, there would be no one to hold responsible when necessary decisions are not made. No decision is a decision. It is a decision favoring the status quo. This is not a good long-term adaptation strategy.

With his selection and mentoring of Dr. Chu, HPMG's first president, Dr. Saward set HPMG on its way toward a strong executive. In a "strong chief system," the executive *has the responsibility and the authority* to carry out necessary initiatives. If it does not, there are no excuses—the blame is squarely on the executive. It promotes political stability, which gives the executive time to nurture careful development of culture-changing programs of excellence.

The president is elected for a six-year term and only needs to be ratified for additional terms. There have been only four HPMG presidents—Philip Chu, MD (1960–1970), William Dung, MD (1970–1992), Michael Chaffin (1992–2007), and Geoffrey Sewell, MD, (2007–present)—in the first sixty years. Presidents get to appoint their associate medical directors. These are subject to ratification, but not to popular or board election, and then are re-ratified by the elected board only every three years. The president also gets to appoint the chiefs and PICS who are ratified in the same way. These chiefs are then free to appoint their section chiefs and assistant chiefs who serve at the pleasure of the chief or PIC. There is no ratification of these subordinate chiefs except for the ratification of the chief every three years. Thus, no chief can complain that they are not responsible for the poor performance of one of their sections because they have the *responsibility* and *authority* to replace that section chief without outside review. If enough of a chief's sections are functioning poorly or if a chief is abusing power, it is the responsibility of the president to remove that chief. If the president does not do so, then the elected board must at the time of that chief's ratification—and it has but rarely. *No excuses*—that is the power of a strong chief system.

The Elected Board Controls Policy—The Executive Controls Day-to-Day Operations

It took fifteen years of debate to establish this policy. Bill Dung, HPMG's second and longest-serving president, regarded it as his greatest achievement. Leadership is about making often painful decisions. The win-win decisions have usually been made at a lower level. *If leaders are to have the responsibility for decisions, they must have authority to make those decisions*—or no decisions will be made.

The reason for an executive hierarchy is to make administrative workload manageable by dividing it up and giving direct responsibility to those with direct, local knowledge of operations. For example, the best person to make up the orthopedic on-call schedule is the section chief of orthopedics who is aware of the day-to-day operations of the department and the subspecialty capabilities of the orthopedic surgeons. The resulting schedule is likely to be elegant and nuanced.

If the associate medical director (AMD) of surgical services is forced to make up the schedule, it is likely to be simplistic and crude because the AMD of surgical services, who may not be in the Orthopedics Department, is less aware of day-to-day orthopedic operations. If the medical director or the board of directors is doing it, it would be even worse. More important—the AMD of surgical services or worse executive medical director would be distracting themselves from their primary job of looking after the larger-scale interests of HPMG. This is why micromanagers fail.

From the standpoint of the section chief of orthopedics, it is likely that some popularity was expended to enact that on-call schedule. If a disgruntled faction were to go over the head of the section chief to the chief of surgery, short of illegal, immoral, or patently unfair policy, the associate medical director (AMD) of surgical services should back the section chief of orthopedics. If the AMD of surgical services were to repeatedly overrule the section chief, it wouldn't be long before the section chief is referring all decisions to the AMD. The AMD of surgery is then distracted from the job of running the surgery department. This logic applies up the line to the medical director and especially to the elected board of directors. They do not and should not want to be managing the day-to-day functions of orthopedics or any other department. Fortunately, in HPMG, it is not uncommon to have an elected board of director state in debate: "This is an operational matter, and we should be supporting the decision of the chief."

Amnesty

"Friends may come and go but enemies accumulate" (Thomas Jones 1892–1969). Physician leaders are often called upon to do difficult things. They have the burden of explaining unpopular Medical Group resource and staffing decisions. They are primarily responsible for service and quality discipline within their departments, and they are on the line for their hiring decisions. In addition to the added administrative workload, they acquire (and keep) difficult patients who only want to "see the chief." Because of the "citizen chief" policies, physician leaders may rationally wish to return to full-time clinical care before they retire.

Potential physician leaders are well trained as physicians to accurately assess risk-benefit. If a stint in leadership presents too great a career risk, they will avoid it. Good leaders are a scarce resource. Anything that increases this scarcity is bad policy. For this reason, it has been HPMG's wise policy to treat ex-leaders kindly. Observing this, over the years, potential leaders have been more willing to "chance it."

HPMG has grown steadily in size, prosperity, and accountability. This could not have happened without an effective governing structure that is considered legitimate by the group's physicians.

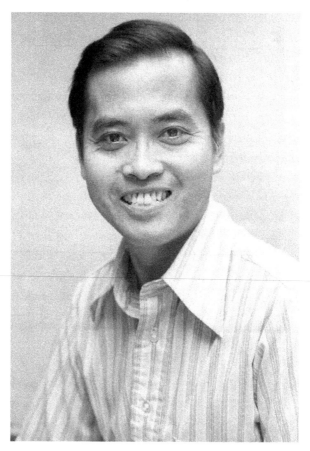

William M.H. Dung, MD, medical director 1970–1992.

CHAPTER 7

WILLIAM M. H. DUNG, MD: THE SECOND PRESIDENT OF HPMG

D
r. Bill Dung was the second and longest-serving medical director in HPMG history. He led the program during a critical time when the very survival of the Medical Group hung in the balance. Bill related to the author about how he joined the program. He spent his time in Honolulu when he wasn't actually in attendance at the University of Washington Medical School. As such, he became familiar with the Honolulu medical community. After graduating from medical school and completing his internship, he went on to complete mandatory military service as a regimental surgeon in the Fourth Marine Regiment First Marine Brigade.

Upon his return to Hawaii, he was searching for a position in Honolulu while awaiting discharge. He heard that Henry Kaiser was planning to establish a Health Plan in Hawaii, but he also heard nothing but bad things about the program even though it had not even begun operations. He therefore went to Drs. Yee and Izumi, who he knew from his previous time in Honolulu, to find out more. They were later to become original partners of the Pacific Medical Associates. They recommended that he ask "Henry" himself since Mr. Kaiser was recruiting "his" doctors personally.

Bill described to the author the interview that changed his life. He was in naval uniform nervously fidgeting with his uniform cap when on June 16, 1958 he was ushered into Mr. Kaiser's ground-floor office in the Kaiser (now Hilton) Hawaiian Village Hotel. He had Mr. Kaiser's undivided attention. Mr. Kaiser told him the apocryphal story of how his mother had died in his arms because of inadequate medical care. He went on to say that the Kaiser Health Care program was what he would be remembered for.

Bill was inspired by that conversation and impressed with the great man's vision. He was from then on determined to be part of this vision. He ignored the advice of community doctors who told him that he would be committing professional suicide if he did. He was hired as a contract physician by the Pacific Medical Associates in April 1959. He was still employed by them when Dr. Keene canceled the Pacific Medical Associates contract on August 20, 1960, and formed HPMG from thirty-one of the thirty-three contract doctors. Thus, Bill Dung was one of the thirty-one founding members of HPMG.

During the decade of Dr. Chu's leadership, in addition to his general medical practice duties, Bill quietly and competently performed administrative positions of increasing responsibility. In 1963, he served on a task force studying patient-physician relationships where he emphasized the importance of quality of care and service.

In May 1966, he was appointed the first chief of the Emergency Department, which also included the urgent care clinic. As part of these duties, he organized the KP Hawaii Multiphasic Clinic—a popular, well-patient preventive screening program based upon the already established Northern California program organized by Morris Collin, MD, in 1962.

By 1968, in Northern California, the multiphasic program had screened more than half a million patients and had provided the data for more than 150 medical publications. The Hawaii Multiphasic Screening program began in January 1968 and lasted almost twenty years. Through this program, hundreds of apparently healthy patients were screened every week with a focused history and physical examination, basic laboratory tests, a chest x-ray, and an electrocardiogram. In contrast to the popular, time-consuming, and relatively unfocused yearly physicals and expensive "executive physicals," it was designed specifically around the efficient, early diagnosis of treatable conditions. Every week, potentially serious conditions were detected, including hypertension, cardiac arrhythmias, cardiac murmurs, thyroid, abdominal, breast and prostate masses, suspicious skin lesions, kidney disease, blood in the urine or stool, urinary tract infections, anemia, leukemia, diabetes, and others. These patients would then be referred back to their personal physicians for further evaluation and treatment. It was popular with patients, and lives were saved. Scientific papers were generated from the data.

In one 1981 KP Hawaii study published by the *Hawaii Medical Journal*, at a time when up to half of all prostate cancer patients presented with metastatic bone spread, the figure for the Hawaii KP prostate cancer patients was only 17 percent. As preventive care became more established scientifically, the best parts of the multiphasic exam were incorporated into individual primary care practices and the many organized screening programs that distinguish Kaiser Permanente care to this day.

In January 1968, Dr. Dung was elected with more votes than the other two candidates combined to the ruling executive committee of HPMG. He went on to be appointed as physician in charge of the new Punawai (Hawaiian for "Spring of Life") Clinic in central Oahu—at that time the largest clinic outside of the medical center. In January 1969, he was appointed secretary of the executive committee.

HPMG was completely unprepared for the sudden death of Dr. Chu in July 1970. There was no succession plan in place. Two assistant medical directors, Dr. Hau Vu, an obstetrician-gynecologist, and Dr. Tom Brown, a radiologist, had served in high-level administrative roles under him. Both had their own following, but Dr. Chu's strong leadership had inhibited the formation of factions around each of them. In the power vacuum of his sudden death, powerful factions quickly emerged.

Dr. Chu died at seven o'clock on Friday morning, July 18, 1970. The next day, Dr. Keene flew to Hawaii to address the executive committee. He advised them to take their time selecting the next medical director and to consult experienced PMG leaders such as Dr. Ray Kaye, the recently retired medical director of the Southern California PMG. Dr. Kaye provided valuable guidance and helped the Medical Group through a difficult power transition.

Between July and December, Paul McCallin, MD, served as "acting executive chairman." As such, he presided over the executive committee meetings and represented HPMG at the Kai-Perm meeting in October 1970.

One of the last and most important achievements of Dr. Chu was his work to pass a Hawaii law allowing professional corporations in Hawaii. HPMG existing as a professional corporation would have a legal framework for tax protection of what would become the generous benefit program of HPMG. To apply for professional corporate status, the Medical Group had to develop articles of association. Despite the political rivalries, this was accomplished under the leadership of Dr. McCallin by the beginning of December.

Five months had passed since the sudden death of Dr. Chu. It was time to elect a new HPMG president. On December 7, Dr. Keene came to Hawaii for a week to guide HPMG through its first medical director succession. What he found was disturbing. There was no consensus. Both of the interested leading candidates—Vu and Brown—and their followers were far apart. He initially favored T. K. Lin, MD, a more neutral party, a respected cardiologist, and a founder of HPMG, but Dr. Lin was not interested. He preferred clinical practice over leadership.

Dr. Keene needed to find a candidate who was capable of the job, but more important, who would be accepted by both factions. On the recommendation of Ray Kaye, he approached Bill Dung. Bill had not considered himself a candidate for medical director. He was happy with his position managing the Punawai Clinic and his other clinical duties. He described the call from Dr. Keene's office to his clinic in Punawai to the author as a turning point in his life. He was reluctant to run, but he was willing to do it for the good of the program.

Bill's humility, honesty, solid administrative performance, and quiet but positive demeanor made him an attractive candidate. In an acrimonious general membership meeting on December 14, 1970, the Medical Group could not even agree on an election process. It was therefore decided to present all eleven members of the executive committee as potential candidates. On the first ballot, it was Drs. Dung 16, Vu 14, Brown 8, while Drs. Huitt, Roth, Kim and McCallin got one to three votes. These four withdrew their candidacy. On the second round, it was Dung 19, Vu 18, and Brown 9. Dr. Brown withdrew his candidacy. On the third round, it was Dung 26 and Vu 20. William Dung, MD, was thus elected the second medical director of HPMG with a 57 percent majority.

He was under no illusions about how difficult the job would be. He said it best in his own words from his confidential administrative diary. In the first entry made on the day after his election he wrote:

> Lord knows, I do not need the "job" as an ego trip—and am well satisfied with my life, contribution to society, to health [care], and to my family. Yet now I am in this position—not one of my own choosing—but I enter it with confidence and commitment that I will do everything that I can to make the Kaiser Permanente type of program in Hawaii the best. Since speaking with Henry Kaiser in the summer of 1958 and entering the program in April 1959—I have a profound and deep belief that our method of health care-delivery is the only way quality health care can survive in the future. To this end, I direct my energy and thoughts during the coming years.

December 17, 1970, four days after he was elected president, he wrote in the administrative diary:

> I have inherited a completely disorganized and factionalized Medical Group. It is leaderless and I do not see how morale can be any poorer. I have never seen as deep a rift between the Health Plan organization and HPMG. It borders on a distrust so deep that it seems to touch nearly on hate. This I have not seen since September of 1960 when the original Pacific Medical Associates was dissolved.

In this entry, he went on to set out his long-term plan. He set out ethical standards and long-term Medical Group and program goals. Remarkably, he did not deviate from these standards and goals during the next twenty-one years of his administration.

Regarding ethics he wrote in the diary:

> Three more important principles—never forget!!! 1. Communication—always work at it. 2. Be scrupulously honest 3. Never break a confidence.

He remained true to these principles, and as a result, people trusted him during good times and bad.

Regarding Medical Group goals in the diary he wrote:

> 1. Board controls policy—chiefs control operations. 2. Clinics need to be under the control of HPMG. 3. HPMG needs to become more of a participatory democracy. 4. Morale must be addressed with greater communication and a fairer and more realistic compensation package.

Over the next two decades, these objectives were largely achieved.

Finally, he set down his regional goals:

> 1. The program should be statewide—growth is good. 2. The program should participate meaningfully in medical social welfare programs. 3. Most important, the success or failure of the program will depend upon the quality of the partnership between Health Plan and Medical Group. The success of the program in Hawaii continues to depend upon the attainment of these objectives.

The centerpiece of his communications effort was the chairman's comments that began in January 1971 and were issued every two months for twenty-one years without missing a single issue. The president's newsletter was continued by Bill's successor, Mike Chaffin. In it, there would be an overview statement and then a summary of executive committee and operations committee activities. The newsletter was carefully prepared and comprehensive. This was to be the president's antidote to what he called the NETMA ("No one ever tells me anything") syndrome. From then on, no HPMG doctor could reasonably claim that they didn't know what was going on. This had been a growing criticism of Dr. Chu's presidency.

Unifying HPMG Leadership

Bill's first administrative attempt to break up the factions was stopped cold. He proposed Alex Roth, MD, as his executive medical director at the January 7, 1971, general staff meeting. Dr. Roth was an allergist who had been recruited from the faculty of the University of Kansas by Dr. T. K. Lin who had known him there. He became chief of pediatrics and had served capably and positively in many administrative roles. Bill described him as cool, efficient, and methodical.

Bill's nomination of Dr. Roth was promptly defeated by the executive board in a 5–4 vote. It was the only appointment during Bill's twenty-one years as medical director that was rejected by the board of directors. Disappointed and bowing to political necessity, at the next general staff meeting a week later, he fashioned a compromise. He appointed the two faction leaders Drs. Vu and Brown as co-vice presidents since neither candidate could achieve consensus support. The level of trust was so low that both factions insisted that both candidates be presented in the same motion to prevent one side or the other from reneging on the deal. Dr. Vu was to concentrate on Medical Group general policy and finances, and Dr. Brown was to concentrate on operations. Bill hoped, vainly it turned out, that they would learn to work together. It would take four years of divided leadership, an attempt on his presidency, and the resignation of both vice presidents from the Medical Group before Bill achieved undisputed leadership of HPMG.

Despite the divided leadership, Bill held HPMG together, and real progress was made during the first eighteen months of his administration. Successfully enacted was a standardization of chief's pay, sabbatical policy, a permanent pay increase for board certification, profit sharing after three years, and an education leave policy. He greatly strengthened the "chiefs are operations and the board is policy" strategy by establishing that chiefs would be appointed by the president with board ratification every three years. Good progress was made with the University of Hawaii affiliation, and program membership continued to grow.

Bill patiently and methodically worked his objectives, making slow progress. He had written in the first entry of his administrative diary that he would perform an eighteen-month private personal reassessment of his performance, which he would confine to the diary. In May 1972, he made such an assessment. He felt that doctor morale was better and that his leadership style was increasingly accepted. He felt that if an election were held, he would be reelected. The HPMG—Health Plan distrust had only somewhat improved. While he had successfully quashed the divisive idea of an HPMG audit of Health Plan finances, he was having increasing difficulty working with the current regional president, Conrad Bohuslav. Operationally he felt that he was making slow but steady progress with his plan to make the elected board policy and the chiefs' operations. His greatest accomplishment was the agreement that HPMG would assume clinic operations, which previously had been under Health Plan management. This would greatly increase the accountability of the clinic staff to the doctors they were supposed to be assisting. He gave himself good grades for establishing the respect of HPMG in central office in Oakland and in the local community. The community was coming to understand that HPMG was a physician-driven organization.

Partnership Stressed

Since the founding of the Hawaii KP program, there had been a single medical director—Phil Chu—but several regional Health Plan presidents. Because of his continuity, strong personality, and clear program direction, Dr. Chu had dominated the partnership. The regional presidents and Central Office in Oakland, for the most part, had followed his lead.

Conrad Bohuslav, the regional Health Plan president at the time of Dr. Chu's death, had done the same. When Dr. Dung became president, he resolved to make Bohuslav a true partner and not to go through or around him on Health Plan concerns either locally or in Oakland as had Chu. While well intentioned, Bill acknowledged this to be one of the two major errors of his first term. Without strong direction, Bohuslav never really accepted Dr. Dung as an equal partner; he micromanaged issues and had difficulty making decisions.

The 1971 medical services contract had been delayed at least three months, and the 1972 contract was still not finalized five months into the year. Bohuslav was called before the HPMG board in August 1972 by Dr.

Dung to explain the delays. They and Bill remained unsatisfied. The board submitted to Bohuslav a written "bill of particulars." Bill had privately and clearly warned Bohuslav that the crisis was building in a series of contentious one-on-one meetings in March, April, and May 1972.

Bill had also learned through back channels that his partnership strategy with Bohuslav was not mutual. Bohuslav was critical of Bill's leadership and the performance of HPMG to his Health Plan superiors. Bill had hoped to keep the disagreements within the Hawaii region, but in October 1972, Bohuslav presented it as a surprise attack to his superior Jim Vohs, the soon-to-be full CEO of Kaiser Permanente. This was the turning point in the relationship. Bill was now prepared to go through and around Bohuslav at Central Office during Bohuslav's remaining two years in Hawaii as had Dr. Chu before him. This did have the effect of on-time medical service contracts for 1973 and 1974, but the conflict would only be resolved by the resignation of one or the other.

The Second Salary Crisis

The 1970s were a bad time for the US economy. There was an 88 percent devaluation of the buying power of a dollar between 1971 and 1981 due to two "gas crises," a fiscal hangover from the Vietnam War, and poor performance of the economy. During this decade, there was an actual stock market loss when inflation corrected. The top federal income tax bracket was 70 percent—exclusive of state and local taxes. The 50 percent federal tax bracket was at $44,000. Tax brackets were not corrected for inflation and were riddled with loopholes. As salaries went up in a losing attempt to compensate for the rapidly decreasing buying power, taxes went up even faster as workers were driven into higher non-inflation-corrected tax brackets. This was known as "bracket creep." The combination of a slow economy and rapid inflation was called "stagflation" by pundits. With continuing program austerity to remain competitive with HMSA, poor communication between Health Plan and HPMG, and ill-advised government and then program salary-price freezes, HPMG doctor salaries fell far behind. On top of everything, Hawaii had—and has—one of the highest cost of living indices in the United States. This brought on the second

HPMG salary crisis, the first one having been in 1960. This crisis threatened both Dr. Dung's presidency and the survival of the Medical Group.

So 1975 was another critical year for HPMG, similar to the 1960 traumatic founding and the 1970 Phil Chu succession crisis. Between February and May 1974, Dr. Dung was assigned by the program to attend the Harvard Advanced Executive Training Program. During this time, away from the hustle and bustle of the daily HPMG mini crises, he was able to concentrate on long-term strategy. His sense that the divided coalition leadership was not in the long-term interests of HPMG was strongly reinforced by the instructors. He resolved to settle the issue once and for all upon his return—even if it cost him the HPMG presidency.

He returned to work on May 8, 1974. On the next day, at the board of directors meeting, he announced his planned reorganization. The two vice presidents—Drs. Tom Brown and Hau Vu—would no longer have independent authority. They would now be staff to Dr. Dung. All HPMG administrators would now report directly or indirectly to Dr. Dung. Dr. Brown eventually accepted the change gracefully, but Dr. Vu did not.

During the rest of 1974 and early 1975, the salaries became progressively less and less competitive, and well-respected staff were leaving HPMG for this reason. In February 1975, the crisis was coming to a head as two HPMG stalwarts announced they were leaving. Dr. Brown applied for a six-month leave of absence to try a position in Indiana for financial reasons. He resigned when the six months was up to take that position. T. K. Lin resigned for financial reasons and for dissatisfaction with the direction of HPMG. Losses peaked during April and May 1975 when 10 percent of the Medical Group announced forthcoming resignation dates.

Dr. Dung's opposition centered around Dr. Vu who presented all this as evidence of a failing administration. Word got back to Dung. Bill confided to his administrative diary that was no longer sure that he would be re-ratified as president in 1976. Rumors got back to him that Dr. Vu and his allies were not going to wait that long. Bill decided to strike first.

On March 6, 1975, Dung had a private meeting with Vu to announce that he was planning another reorganization. He intended to appoint Alex Roth executive vice president. Vu told him that he would oppose this, and if he didn't prevail, he would resign. Bill went forward with the plan anyway. It was a test of strength.

In a contentious meeting on March 20, 1975, Dr. Roth was ratified by five yes votes, one no vote, and three abstentions. Dr. Vu did not resign. Instead, he stepped up his efforts. Reports again got back to Bill. The showdown was to occur at the board meeting on May 1, 1975. Vu and his supporters proposed that the present administration and board of directors should resign and submit themselves to a vote of confidence by the associates, and if they lost, they should all step down.

With the help of allies, such as Tom Brown, still vice president until his planned resignation, Clifford Straehley chief of surgery, and Alfred Scottolini, chief of pathology, the effort was blocked. Bill noted correctly during the debate that a complete change of governance would be very disruptive during this time of crisis. He pointed out that he had been elected president until 1976. If the associates wanted to remove him, they could do it then by refusing to ratify him. He also stated that he would accept the resignation of any members of the board who wished to resign if they felt they did not have the confidence of the group. He went on to state that he would then hold a prompt board elections to replace them. No board member resigned. Bill's opponents had taken their shot and missed.

Dr. Dung met with Dr. Vu on May 12 to tell him that he needed a vice president who would be working with him and not against him and that he was planning to announce his removal as vice president at the May 15 board meeting. There was no need for this announcement as Dr. Vu subsequently announced his resignation from HPMG effective August 1. Dr. Vu moved to California and practiced in Modesto and then in Riverside. He retired to Coronado, California, and died on September 19, 2017 at the age of eighty-eight. Bill personally considered this political crisis the low point of his entire twenty-one-year administration, but it was also a turning point. Since 1967, an increasingly disruptive divided leadership crisis had been brewing. At great emotional and political cost, it was now resolved.

1975: The Turning Point

In retrospect, 1975 was a turning point year for HPMG and Health Plan. In January, Jim Vohs was appointed the CEO of Kaiser Permanente. He succeeded another friend of the Hawaii region, Cliff Keene. Both felt strongly that Kaiser Permanente had the potential to be a national and international model "third way" of providing high-quality, efficient health care. As such, they both gave the regions outside of California administrative attention out of proportion to their size when compared to the California regions. They saw them as KP "missions." They understood that if the program could only survive in California, it would not have the standing to be considered a health care model. It would forever be seen as a California social experiment—surviving as a "one-off" Henry Kaiser specific historical accident. For this reason, even though the Hawaii region represented less than 3 percent of the KP membership, one of the first things that Vohs did as CEO was to come to Hawaii to investigate the dysfunctional partnership firsthand. He decided to replace Bohuslav.

On February 12, 1975, Vohs called Dung and told him that he was replacing Bohuslav with Ron Wyatt. Bill wished "Connie" Bohuslav well in his presidential newsletter of March 1975. Bill stated gracefully that he had served the region loyally first as comptroller for seven years and the regional Health Plan president for seven more years. Bohuslav went on to an administrative Medicare position in Central Office in Oakland.

Wyatt came with outstanding credentials. He had bachelor's and master's degrees in Public Health from the University of California at Berkeley. He had joined KP in 1962 as the hospital administrator of the Panorama City Hospital. He was then promoted to the Northern California regional hospital administrator and then in 1970 to regional president in Ohio. He and Dung had a productive thirteen-year partnership, which ended in 1988 when he retired from the position of Hawaii regional president.

In 1975, two important additions to Dr. Dung's administrative staff joined HPMG. Up to that time, Bill felt that the Medical Group was too small to afford a business manager, but the difficult medical services agreement negotiations had convinced him to change his mind. In June 1975, Mike Linderman began his twenty-five-year tenure as business manager. He had obtained his MBA at Stanford University and had a successful career in finance. He was to assume the management of the nonphysician staff of the Laboratory, Diagnostic Imaging, and Optical Departments as well as the clinic staff. He was instrumental in establishing policies and procedures that placed HPMG on a sound financial footing. He was most valuable as the partner first of Dr. Dung and then his successor, Dr. Chaffin, in the often-contentious yearly medical service agreement contract negotiations.

In the same month, Gladys Ching, RN, Began her thirty-one-year career with HPMG as the director of clinic nursing. She replaced Mr. Joseph Paek who had been long-term administrator of the clinic staff first under Health Plan and then HPMG. He left Hawaii to take a position in Kaiser Permanente International. Initially, Gladys reported to Mike Linderman, but she eventually had a direct reporting relationship to the medical director. While Bill had successfully negotiated with Health Plan to obtain administrative control of the clinic staff, Gladys—over her long thirty-one-year HPMG career—gently, consistently, and persistently successfully established a culture of service and accountability to physicians and patients among the clinic staff. Gladys retired in 2006 at the end of Dr. Chaffin's administration. Both of these dedicated and capable administrators were to take an enormous management burden off of the shoulders of two medical directors: Bill Dung and then Mike Chaffin.

With the Medical Group leadership crisis resolved, a new capable regional Health Plan president—and revitalized Medical Group finance and nursing administration—Dr. Dung patiently pursued his administrative goals with increasing success. Morale steadily improved. During 1975, the program broke through the hundred thousand-member mark and was at more than 105,000 by the end of the year.

Progress continued in 1976. On October 10, on the eve of the reaffirmation balloting, Bill wrote in his administrative diary that he estimated forty-eight votes in favor and eighteen against. He was wrong. Bill Dung was easily ratified for another term with 88 percent of the associates voting in favor of him. On Thursday, October 21, the final vote count was fifty-seven yes, seven no, and one abstention. As he wrote in his administrative diary on October 25, 1976: "Thank you Lord! I am now my own man." The eight-year divided leadership crisis had been a costly drain on the vitality of HPMG. With the emergence of Dr. Dung as undisputed leader of the Medical Group, that wasted energy was now directed toward the external competition.

Dr. Dung's Second Term

His second term was one of growth, prosperity, and the stabilization of the group with policies and procedures that persist to this day. Between 1976 and 1982, the program grew more than 20 percent, and the Medical Group grew even faster, resulting in significant service improvements. The doctor patient ratio had dropped from 1:1,116 in 1970 to 1:868 in 1982. This was at a time when the doctor patient national ratio was 1:680. This disproportionate growth of HPMG was made possible by the membership growth and the stabilization of HPMG finances under the leadership of Mike Linderman as business manager. By the end of the term, the doctors were seeing some of the largest divisible surpluses to date. Salaries were catching up with the fee-for-service doctors, and the benefit package exceeded them.

During Dr. Chu's administration (1960–1970), the group grew from thirty-one to seventy-six doctors, and almost all of them were at the medical center. Everyone knew each other and often socialized together since they were socially ostracized by the outside medical community. In this environment, Dr. Chu could make the necessary ad hoc policy decisions with relative ease, but by the end of his term, as the group grew and became more geographically dispersed, factionalism was growing and demands for a greater voice in HPMG governance were being heard. These issues were clearly recognized by Dr. Chu, but he died suddenly and unexpectedly before he could address them.

By the beginning Dr. Dung's second term, there were 117 doctors in HPMG, dispersed to six clinics on Oahu and two on Maui. Dr. Dung understood from the beginning that addressing the communication issue was a priority. It was for this reason he had published the presidential newsletter every two months. He also understood that the governance structure needed to be opened up. This had been accomplished during his first term despite the divided leadership. With unified leadership and well-accepted democratic processes, there was a governing framework that methodically began to develop the policies and procedures that could be scaled up to an HPMG of any size.

In November 1976, the framework of a generous retirement program was established. In February 1977, an incentive plan was established for physicians who had made exceptional contributions to the program. In July 1977, full retirement vesting was dropped from fifteen to ten years. Later, it would be reduced to five years.

In January 1978, the principles of compensatory time for off-hours services were established. This eliminated the resistance of staff to come in the middle of the night for consultations. In February 1978, rules were clarified for future presidential elections. Bill's term had another four years to run, thus no elections were imminent, which kept partisan politics out of the discussion. In May, education leave with an education allowance was standardized at one week for the first two years and then two weeks a year thereafter on a use-it-or-lose-it basis. This almost guaranteed self-directed continuing medical education.

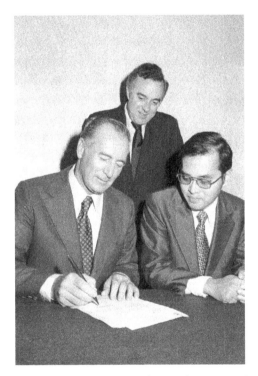

(L to R) Ron Wyatt, Hawaii regional president, Joseph Califano, secretary of health, education, and welfare, and William Dung, Hawaii Permanente Medical Group medical director at the signing of the first HMO contract in Hawaii.

In September, 1978 the "rule of 80" was established. The program had traditionally provided full medical coverage during their careers and after retirement, but what qualified for retirement coverage was unclear. The "rule of 80" promised lifetime health care retirement coverage for all HMPG physicians whose age and years of service added up to more than eighty. Very few medical groups or private practices provide postretirement health care coverage at all. These policies greatly increased the security and attractiveness of the HPMG compensation package. HPMG was greatly strengthened by these policies, and they exist to this day largely unchanged having withstood the test of time.

The Next Generation of HPMG Leadership

By the late seventies, the spearhead of the baby boom generation born in the late 1940s were completing their medical training and entering the medical marketplace. They had matured and obtained their college education during the turbulent late sixties and early seventies. The baby boomers were the largest, richest, best-educated, and most self-confident generation up to that time in American history. This had been a time of great social change in America. The Peace Corps, civil rights reforms, and the antipoverty programs had increased their social consciousness.

At the same time, the Vietnam War and its anti-war protests, urban racial riots, and a string of assassinations and political scandals collectively increased their skepticism of established norms. Nothing represented the establishment in medicine more than the AMA. As such, this generation was far more open to a different way of health care-delivery no matter what the AMA said about managed care programs such as Kaiser Permanente. Between 1977 and 1980, a period of relative prosperity and stability for HPMG, a disproportionate number of future HPMG leaders joined the group. At least some of them saw the anti-managed care positions of the AMA position as a personal challenge and as an opportunity to join an organization that would represent the future of medicine. By 1981, they would be the operational chiefs of more than 70 percent of the Medical Group and would go on to career-long leadership contributions to HPMG.

Karl Pregitzer, MD, joined the group in 1977. Prior to that era, most

Emergency Department doctors were doctors who were between training programs or between jobs. Karl graduated from the second class of residents at the University of Southern California who formally trained in emergency medicine, which was emerging as a specialty in its own right with its own board certification. By 1978, he was chief of the HPMG Emergency Department (ED) after a failed department attempt to rotate chiefs by the members of the department. During the next thirteen years, he reorganized the department as its own specialty and increased its professionalism by demanding board certification of all of the department members.

In the early 1980s, during his tenure, the Industrial Medicine Department was established as a section of emergency medicine. Once it had matured, he assisted in its establishment as an independent department. The Industrial Medicine Department has since made a significant contribution to the program both for non-plan income and marketing to businesses. During the fifteen-year Chaffin administration, he was promoted to vice president of outside services and special non-plan products. He was made an associate medical director when Dr. Sewell became medical director in 2007. He served as such until his retirement. He was a nationally recognized coding and billing expert. Prior to his time, more than 95 percent of program income was prepaid. Few, if any, resources were assigned to non-prepaid plan services, which were being delivered essentially for free because of poor collection and billing mechanisms. As cost sharing became an important part of medical financing, the ability to collect co-pays was essential to the survival of the program. Having a robust billing and collection mechanism in place positioned the program to bid successfully for the Maui Hospital contract, which would have a large non-Kaiser, non-prepaid component. Upon his retirement in October 2015, he had been the longest-serving full-time physician (thirty-eight years) in HPMG history. This record is unlikely ever to be surpassed.

Peter Clapp, MD, also joined HPMG in 1977. He came from a distinguished academic background, having trained at the Tufts and Harvard programs and having served on the full-time faculty at Boston University Medical School. He was a pioneer in interventional radiology, and he established the interventional radiology subsection in HPMG. This state-of-the-art subsection remains one of the strongest in the medical program.

One of the first things he did when he was appointed chief in 1978 was modernize the name of the Department of Radiology to the Department of Diagnostic Imaging. For the first half of the twentieth century until the early 1960s, diagnostic imaging was mostly x-ray flat-plate film hard copy images sometimes enhanced using contrast agents. By the 1970s, the name of the specialty "radiology" was out of date with rapid advances in video fluoroscopy, radioactive tracer scans, ultrasound, computerized tomography, and finally magnetic resonance imaging (MRI). Dr. Clapp's renaming of the department was to presage a decade of department modernization along its present lines. Especially valuable was his skill at diagnostic imaging facility design during the move to the new hospital.

In 1978, Michael Chaffin, MD, joined HPMG. Even before he joined, it was clear that "other-centered" service was to be the hallmark of his life and career. Out of high school, he served in the Peace Corps in Brazil. After his medical education, he was a National Health Service physician serving remote Micronesian communities where often he was the only the health care. All this was done while raising a young family with Rhonda, his wife of more than fifty years. Once in HPMG, he proved to be an outstanding internist, popular with patients, doctors, and staff. During the lead-up to his election as medical director, he had served as interim chief of medicine and physician in charge of the Windward Clinic, quality assurance director, and finally vice president and executive vice president in 1987–8. His fifteen years as president of HPMG is worthy of its own chapter.

In 1979, Stephen D. Miller, MD, joined HPMG. He was a well-trained, popular ophthalmologist with a retinal surgery subspecialty. He was soon section chief of ophthalmology and then chief of surgical services.

At the end of 1982, he resigned from this position to become vice president of finance under Dr. Dung. It was a position that he held during the Dung and Chaffin administrations until his retirement. He was instrumental in developing the compensation policy based upon the external standard of national average salaries. It was a policy that successfully enabled the hiring and retention of outstanding HPMG doctors. He was also instrumental in the development of a sustainable staffing policy that made these competitive salaries possible. Both have stood the test of time for over a quarter of a century.

Toward the end of Steve's career, his involvement in the SEVA Foundation increased. The SEVA Foundation is an internationally acclaimed charitable organization that establishes self-sustaining ophthalmologic hospitals in underserved areas of the world. As of 2016, they were increasing the quality and efficiency of sixty-six eye hospitals in twenty-two countries. Through its activities, every year, tens of thousands of patients have their eyesight restored. Steve retired early to further increase his involvement with SEVA, and from 2014–6, he served as chairman of the board of directors. In 2015, SEVA won the Champalimaud Award—the Nobel Prize equivalent for international eye care.

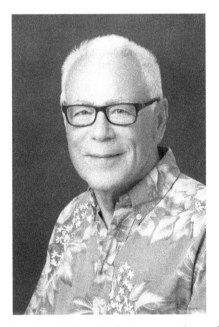

Stephen D. Miller, MD, HPMG vice president of finance (1983–2001). Later he was chairman of the board of directors of the SEVA Eye Foundation (2014-2016).

In 1980, Lee Jacobs, MD, joined the program directly from a fellowship in infectious disease. He was a well-liked, natural leader. By 1981, he was the chief of medicine and medical subspecialties. At that time, primary care doctor-patient relationships were informal. While many patients identified with a specific primary care doctor, there was still much medical care that was delivered randomly on the basis of doctor availability. This lack of continuity of care had the potential to weaken the doctor-patient relationship, delay diagnosis and treatment, and diffuse accountability. This was in contrast to typically stronger doctor-patient relationships in fee-for-service medicine: the KP competition.

Marketing data clearly demonstrated that patients without a personal care physician were most likely to leave the program. He began the reorganization of the department so that every primary care physician would have a "panel" of patients for which they would be responsible. This policy clarified the lines of accountability that made measurement of quality assurance, patient satisfaction, and peer satisfaction possible. It was the first such program in KP.

In 1985, he was recruited away from HPMG by the medical director of the new Georgia region, which was based in Atlanta, to become their associate medical director. He served in executive positions in the Georgia region and nationally until his retirement in 2007. He had a rich administrative career, including missionary efforts outside of KP. As of 2017, he continued his service to the program as coeditor of the medical journal *Permanente Medicine*.

In 1980, the author joined HPMG directly from a Mayo Clinic residency in urologic surgery. The five-year Mayo Clinic experience had a strong influence. He had been impressed with Mayo's relentless patient-centered efficiency, which drove democratically, physician-directed, well-thought-out policies and procedures administered by competent managers. This structure, in turn, supported well-coordinated, subspecialized medical care-delivery. He had a strong interest in change agency leadership since high school and succeeded Steve Miller as chief of surgical services in early 1983.

With a special administrative interest in clinical operations, he served in various executive positions within HPMG, the hospital, and the program for the next twenty-seven years. These activities included the prospective Quality Assurance Program, the Specialty Care Model, the KP Hawaii Heart Program, and a twenty-year campaign to develop standardized, data-driven, Medical Group performance standards and finally HPMG Clinical Grand Rounds. He served as chief of surgical services from 1983 to 2005 and then from 2005 until his late 2009 retirement as the associate medical director of hospital, surgical, and medical specialties as well as chief of staff of the Kaiser Moanalua Hospital twice. He felt strongly that the current generation of HPMG leaders should understand that mentoring the next generation of leaders as one of their most important duties.

Also in 1980, Christine Fukui, MD, joined HPMG directly from her fellowship in pulmonary medicine from the prestigious University of California in San Francisco. She was a popular, very capable, hardworking clinician who founded the high-performance section of pulmonary medicine and remained its chief for her entire HPMG career. She was consistently listed in the "Best Doctors in Hawaii" in *Honolulu Magazine*. She was elected to three terms on the board of directors. In 2005, she was appointed the chief of medical subspecialties and because of her success in that role the vice president of hospital quality and patient safety. Between 2007 and the end of 2009 when she retired, she served as associate medical director of quality assurance safety and risk. She was long active in the American Lung Association of Hawaii and the Hawaii Thoracic Society. In 2006, she was named Outstanding Clinician of the Year by the American Thoracic Society.

With the operational and financial accomplishments of Dr. Dung's second term and the so-far-successful recruitment of a new generation of future leaders to replace the pioneers, things were looking up for HPMG. Thus, on September 1, 1982, William Dung, MD, was easily reaffirmed with sixty-nine yes and twenty-two no votes (75 percent) to a third term as president and medical director of HPMG.

The Building Program

The original Kaiser Hospital in Waikiki, built in 1958, had been planned for a capacity of seventy-five thousand Health Plan members. It was scheduled for replacement in 1975, but it continued to serve the program for another decade with a few additions. When it closed in 1985, it was serving 138,000 members.

Planning for the replacement hospital began as early as 1967. In that year, the master plan was to have two hospitals: the original hospital in Waikiki and a small hospital on the site of the Punawai Clinic. By the mid-1970s, it was apparent that this was not a practical solution because the

Punawai site in Waipahu would be too small and too far from the projected population center of Oahu. Consideration was then given to building a second tower next to the existing ten-story hospital tower in Waikiki. This option was soon precluded by city building code and zoning changes. In retrospect, that was fortuitous.

In subsequent years, the population center of Oahu shifted farther to the west and center of the island. Furthermore, Oahu traffic progressively worsened. Access to the medical center would have had to have been through traffic-choked side streets.

By 1975, the decision was made to purchase a site for a completely new hospital near the projected geographic population center of the island with easy access to all three island freeways. By late 1976, the search was on. In October 1977, an agreement was reached with the Damon Estate for KP to purchase fifteen acres adjacent to the Moanalua Golf Course. This site had easy access to the Moanalua Freeway and was near the correctly forecasted Oahu population center.

During 1978, program leaders worked their way successfully through the thicket of federal, state, and city approvals required for the new hospital. The design contract was awarded to Payette Associates of Boston, which was internationally known for its hospitals. Architects Hawaii, a well-established local firm, was awarded the architectural contract for what was to become an award-winning building.

During 1979 and 1980, detailed design and planning proceeded. The construction contract was awarded to Pacific Construction, a well-established local contractor. Throughout the planning and building process, HPMG physicians were heavily involved. They contributed especially to the locations of departments, for example the diagnostic imaging and lab suites were located close to the Emergency Department, and also to department design to facilitate workflow. This was especially important for operating room design and clinic procedure rooms, diagnostic imaging, and the laboratory. Large and small improvements were suggested and implemented even down to the idea of child safety covers for electrical outlets in pediatrics.

The initial plan was a two-phase construction of the new hospital as there were not sufficient funds to build the hospital in one phase. In this plan, the first phase would be completed at Moanalua with all of the surgical and technology-dependent hospital services, such as lab and diagnostic imaging, being delivered there. The original Kaiser Hospital would have an emergency department, basic lab and diagnostic imaging services, and ambulatory surgery and primary care medical services. Maintaining two hospitals simultaneously would have been an expensive, logistical, operational and staffing nightmare.

Fortunately, in September 1982, the original Kaiser Hospital site, built on prime land in Waikiki, was sold for $29 million. The original cost of the land had been $800,000. This was enough to finance the hospital construction in one phase—to the relief of all.

With local control, construction proceeded on time and under budget. This was in sharp contradistinction to the first major renovation and expansion of the hospital, which was not required for another twenty years and was managed from the Facilities Department at Program Office in Oakland. On September 30, 1985, the award-winning new Kaiser Moanalua Medical Center was dedicated. The day before, on September 29, a smooth transfer of all the patients at the original Kaiser Hospital to the new hospital was completed without incident. This major logistic effort was coordinated by Dr. Bob Poole, an ambulatory surgeon who had experience with medical mass transfers as a colonel in the Medical Corps prior to joining HPMG. He was assisted by Irene Lee, an experienced, loyal, and respected operations manager.

The hospital wasn't the only facilities-modernization project. With the hospital and clinics moving out of Waikiki, the downtown center city population would be left unserved. This problem was solved by the simultaneously constructed Honolulu Clinic. The Honolulu Clinic was a modern, attractive fifty-physician office surrounded by three main thoroughfares: Pensacola, King, and Beretania Streets. In addition to good automobile access, this densely populated location was served by multiple bus routes. It was approximately a mile and a half and halfway between the tourist and business centers of Waikiki and downtown. It opened in the summer of 1986.

Dictated by the island geography, road networks, traffic, and a strong sense of neighborhood, the Hawaii region has a much higher clinic density than any other KP region. The Maili clinic was opened in 1960, then the Koolau (Windward – Kaneohe, Kailua, and Waimanalo) Clinic in 1966, and the Lahaina and Wailuku Clinic on Maui in 1968 and 1969. By the early 1980s, these clinics were badly in need of expansion, replacement, or renovation.

In 1976, Lahaina Clinic, the first of the neighbor island clinics, was replaced by a new facility as was the expanded and modernized Wailuku Clinic. Modern Oahu expansion clinics were built in Mililani in central Oahu in 1983 and Hawaii Kai at the eastern extreme of Oahu in 1984. By 1987, KP Hawaii had the most modern medical facilities in the state—but also the highest level of debt in its history. Ironically, before the end of the decade, this successful building program was to contribute to the third and worst HPMG salary crisis in its history.

Medical Economics—New Rules of the Game

"There is nothing permanent except change" (Heraclitus). People, and the businesses they operate, don't like to change. When they don't change, change eventually overwhelms them. This explains the brisk turnover in the *Forbes* top 100 companies. The frequently painful, but ultimately successful, adaptation to the consequences of external market changes characterized the remainder of Dr. Dung's administration.

Prior to 1980, the economics of US medicine were relatively simple. Nationally, it was dominated by fee-for-service medical care with Blue Cross and Blue Shield as the pass-through mechanism. Only a small percentage of the care was delivered through prepayment mechanisms, mostly Kaiser Permanente. Though it was a close-run thing, during the previous three decades, prepaid health care proved that it could survive in the face of great political and economic threats—albeit as a niche player. Both types of health care-delivery were predominantly nonprofit.

In 1965, Medicare and Medicaid became the law of the land, which enabled a backlog of unmet health care needs to be met, but also allowed unrestricted growth of health care services, most of which were fee-for-service. It was a bonanza for health care providers, hospitals, medical equipment vendors, and pharmaceutical companies. As stated earlier, the need for health care can be infinite, but the resources will always be finite—even in a country as rich as the United States.

By the early seventies, health care costs were already accelerating much faster than the growth of the economy. Health care which consumed 4.7 percent of the nation's productivity in 1950 was up to 7.7 percent in 1965, 11 percent by 1991, and 17.5 percent in 2016. From 1947 to 2016, the US economy as a whole had a yearly growth rate of approximately 3.2 percent. This medical cost trend was clearly unsustainable. It was quickly recognized that the unchecked rapidly rising cost of health care would eventually crowd out other societal needs. Understandably, politicians did not want to get into the business of rationing health care. At the same time, the voting public was skeptical that the same government that gave them the Post Office and Amtrak could manage the complexities of health care-delivery. The bipartisan solution was the 1973 Health Maintenance Organization (HMO) act. It seemed to address the problem.

Fee-for-service care ensures accelerating medical costs. Because the amount of care delivered determines reimbursement, there is an unchecked, powerful incentive to deliver ever more and more care—whether it is cost effective or not. Thus, medical care captures more and more of the economic output of the country. On the other hand, HMOs, as then defined, were prepaid models. Prepaid meant a free market based, fixed budget for services. The hope was that a fixed budget would incentivize HMO professionals and administrators to work together to make informed resource (budget) allocations based upon clinical necessity and effectiveness.

In 1998, the KP pharmacy budget was fixed as always and then sildenafil (Viagra) became available. Unrestricted coverage of Viagra would have cost about the same as the entire antibiotic budget. Since there wasn't funding for both, a decision had to be made: Should resources (coverage) directed to infectious disease by covering antibiotics or erectile dysfunction (impotence) by covering sildenafil (Viagra)? KP chose antibiotics. While Viagra was available, it was not a routinely covered benefit. Thus, these health care "experts" were doing the "rationing" instead of the government. As expected, KP and not the political process had to absorb the criticism.

The federal HMO Act cleared out a thicket of state and local laws, often AMA-sponsored ones, which had inhibited the establishment of prepaid HMOs. The act also provided startup funds and a readymade customer base. Any employer with more than twenty-five employees was required to offer at least one prepaid HMO on a dual-choice basis (until 1995) to their workers.

Two problems were unaddressed by the law. The intention of the law was to make the HMOs responsible for the health of their patients (customers). The title was, after all, the "Health Maintenance Organization Act." However, this mandated health maintenance was poorly defined. Kaiser Permanente, as founded, saw nonprofit health maintenance as its reason to exist and prepayment was simply a means to provide stable funding to obtain the resources to accomplish this mission. Unfortunately, most HMOs saw the act as a way to corral large numbers of patients, which they now controlled, and then leverage this control against providers of health care. This would allow them to bargain down the cost of hospitals, doctors, pharmaceutical companies, and other health care providers by denying higher-cost providers access to these patients. Market share, driving down provider costs and services, and increasing profits, if for-profit, became HMO priorities. It wasn't until the 2000s that federal government "pay-for-quality" policies ("P for Q") suddenly increased their interest in promoting prevention and quality.

More important, the HMOs were not required to be nonprofit. The business case of for-profit health care plans was that there was so much inefficiency in health care that good management could lower the cost of medical care, and the cost savings would fund profits that investors would find attractive. This, in turn, could attract more investor capital, which would provide more resources for more innovative high-quality, good service, cost-effective care. The companies that did not provide a good value product would fail, leaving more resources on the table to fund the more efficient companies, which would grow. Stock prices are based upon growth potential. That is how true capitalism works. For capitalism to do its magic, however, there must be true competition: a level playing field, no corporate welfare, no monopolistic sharp practices, and especially no medically indefensible denial of care. The beneficiaries of the competition must be carefully defined. Are the beneficiaries the stockholders who invest their money expecting a profitable return, the managers they pay to get that return (for-profit model), the providers who deliver the care, the employers who are footing most of the insurance bill—or the patients being served? The original thesis of Henry Kaiser and Sidney Garfield for the Kaiser Health Plan was that patients should be the primary beneficiaries of health care. The interests of the other beneficiaries should be at best secondary. This policy was established early on by Edgar Kaiser at the Grand Coulee Dam site where he decreed that medical care for labor would not be a profit center.

Medical care reform is a question that society is grappling with to this day. If the political process does not finally define who should be the primary beneficiaries of health care, enact rules that set a level playing field, establish a free market solution based upon honest competition with the objective of the best quality and lowest cost for patients will not be forthcoming. It would then fall to a government monopoly to control medical reimbursement. Bureaucratic monopoly has its own problems that are at least as great. Would a government single-payer health care look like the Medicare model, based upon free market principles, or the Veterans Health Administration (VA) and the Indian Health Service models, which were designed as single-payer government bureaucracies? Because the original HMO Act did not address these questions, they must be addressed now.

There were indeed huge inefficiencies in health care to be exploited. Growth of prepaid care was slow at first. Then it accelerated as more and more for-profit companies saw that they could enter the health care markets and make huge profits. For-profit health plans quickly dominated US health care. The initial effect was to slow the growth of health care costs.

The worst of the inefficiencies were wrung out of health care by the early 1990s. The low-hanging fruit—the breakup of provider monopolies and the failure of inefficient hospitals and medical care businesses—had been plucked. As competition tightened, corporate management was open to sharp, but legal, business practices. These practices went well beyond the efficient provision of appropriate care and strayed into the denial of appropriate care. Prior authorization policies originally designed to ensure appropriate use of medical resources were now weaponized to deny care for clearly indicated surgery, cancer treatment, and other expensive diagnostic tests and therapies. Cynically the cheapest care is the care that doesn't happen and the patient dies.

Doctors were required to waste inordinate amounts of time overcoming intentional and unnecessary bureaucratic obstacles to the delivery of clearly appropriate care. Doctors called it the "hassle factor." When doctors pushed back, health plans wrote "gag" orders into their contracts, which meant that the doctors could not advise patients about denied but needed treatment or even criticize the Health Plan without losing their contract. Another abuse was cherry-picking. Community rating, where everyone in a geographic region has the same rate structure for care, wasn't built into the HMO Act.

For-profit health plans figured out that they could make even greater profits if they didn't have to provide the care at all by cherry-picking healthy patients. Marketing was designed to discourage sick patients from joining their plans by enacting high co-pays and selectively marketing their plans to young, healthy customers. This, of course, increased the cost of health insurance for those who really needed it—if they could get insurance at all.

Uncovered medical care became the most common cause of personal bankruptcy. By the early nineties, these abuses had given HMOs a very bad name. For many HMOs, there was little about health maintenance and a lot about profits. This became a major public relations problem for Kaiser Permanente as patients had difficulty distinguishing KP, the original HMO pioneer, from the abuses of other, often for-profit, HMOs. KP was being tarred with the same brush. The HMO Act did slow the growth of health care costs—but not enough. Like all attempts at reform, it had its unintended consequences: market chaos, many failed care-delivery experiments, unaddressed abuses, and a growing uninsured population who couldn't get affordable insurance or any insurance because of preexisting conditions. Many of the worst abuses were corrected by spotty attempts at legislation, but they did continue. By the 2000s, there was a widely perceived need for comprehensive health care reform.

Hawaii Medical Economics

For decades, there were really just two health care players in Hawaii: HMSA and Kaiser Permanente. They competed toe to toe with each other, keeping costs down and service up. With the new federal HMO Act, there was now wide latitude about who could call themselves an HMO in Hawaii. With the local legal and legislative barriers to entry lowered, a number of new players positioned themselves to market competing plans in Hawaii, but Hawaii was different.

In the eighties and nineties, many health plans tried their hand at the Hawaii market. They either failed outright or struggled on as minor players. Hawaii was a harder target than it appeared. It was a small, isolated market. The population of the state was about the same as Maine or New Hampshire, but the population was much more diverse. It was separated from the rest of the country by an ocean. No other state had two dominant, well-established, popular health plans with radically different but proven health care-delivery models. The competition between KP and HMSA had been direct since the late fifties. KP's low prices kept HMSA rates down, while HMSA's fee-for-service private physician care-delivery model forced Kaiser Permanente to provide good service. By the 1980s, medical care costs in Hawaii were among the lowest in the country—while the quality and service were among the highest. Hawaii is routinely rated as one of the healthiest states in the nation. As of 2018, the cost of medical care represented 13.8 percent of the economy of Hawaii versus 17.8 percent for the nation. HMSA and KP continue to cover more than 70 percent of the population of the state.

Starting in the early 1980s, a flock of new players tried to enter the Hawaii health care market, but they had little idea of how to price their plans. Most "shadow-priced" KP and HMSA with slightly lower rates without knowing what their operating costs would be. Some even tried "buying business" with unrealistically low rates to get a toehold in Hawaii.

In the face of the HMSA-KP-dominated, already efficient Hawaii market, their reimbursements did not offset their costs. Most eventually went out of business or left the state, but this typically took at least a few years. During that interval, HMSA and KP were challenged as both lost members to these underpriced, often temporary, competitors. The response by HMSA and KP was to lower rates to maintain membership. This forced sharp cuts in care-delivery budgets.

Setting rates correctly is always difficult. Overshoot, and membership—and the income it generates—drops. Undershoot, and there are not enough resources to deliver care to the members you already have. From 1986 to 1989, KP seriously undershot. The resulting patient care resource starvation affected, among other things, physician salaries, which were frozen by 1986.

The Third HPMG Salary Crisis

Lagging physician salaries had been the root cause of the 1960 and 1975 political crises that threatened the existence of HPMG. An even worse crisis was to come in 1988 and 1989. In the sixties and seventies, HPMG salaries were significantly lower than the competition; however, the effect was blunted by very high income tax rates.

The author recalls during a job interview in 1980 about how the fee-for-service urologists in that group limited their work hours to a taxable income of about $90,000 because anything more than that went disproportionally to taxes. It was not unusual for physicians to take Wednesdays and weekends off in lieu of "working for the government." The late 1970s strides made by HPMG to improve retirement and disability benefits, the standardization of overtime benefits, as well as vacation and education leave, coupled with quality of life practice improvements further blunted the effect of the lower salaries. Benefits for the most part were not taxed.

By the early 1980s, HPMG leaders were optimistic that the increasing success of the program both clinically and financially would fund salary increases to competitive levels. With competitive salaries, a robust benefit structure, and a cooperative, multispecialty, high-quality practice style, an HPMG career would be more desirable than one with the competition. HPMG would then have its pick of the best doctors. That dream was to be delayed for more than a decade by two external events: 1980s prosperity and incorrect federal staffing models.

The top marginal federal income tax rate stood at 70 percent in 1981. Between 1982 and 1988, the Reagan tax cuts lowered the top rate to 28 percent. This and falling interest rates ushered in period of unprecedented national prosperity. Whether the tax cuts caused this prosperity is a partisan debate, but what was undebatable was that taxpayers could keep more of what they earned, and they were earning more, especially physicians. Now taking Wednesdays and weekends off was much less attractive than the loss of substantial after-tax income.

During the 1980s, national physician salaries increased rapidly—while the HPMG salaries stagnated. In the early eighties, there were a few good HPMG divisible surplus years that blunted the increasing salary disparity, but by the mid-eighties, the divisible surpluses dried up because of the excessive rate cuts in the panic to maintain market share. The physician salary freeze in 1986 and again in 1987 accelerated the salary disparity. By 1988, HPMG salaries were clearly uncompetitive. To make matters worse, the widening salary discrepancy was not evenly distributed among the HPMG specialties, which reignited interdepartmental conflicts.

In 1980, Congress commissioned the GEMENAC (Graduate Medical Education National Advisory Committee) study to assess future physician needs by specialty. It concluded that the country was facing a severe doctor surplus in the specialties, especially surgical specialties—and that doctors should be encouraged to train in the primary care specialties. This was big news. The response by the specialty professional organizations was immediate. Specialty training programs were cut back drastically. For example, in the space of a few years, the American Board of Urology reduced residency positions from more than 720 per year to less than 250. The GEMENAC study was never repeated, and today, most regard it as having been a poor predictor of future trends, but it had its effect. The economic law of supply and demand dictates that making something scarcer increases its value. The unintended consequence pf GEMENAC was that during the eighties and nineties, specialty compensation went up much faster than primary care compensation.

In 1980, the highest HPMG specialty physician scale peaked at $90,000, while the lowest-paid physician specialty scale peaked at $60,000. Even then, the 50 percent premium for the highest-paid specialties, such as orthopedics and neurosurgery, was much less than that of the competition where the premiums for premium specialties were more typically 250 percent. At the end of the decade, it was more like 400 percent versus 200 percent within the HPMG salary scale.

By 1987, excellent clinicians were leaving HPMG for much better-paying positions elsewhere. It was increasingly difficult—and finally impossible—to replace these physicians because recruiting salaries were simply too low.

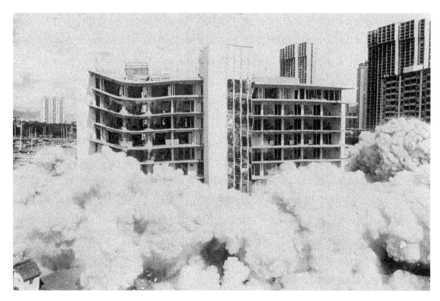

Demolition of the Kaiser Waikiki Hospital in October 1985.
It was featured in the last season episode of *Magnum P.I.*
New facilities increased membership but also debt, which
led to the second HPMG compensation crisis.

To add insult to injury, because the mid-eighties rate cuts overshot what was needed to be competitive, KP suddenly had the lowest rates in Hawaii. That coincided with the modernization costs of almost all facilities, which was complete by 1987. KP medical facilities were now the most modern in Hawaii. This combined with the low membership rates resulted in unprecedented membership growth in the face of accelerating physician losses. With fewer doctors and less clinical support to service the new members, service declined—while the clinical stress on the doctors increased. To maintain service, more cases were sent out for care to the fee-for-service competition. Externalized care typically costs three to five times more than the previously internalized care with far less quality control. This skyrocketed the outside services budget so that the increased membership dues that should have been used to restore internal clinical budgets were instead being diverted to pay for expensive outside services. KP Hawaii was in effect subsidizing the competition at the expense of its own clinical infrastructure.

By the late 1980s, KP Hawaii was facing a financial and operational death spiral in the face of this unsustainable membership growth. There was accelerating membership growth in the face of unreplaceable accelerating physician losses and worsening service. Expensive outside services were subsidizing the competition while diverting funds away from internal clinical budgetary needs, especially correction of the uncompetitive physician compensation package. Eventually, even these new members would leave the program because of service issues. A newly declining KP reputation, which had been recovering nicely from its early days, would again be damaging for a generation. Into this inauspicious environment, the Medical Group faced the first major change in leadership in twenty years with the coming election of a new president.

The Second Presidential Election

In 1980, Dr. Dung initiated the "HPMG Climate Survey." The same questions were asked every year so that trends could be followed. The three questions were simple and straightforward and measured on a 1 (happy) to 10 (unhappy) scale: "Are you happy with being a member of HPMG?" "Are you happy with the quality of care provided by HPMG?" "Are you happy with the compensation package of HPMG."

From 1980 to 1991, when the survey ran, "happiness" peaked in 1984 and then declined at an accelerating pace with 1988 as the nadir year—the year that the election process was to begin. In terms of dissatisfaction, low compensation always led the way by a large margin. Morale had still not recovered to early eighties levels by the end of Dr. Dung's administration in 1991.

Dr. Dung had done everything that he could do to prepare for an orderly transition. He ensured that the presidential election rules were modernized and ratified by the board of directors in 1977—eleven years before the actual election. The process was made demagogue and special interest resistant by having search committee members elected from the elected board of directors, chiefs, and associates. The search committee process was intended to be deliberate. A single candidate recommendation by the search committee was required, and that candidate had to be approved by a majority of the elected board of directors before being presented to the general staff for ratification by 50 percent plus one of the associates. Outside candidates would be considered only after agreement could not be reached on an internal candidate. The search committee had only two chances to get a candidate ratified. If it failed, it would be dissolved—and the process would have to start all over again.

Dr. Alex Roth had been the executive vice president, loyally and capably reporting to Bill Dung, since the 1975 leadership crisis. By the mid-1980s, Dr. Roth was approaching retirement age, and Dr. Dung decided to replace him with a succession of potential medical director candidates. Each appointee would be made vice president the first year during which they participated in the executive-level decisions made at the weekly HPMG executive committee meetings. The second year, they would become executive vice president, during which time they were assigned an administrative project and served in a true executive capacity at the HPMG executive committee and as acting medical director during Dr. Dung's absences.

The first vice president-executive vice president (1985–6) was Ulrich Stams, MD, the chief of urology and an elected board member. His assignment was to sort out the role of family practice vis-à-vis internal medicine and pediatrics. Next (1985–6) was Stephen Miller, MD, chief of ophthalmology and former chief of surgical services and elected board member. His assignment was HPMG financial policy. Next (1986–7) was the author, then chief of surgical services and hospital chief of staff. His assignment was to organize and implement the Medical Management Analysis Prospective Quality Assurance program. The final candidate before the election was Michael Chaffin, MD (1987–8), the physician in charge of the Windward Oahu Koolau Clinic and a former chief of medicine. His assignment was primary care-delivery.

During their two-year terms, each candidate was enrolled in the joint KP-Stanford University Kaiser Permanente Executive Training Program (KPEP). It was like a mini-MBA for future executive leaders of both Health Plan and Medical Groups. This six-week course, split into three two-week sessions, included instruction in management psychology, marketing, basic economics, medical and business ethics, as well as the Kaiser Permanente history and philosophy. Lectures were given by Stanford professors as well as past and present Kaiser Permanente executives, including the current president, Jim Vohs. There were presentations from personalities who had worked closely with Dr. Garfield and Henry Kaiser, such as Cecil Cutting, MD, a key founder of the program. On one Sunday, there was an optional trip to the wine country as well as to the Permanente Creek. This course was designed to whet the management appetite of physicians so inclined and to provide a basic KP-themed business education. Most found it a valuable learning experience and established program wide networking relationships that often lasted for decades.

Dr. Dung's intention was to expose potential medical director candidates to the responsibilities of HPMG president, test their interest and ability, provide basic management education, and provide exposure to HPMG membership as a whole. Clearly some were more interested than others, and all did useful work that could validate their candidacy. Most found KPEP inspirational.

Unfortunately, HPMG was headed into the worst salary crisis of its history, and operationally things were coming apart. For the actual candidates, while the vice president appointments provided valuable experience and were a good test of their management skills, it did not help their candidacy. As each one dealt with crisis after crisis, they were high-profile representatives of Dr. Dung's administration, especially from 1986 on. Not unexpectedly, they were identified with the deteriorating compensation program and subsequent operational problems even though these events were for the most part entirely outside of their control.

Presidential elections are perilous times for Permanente Medical Groups. Politics can bring out the worst in people. People say and do things that they would never say or do in other circumstances, especially during times of crisis. Loose talk, anger, misunderstandings, rumors, and treacherous behavior can break long-term friendships permanently and inspire feuds that can last for decades. Good doctors and potential future leaders may leave or even drop out.

During and after the elections, the serious business of the Medical Group must go on. The damage caused by a fiercely contested election can get in the way of the necessary healing process for years or even decades. Anyone aspiring to be a medical director or any high-level executive position must have thick skin. The saying goes that you can't take politics personally if you want to be an effective leader. In reality, sometimes the political nastiness is personal. A true leader must always be prepared to forgive, but it is much harder to forget. While Dr. Dung had done everything he could to plan for a smooth transition - that was not to be.

In the spring and summer of 1988, a representative of the chiefs, the elected board of directors, and three at-large representatives were elected to the search committee. Once it was selected, Bill Dung, understanding the danger of a divided HPMG based upon his own previous experience, appealed to the search committee to succeed in their mission and then to support the chosen candidate with the board and HPMG associates. That was also not to be.

The search committee meetings began in the summer of 1988. They were contentious from the start. There was an atmosphere of rising distrust and anger in HPMG because of the low salaries. Rifts had reopened between primary and specialty care, neighbor islands versus the medical centers, and chiefs versus non-chiefs. Negativism was at a very high level. As a result of the skepticism, candidates were submitted to a gauntlet of tests. Each candidate was required to present three years of income tax statements for examination by the search committee—some of whom actively opposed their candidacy. They were subject to a surprise urine drug test and—worst of all—an HIV blood test. At the time, AIDS (Acquired Immune Deficiency Syndrome) as it was then called, was an incurable, increasingly common, slowly fatal disease. It was still poorly understood thanks to insufficient scientific knowledge and media-fueled hysteria. There was no reliable treatment, and AIDS could take months to years to manifest itself after a positive HIV test. The public associated AIDS with homosexuality and intravenous drug use. It was only later understood that it could be transmitted by exposure to any bodily fluid, including tears, blood, and urine. Doctors are routinely exposed to bodily fluids in the course of their work. At the time, HIV test information was considered to be so sensitive that informed consent was required to even perform the test, and there were criminal penalties for revealing results without permission. A positive HIV test would end a candidate physician's career even if the bid for president failed.

The author and Steve Miller were activists who believed strongly that medicine was going to change at an accelerating pace and that the Medical Group leadership should proactively confront the coming changes by instituting and acting on quality of care and service measurements, fiscally responsible formulas for staffing and compensation, improving the quality of the doctors in the Medical Group, and a more activist stance in the partnership with the Health Plan. They were also closely associated with the Dung administration as vice presidents and then executive vice presidents between 1985–7. They were seen as strong supporters of an increasingly unpopular Bill Dung, which they were. During the worsening salary crisis, they had served in high-profile positions of executive leadership. As such, they were required to make difficult, often unpopular, decisions just to keep the Medical Group functioning. With the morale of HPMG at its lowest ebb, this hurt their candidacy.

The third candidate, Herb Young, MD, was a pediatrician, the longest-serving member of HPMG among the candidates, the physician in charge of the Punawai Clinic, and an elected member of the board of directors. He had not served as one of the rotating vice president-executive vice presidents, and he was quiet about change. This aided his largely passive campaign as he had not served as a vice president during the salary crisis and its attendant problems. That he was the only primary care physician in the running was attractive to many of the numerous primary care physicians.

The author ran the hardest. In the summer, he sent out three comprehensive position papers by direct mail to all HPMG physicians two weeks apart. This generated support, but it was clearly an activist agenda. By December, he was the frontrunner. On the Friday before Christmas 1988, the three candidates were presented with sixteen difficult questions to be answered in writing with a deadline of January 2 for submission to the committee. The author submitted a thirty-page response that was significantly more detailed than the other two responses. The committee was prepared to present him to the board of directors as their choice, but there was one holdout. The search committee had hoped for a unanimous choice. The only remaining option was to go outside of HPMG.

Lee Jacobs, MD, former HPMG chief of medicine and now associate medical director of the relatively new Georgia Region Permanente Medical Group was contacted and flown out for an interview by the search committee. He had all the advantages of an outsider and was favorably remembered by the Medical Group. He had been recruited to the Georgia region in 1985 by its aggressive medical director with the idea that he would soon succeed him. It was four years later, and this had not happened. He was still associate medical director in Georgia. In 1985, when he left, HPMG morale was at its height, and the salary crisis had not yet emerged as an issue. He had been popular and effective during his three years as chief of medicine. He underwent an afternoon interview with the search committee after which they chose him as a compromise candidate that they could all support. The search committee added that if for some reason Jacobs did not make it through the process, the author would be the internal choice. The local candidates, having gone through a demanding one-year process, were chagrined but supportive of his candidacy. Miller and the author were his friends and had worked closely with Lee during his time in Hawaii. Unfortunately, the election process was by no means over.

Lee expressed interest in the position and then met with representatives of the search committee to work out the financial details. On the morning of Thursday, March 16, 1989, the day he was to be ratified by the elected board of directors, he sent a fax from Georgia declining the nomination, citing lack of progress in the financial negotiations as well as family ties in Georgia and mission work obligations as the reasons. In an interview almost three decades later, he noted that the real reason was that the process had moved suspiciously fast and that he wasn't comfortable with his understanding about what was then going on in Hawaii. The author was now the default candidate.

At the April 6 board meeting, the author answered questions prior to a scheduled vote on approval of his candidacy to be presented to the associateship for ratification. It was expected to be approved. An opposition-elected board member left the meeting to prevent a vote from being taken that night. It was decided to make the vote a secret paper ballot to be opened on Monday morning, April 10, in Dr. Dung's office. This bought time for the opposition.

Dr. Dung knew something was up. He came to the author's office the next day—Friday—with a paper ballot. As chairman of the board, Bill had one vote. He ominously marked his yes vote in front of the author, sealed it, and signed over the seal. There was intensive lobbying by the opposition over the weekend, and it bore fruit.

On Monday, during the lunch hour, Dr. Dung came to the author's office. With tears in his eyes, he presented the bad news personally. The vote not to approve presentation to the associateship had been decisive: five against, three for, and one abstention. The search committee, having failed to produce a candidate after two attempts, was dissolved as per the bylaws. The process, which had taken over a year so far, had to start all over again. The sense of a succession crisis was building in the Medical Group, which put pressure on the elected board and next search committee to find a successor—soon.

The second time around, the search process went much smoother. By the beginning of September, a new search committee was elected. Nominations were opened. Letters were sent to the three previous candidates inviting them to run. The author politely declined. He had run hard in the first round at the personal request of Dr. Dung, and he felt that he had discharged his duty. He was relieved to able to get back to clinical medicine and his duties as chief of surgical services. Miller similarly declined, which left Dr. Young as the sole candidate.

Dr. Pregitzer, a strong supporter of the author, entered the contest. Like the author, he had been an outspoken, activist, supporter of Dr. Dung's policies and had served effectively as chief of the Emergency Department since 1978. He had the support of the Dung supporters, but like the author, he was unacceptable to Dr. Dung's opposition. The second round was shaping up to be a replay of the first.

Michael Chaffin, MD, had joined HPMG in 1978. He was successfully recruited to be the chief of the Intensive Care Unit at the University of California at Davis near Sacramento in May 1981, which speaks eloquently to his clinical skills. Sacramento had been his hometown. Before the year had ended, he returned to HPMG because of unresolved political conflicts at Davis, which he wanted no part of. Soon after his return, he was appointed physician in charge of the Windward Clinic. He lived in Kaneohe on the windward side of Oahu, only a few miles from the clinic. The clinic management problems were few, and his practice was a happy one. He later said that it was the happiest time of his career. Therefore, when the author, in 1986, asked him to consider running for medical director in 1988 when Dr. Dung finished his last term, it was no surprise when he declined. He was nevertheless a quiet but strong supporter of Dr. Dung's policies and had partnered with the author during the establishment of the new quality assurance program as quality assurance director.

During his time as vice president and executive vice president (1987–8), the worst of the conflicts had passed, and he had the opportunity to apply his thoughtful, kind, and moderating approach to the problems that remained. Dr. Dung's supporters considered him as one of their own. Being in a peripheral clinic, he had avoided the worst of the conflicts, and as such, he was acceptable to Dr. Dung's opponents. He was reluctant to give up his nearly ideal practice situation for what would be the unceasing conflict associated with being medical director. Like Dr. Dung before him, he was finally convinced to run as the solution to an emerging and serious leadership crisis.

There were two search committee meetings where the candidates presented. Pregitzer had provided more detail in the first meeting, and thus was quite competitive, but after the second round, Chaffin emerged as the unanimous choice of the committee. Relieved, on November 2, the board of directors unanimously approved his presentation to the associates for ratification as the third president of HPMG. He made the required five clinic presentations and was handily ratified by the associates with a vote of 135–7 (95 percent).

The author had been seen as a change agent-activist, a polarizing figure with strong supporters and opponents. Ironically, the supporters and opponents were for and against him for these same reasons. While a policy of proactively addressing the coming change was a good plan, in retrospect, HPMG in 1989 did not need more conflict. Mike Chaffin, on the other hand, was exactly what HPMG needed: a thoughtful, deliberate, peacemaker. The change agent-activists, very happy with Mike Chaffin, remained with the program and were soon to continue the pursuit of their agendas with the encouragement and support of Mike, but the Medical Group needed to reunite and settle down first.

The Interregnum

Bill Dung was to serve as medical director for another two years. In keeping with the succession process he had established in his presidential newsletter of September 1987, Mike Chaffin would serve as the executive vice president and chief operating officer (COO) with increasing responsibilities during that time. As COO, chiefs would report directly to him after January 1, 1990. Dung presided over board meetings during the first year, and Chaffin presided during the second.

Within weeks of the election, some members of the elected board of directors approached Chaffin about prematurely ending Dung's presidency and putting his salary back into the general fund. Bill Dung was clearly hurt by this action. In his January 1991 president's newsletter, he wrote an uncharacteristic, detailed defense of his remaining presidential term and how he had served HPMG in 1990. Initially, Chaffin had politely put off the involved board members, but the issue wouldn't die.

When word got out about the attempt on Bill's employment, influential supporters of Dung let the involved board members know that any attempt to remove Bill would be vigorously opposed. Chaffin finally had to put the issue to rest by telling the involved elected board members that if they succeeded in removing Bill, he would resign from the presidency. This decisive action not only preserved the peace it greatly strengthened the "leadership amnesty" tradition of HPMG.

Both Mike Chaffin and the subsequent regional Hawaii Health Plan president, Cora Tellez, later acknowledged that the premature removal of Dr. Dung by the elected board would have been a grave mistake as he provided valuable mentoring to them, especially during the 1990 and 1991 medical service agreement (MSA) negotiations. He served as a moderating interface with the difficult new regional Health Plan president Dan Wagster. This yearly negotiation between Health Plan and the Medical Group was where conflicts between the cultures of medicine and business were most likely to collide. Trust, patience, understanding, and dedication to the partnership and program ideals were required on both sides to make them successful. When successful, the program is unbeatable.

In mid-1988, Ron Wyatt, the regional Health Plan president since 1977, retired. He had worked closely and cooperatively with Dr. Dung during that period. His smooth, non-confrontational style had earned him respect among HPMG leaders. He was replaced by Dan Wagster. Dan was a thirty-eight-year veteran of the Kaiser organization: ten years in Kaiser Industries and then twenty-eight years in Kaiser Permanente. He was very experienced and had served as the regional president of Southern California. Jim Vohs had appointed him to succeed Ron Wyatt as a pre-retirement position.

Wagster had a much rougher style than Wyatt. He got his start with Kaiser Industries as a manager dealing with militant unions. He appeared to view Permanente Medical Groups as doctor unions, and he dealt with them as such. In many ways, a Permanente Medical Group is union-like to the extent that it represents the collective interests of the physicians, but in KP, it has a much broader function. Its chief role is to balance the medical interests of the patients and the program with the business and financial realities of the program. This partnership is the fundamental strategic advantage of Kaiser Permanente—physicians working actively with Health Plan to achieve the health care ideals of Kaiser Permanente—not with physicians as hourly employees or as oppositional militant union members. To varying degrees, HPMG physicians understand that the failure of the partnership means the failure of the program, which, in turn, would likely result in the failure of HPMG. This is also true for Kaiser Foundation Health Plan. Each side must transcend its parochial interests to do what is best for the program during the medical services agreement negotiations.

Dung was up to the Wagster challenge. Bill had twenty years of experience navigating the small Hawaii region through the rough seas of KP National politics. He had earned great respect at the national level and was now the most senior medical director in the program. At social events associated with the annual Kaiser Permanente national off-site meetings, he and Daisy had developed a twenty-year friendship with the Wagsters.

Dung and Wagster successfully negotiated the 1988 and 1989 medical services agreements during a time of crisis when the morale of HPMG was at its lowest ebb and skepticism of the program by HPMG doctors was at a peak. By 1990, Wagster was familiar with Hawaii issues, and Dung was able to mentor Mike Chaffin directly through the 1990 MSA negotiations and indirectly through the 1991 negotiations.

The bare-knuckle negotiating style of the California KP–PMGs was very different from the indirect, face-saving negotiating style of Hawaii. Wagster's rough, somewhat confrontational style did not sit well with the HPMG leaders who were accustomed to the more cooperative, courtly style of Ron Wyatt. Because of this, he never won over HPMG hearts and minds. It was a good thing for the partnership that Bill Dung was his negotiating partner during this critical time. Jim Vohs understood what was happening in Hawaii, and he had a solution.

It was Cora Tellez. Cora is a remarkable individual. She was born in the Philippines and had immigrated to the United States during childhood with her parents. She graduated from the prestigious Mills College in Oakland, California, on full scholarship and dedicated her life to public service. She was a young rising star in the Oakland city government, when after making a presentation attended by Jim Vohs, he personally recruited her to Kaiser Permanente. He mentored her individually as his administrative assistant.

Correctly recognizing her tremendous executive and leadership potential, by the fall of 1989, having decided that she was ready for her first executive position he appointed her to be the associate regional president of Hawaii to succeed Dan Wagster. Vohs saw this as the first of many KP executive positions of increasing scope and responsibilities. She and Mike Chaffin had a complementary style of leadership, the value of which they both acknowledged. She was aggressive and action oriented. Mike, on the other hand, was thoughtful and cautious. They learned from each other. This balance was ideal for a time of rapid, unpredictable change in the external medical environment. Cora was singularly energetic. When she moved to Hawaii, her husband and children who were well established in Oakland, California remained there. To make this work, she would fly home to the Bay Area every Friday afternoon and spend the weekend fully dedicated to family. She would then fly back to Hawaii early Monday morning where she then fully dedicated her energies to the region working a typical twelve-to-fourteen-hour day. A one-way flight from Hawaii to California is four to five hours during which she did her business reading. She continued this schedule for nearly five years.

During the remainder of 1989 and in 1990, she concentrated on familiarizing herself with the region. She tirelessly met individually on a regular basis with leaders from Health Plan and Medical Group throughout her stay in Hawaii and even after. This went far to neutralize what had been the worsening antagonism between Health Plan and Medical Group. When she became regional president of Kaiser Health Plan in May 1991, the program was well on its way toward healing the partnership breach.

In 1991, Mike and Cora negotiated the medical services agreement successfully. Wagster had moved back to the Bay Area to another position in the KP Central Office. Mike reported to Bill how the negotiations were going. He got advice from Bill, but otherwise, he was in charge. During his last year, Bill reassured the older HPMG doctors who were suspicious of all the change of his total support for Mike.

On September 1, 1991 Bill issued the 125th and last edition of his president's newsletter. This newsletter had started immediately after he became president in 1970 and had been published without fail six times per year for twenty-one years. Encompassing more than 1,500 pages, it remains an invaluable historical source in the HPMG archives detailing events as they occurred as seen through the eyes of President Dung.

On December 10, 1991, there was a celebratory retirement dinner attended by all the regional leaders to honor him. He had already been honored at the national Kai-Perm meeting by the entire program leadership. Especially treasured by Bill was a handwritten letter sent to him by the long-retired Cliff Keene, MD, the first KP CEO, which resides in the HPMG archives:

> Bill, as you know I have had a more than ordinary interest in your career. Since those hectic early days and my personal involvement in selecting you as leader of the Hawaii medical group I have watched with paternal interest your thirty years [actually thirty-one years] of superb leadership and enormous contribution to the entire program. You have done well indeed. With affection, Cliff

On January 1, 1992 Bill Dung retired after twenty-one years as president and thirty-one years as a partner in HPMG.

William Man Hin Dung, MD, died on September 19, 2008, after a long illness at the age of seventy-nine. Together, he and Daisy Pang Dung raised four very accomplished children—Janice, Lili, Mary, and Joseph. The author maintained contact with Daisy Dung, and three months before she died, with the permission of her children, she presented him with a copy of Bill's private administrative diary. It covered the time from his selection as president of HPMG in December 1970 until 1978 after he had been reelected to his second term. In it, he presented his innermost feelings about the position as he went through the ups and downs of his turbulent first term. Especially touching is the expression of the love that he had for his family. It sustained him during the most challenging periods. It is one of the most historically important documents in the HPMG archives.

During his twenty-one years as president (1970–1991), the program more than doubled in size from 87,000 to 183,000 members. A beachhead on the Big Island of Hawaii was established in Kona. As of 2016, 25 percent of the Big Island population was served by Kaiser Permanente. A stable, balanced, and accountable governance structure, which has survived largely unchanged to this day, was established. A quality assurance program, which became a model for the national program was established and also remains largely unchanged. The members were now served by among the most modern medical facilities in Hawaii. Finances were stabilized, and the foundation was laid for a sustainable staffing and compensation model that was successfully implemented during the next administration of Mike Chaffin. He was a patient mentor and strong supporter of the next generation of HPMG leaders.

Bill Dung's leadership style was built on honesty, principles, humility, and hard work. It is summed up in his stated leadership goal: "The best leader leads a group forward in such a manner that they thought that they did it by themselves." Without his foundational policies, HPMG would not be where it is today.

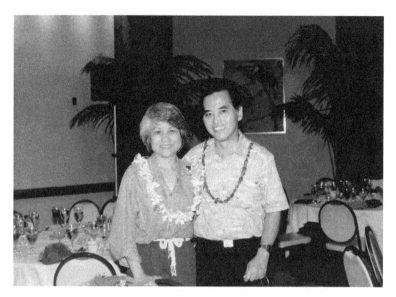

Bill and Daisy Dung.

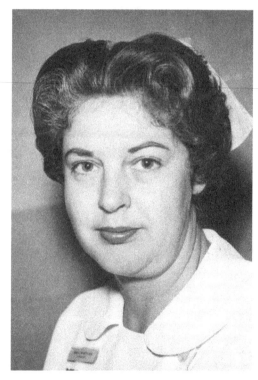

Hospital quality assurance partner Lorraine McVety in her youth.

CHAPTER 8

QUALITY ASSURANCE— FIXING THE JET WHILE IT'S FLYING

I t is with some amusement that physicians responsible for quality assurance (QA) programs hear about medical quality assurance being compared to quality assurance in aviation. Unquestionably, the policies of the Federal Aviation Administration (FAA) have made commercial flight the safest mode of transportation in the United States with a process of continuous quality improvement. However, with some amusement the response by medical QA leaders is:

> Yes, but our jets (patients) are flying while we work on them. They all have expiration dates, and many are at the end of or past their service lives. We have at best about 20 percent of the operating manual (evidence-based medicine), which is millions of pages long and constantly changing at an accelerating pace. Finally, nothing about our jets (patient organ and metabolic functions) or the aviation support services (medical resources) is standardized. At the same time, missiles are being fired at us (by tort lawyers).

Unquestionably all this is true, and the task may appear impossible, but nihilism cannot be the response. Physicians have an ethical imperative to continually improve the quality and effectiveness of care—no matter how impossible the task may seem. Physicians should not shy away from what the FAA and other quality control organizations can teach them, but the limitations must be realistically recognized. Nevertheless, physicians should embrace all the help they can get because quitting is simply not an option.

Quality Assurance Skepticism

To become a physician in the United States, a person must commit themselves to one of the most competitive and arduous of all career paths. While exact numbers are hard to come by, at best, only about 10 percent of students identifying themselves as premeds in their freshman year of college actually make it into medical school. The premed major has a deserved reputation as one of the most difficult and competitive college majors. By senior year, when medical school applications must be submitted, most who started in premed don't bother to apply for or take the Medical College Aptitude Test (MCAT). Understanding their poor competitive positions, they realistically have chosen other career paths. The average successful medical student has an approximate GPA of 3.7 and a MCAT score in the 90th percentile of those who take the test. Of those applicants who go as far as the application process and take the MCAT, only about 30 percent can expect success.

Medical school room and board costs are approximately $40,000–70,000 per year (2017) for four years. Physical, mental, and psychological stress levels are even higher than they were in college. While most entering medical students finish medical school, they face competition throughout medical school for desirable residency positions. Internship and residency last an additional three to seven years. Residents have real life-and-death responsibility, a "see one, do one, teach one" level of learning stress, and long hours. They are, for the first time, paid during this training period—but only at two to three times the minimum wage. Finally, in their late twenties or early to mid-thirties, they become practicing physicians. After finding a practice setting, licensing, paying off education debt, and the years of work that are required to build up a practice, it is very difficult to change positions or to realistically change careers. There is a lot at stake if a poorly designed or unfair QA program sets a physician up for job or even career loss—hence the skepticism.

Unfair quality assurance programs can and have been used to unfairly end careers. The saying is: "A doctor's reputation is only as good as the last three cases." The causes of potential quality assurance abuse are many, but the incentive to stifle economic competition and professional jealousy rank high among them. In a fair quality assurance program, doctors can only be held responsible for what they control. The "captain of the ship" concept of responsibility holds only if the doctor has a captain's authority—and the ship (the medical support system) is sound.

A compromised medical support system characterized by excessive workloads, inadequate assistance with non-doctor tasks, inadequate specialty, laboratory, diagnostic imaging, and hospital and operating room support all mitigate against a doctor being able to properly control the medical management of a patient. For example, it is obviously not fair to expect a doctor's outcomes on a medical mission in Haiti to be as good as that same doctor's outcomes in the big-city home hospital—although the outcomes may be far better than they would otherwise be in Haiti. For physicians to accept a quality assurance program as fair, there needs to be a way to factor in the impact of all these medical support system variables.

In the KP Hawaii region, the solution accepted by physicians was to ensure that all final decisions be consensus driven and made by peers facing the same obstacles to optimal care. That doesn't mean that non-peers shouldn't assist with collecting outcome data. They must because of the volume of quality assurance raw data, but only peers can judge another peer's performance because they all must cope with the same medical support system. Without this fairness safeguard, physicians will not trust a quality assurance program.

ALBERT J. MARIANI, M.D.

The History of Quality Assurance within HPMG

Quality assurance efforts at Kaiser Permanente Hawaii go back to the founding of the program. With medical interventions first in the hundreds of thousands per year, and later with membership growth, in the millions, it is a daunting task. Efforts to improve quality were at first by individual efforts following up hearsay or observation. This worked well when the organization was small, localized to Oahu, and everyone knew everyone else, but as it got larger and geographically dispersed, an informal, anecdotal reporting system was not enough.

Early efforts were spearheaded by Dr. Clifford Straehley. He promoted quality assurance efforts as a priority for HPMG leadership. By the mid-1970s, disease or procedure-specific chart audits against pre-established quality indicators was state of the art for QA programs. For example, after hearing about a couple of common duct injuries that might have occurred during a cholecystectomy (gallbladder) surgery, the decision would be made to do a comprehensive study of all cholecystectomies during the past two years. Results might then be compared to expected national complication rates, including common duct injuries.

The problem, however, was one of scale. There were thousands of potential chart audits. The sampling of millions of medical interventions was necessarily going to be small—too small and too slow to adapt to rapidly changing medical care-delivery. The medical care sampling was necessarily limited by the small number of audits that could be practically performed per year. It was a retrospective program. The problems had already happened.

Another problem was that audits could only be performed on common conditions; otherwise, there would not be enough cases to do statistically meaningful comparisons. Finally, quality assurance results were not well connected to the command structure of the region, which, in turn, controlled resource allocations. Completing this loop would be required to correct systems problems. Thus, the program could identify and correct through the HPMG chiefs individual disease or procedure-based problems, but it was less able to correct the more common systems problems. A comprehensive, prospective program was needed to prevent problems before they happened. It then needed to be tied into the regional command structure of Kaiser Permanente Hawaii. The current program largely accomplishes these goals.

Establishment of the Modern Program

In January 1985, the author was appointed to the newly reorganized position of chief of staff of the hospital. That year, the position was changed from a one-year term to a two-year term. It was expected that the hospital chief of staff would have far greater involvement in hospital policy and be the principal liaison between HPMG and the Kaiser Hospital.

In early 1985, while pondering a way to better coordinate HPMG and hospital activities, Lorraine McVety, RN, entered the office to start a conversation about quality assurance. Lorraine had a sweet, low-key, but persistent personality. She had been serving the program loyally in a variety of responsible roles from its inception. She was now approaching retirement and had been given the preretirement job of hospital quality assurance director—a Joint Commission on Accreditation of Hospitals (then JCAH) requirement. Not much was expected of her, and some just saw it as a reward for her loyal service to the organization. How wrong they were.

She presented a program of quality assurance entitled the Medical Management Analysis (MMA) program. The scientific basis of this program was based upon quality assurance research that had recently been completed at Dartmouth Medical School. The research demonstrated that rather than auditing specific diseases or procedures, which would detect only a small percentage of quality issues, by prospectively monitoring twenty-three generic outcomes, 80 percent of hospital quality issues could be identified. Such outcomes included unplanned hospital readmissions, surgical complications, transfers to higher levels of care such as the intensive care unit, admissions due to failed outpatient treatment, unaddressed abnormal tests, and death.

At the time, since there were approximately ten thousand hospital admissions per year, it was conceivable that a reasonably sized, well-organized quality assurance department could screen all hospitalizations. The Dartmouth research had been adapted to an applicable QA program called Medical Management Analysis, which was marketed by Joyce Craddick,

MD. This was the answer to the QA dilemma of focused prospective screening. Then came the task of adapting it to our program.

Between March 23 and April 17, 1985, three memos were sent a week apart to all HPMG physicians outlining in detail the proposed MMA QA program. Following that, during the summer, the author and Lorraine visited every clinic, department, and section to present the proposed QA program in detail and to answer questions and take suggestions. This went a long way to reassure the physicians of the fairness of the proposed program and its need.

The key to acceptance was the appointment of respected apolitical clinicians from every department, rather than department chiefs, to make quality judgments. The chiefs would then be expected to act on the collective findings. The idea was that these respected clinicians would be fair judges of quality and that these judgments would be at arm's length from the physician managers who had to make decisions about how to deal with any identified quality issues. These handpicked, well-respected clinicians were to make up the Hawaii region quality assurance committee.

Dr. Mike Chaffin, one of these physicians and soon-to-be medical director, was appointed chair of the committee and given a position on the hospital executive committee. QA now had direct hospital executive committee representation—the highest-level hospital governance committee. The hospital executive committee decided overall hospital policy. The QA committee was suddenly a popular and effective interest group, promoting quality assurance, and it was directly represented in the top decision-making body of the hospital. This would prove to be the key to obtaining the resources that would be required to implement and then perpetuate and grow quality assurance in the region—and grow it did.

Because of the respect and collective popularity of the non-chief, apolitical, respected clinician members of the QA committee, there was little resistance. The QA committee met monthly and provided an important, self-correcting, high level of quality control. Among its roles was the responsibility to standardize the quality screening criteria. Each department was expected to submit several department-specific criteria in addition to the standard screening criteria. For example, when one surgical section suggested a 2,500-cc blood loss as the threshold for screening—half the blood supply of an adult human—the committee diplomatically scaled that threshold back by half.

At the monthly QA meetings, there was a general review of all complications, and if one department was internally setting too low a standard of care, it could be challenged. Disputes between departments were also settled at this level—usually by more clearly defining workflow responsibilities.

While the QA governance was being established within HPMG and the hospital administration, Lorraine McVety organized a dedicated QA staff. Initially, they screened every hospital admission against the established criteria. As the department grew in size and effectiveness, eventually both ambulatory clinic care and the coordination of the "blue sheet" program were added. The blue sheet program was one in which anyone could submit a "quality of care concern" form. The blue sheet, which was indeed blue, would then be reviewed by the QA staffers for validity and then sent to the appropriate department representative for review.

An important part of the program was an understanding by the QA staff that this was a peer-review program. The QA staff were **not** peers of the doctors being judged, but the department physician representative was. The QA staff quickly learned how to recognize quality issues and just as quickly developed close working relationships with the quality assurance physician representatives based upon mutual trust.

As respected as they were, even the department physician representatives didn't make the final decision. Any cases of questionable care as well as learning cases were presented at the monthly department QA meeting. No case involving an individual physician could be presented without the physician in attendance and the medical record available.

After department discussion, the physician QA representative was required to grade the care on a six-point severity scale, ranging from bad handwriting – a low bar having been set (1) to death (6). The QA representative was also placed on the spot to decide whether the care was appropriate (+), equivocal (+/-) or inappropriate (-). This data was then recorded and trended by the QA program. All quality data was computerized so that it could be sorted and trended. Negative trends required action by the chiefs, ranging from counseling, to medical education, to reduction of privileges, and even to dismissal from the group. Since the chiefs responsible for making these decisions were acting upon externally generated data, they were well shielded from charges of discrimination.

Principles of Implementation

In the history of HPMG, successfully executed programs were always implemented in a very deliberate fashion. The QA program was a good example. If the time is not taken to do things right before actual implementation, it certainly will be required after—*if* the program survives the subsequent political process. While some of this discussion may be repetitious, it is worth repeating.

Communication

The planners of QA thought through the proposed program very carefully before introducing it. The author, who was the lead physician as president of the hospital executive committee, wrote the three memos distributed to every member of HPMG at two-week intervals introducing the program, the scientific underpinnings, and then explaining the process. Writing these memos clarified the implementation thought process.

Personal Presentation

The written memos piqued physician curiosity as well as skeptical questioning of the proposed quality assurance initiative. The author and Lorraine McVety arranged free lunch meetings with every department and clinic, including those on the neighbor islands. The free lunch almost guaranteed good attendance. The purpose of these meetings was to present the program in person, and more important, to answer questions and address objections. No one has all the answers—even with very careful planning. The questions and most of the objections were legitimate and often highlighted potential program weaknesses. Adjustments made to address those weaknesses strengthened the program.

Evaluation by Peers

From the beginning, the role of the screeners was sharply delineated—they were not empowered to make judgments regarding care. That would be the prerogative of only peer physicians. Screening staff are only to screen charts against screening standards defined and ratified by the quality assurance committee, which is made up of the QA department physician representatives. The original core screening standards were based upon the twenty-three adverse outcomes identified in the Dartmouth study and supplemented by several department specific standards. These standards were reviewed on a regular basis to keep them current.

Final department quality of care judgments are made by the department representative—the respected peer physician subject to the same workload, resource limitations, and specialty patient base as the colleagues to be judged. It is the most important job in the QA program. These individuals are handpicked and actively recruited from each department by the QA program leadership in cooperation with the chief. This should not be left to chance. The most junior member of the department or the last doctor to step back during the call for volunteers are not typically good choices. Even worse would be the selection of a volunteer department member with known weak clinical performance who might want the position for self-protection.

QA department representative is a difficult job that is not suited to a physician who craves popularity. The department QA physician is charged with interpreting the often-contentious consensus of a department quality discussion of a case and then making a clear-cut judgment against a rigid pre-established set of standards. Two judgments are required: one was the severity of the adverse outcome and the second was whether the care meets the standard of care for HPMG and the department. These are then entered into a program QA database. The best QA department representatives were physicians who were not politically active but cared deeply about the quality of care delivered by the department and HPMG.

Fairness

To ensure a level of fairness that any person of goodwill would accept, certain ground rules were explicitly established and have remained largely unchanged. The data is collected the same way for everyone, including chiefs and QA representatives. QA representatives cannot judge their own cases. The chiefs can participate in quality discussions, but they do not make the final quality judgments on individual cases. The chief's HPMG role is to judge cumulative quality department data and to enact action plans for deficient quality performance. This arm's length decision-making provides a level of protection for the individual physician against chief bias. It also protects the chief against accusations of bias. Thus, required action plan decisions by the chiefs are based upon cumulative department data that had been generated not by the chief but by the department as a whole.

For chiefs who might be overly concerned with personal popularity and therefore might not act on adverse quality trends, the QA committee and the HPMG board of directors set explicit numerical thresholds of unacceptable or equivocal quality of care episodes for a given time period—usually one year. Deficient care incidents beyond these thresholds require an action plan by the chief.

When a case is heard by the department, the medical record and any department members involved in the case must be present. Thus, tThe final judgment about case severity and whether it meets the standard of care is available to the individual and the department.

Checks and Balances

Given the frailty of human nature, the best defense against abuse of power is a system of checks and balances. They were built into the quality assurance program.

For the individual physician, the decision of the QA representative has two routes of appeal. The department ruling can be discussed again, or a decision can be appealed to the QA committee made up of all the department QA representatives. Few decisions were appealed, but the availability of an appeal process is reassuring and may prevent abuse.

For individual departments with weak QA leadership, the QA committee is charged with maintaining a program-wide standard of care by reviewing major complications at the monthly QA meetings. The collective wisdom of the handpicked department QA representatives can be expected to see through tricks to standardize quality across departments.

Resolving interdepartmental workflow disputes between departments has been an important function of the QA committee. For example, if the Emergency Department did not ascribe any adverse occurrences to themselves because they put the responsibility on another service, that would require a discussion at the monthly QA department meeting between the Emergency Department and the other involved department. The QA committee as a whole would then define the workflow responsibilities in the debate that followed. That QA committee decision, in turn, could be appealed by any disgruntled departments to the hospital executive committee—the final authority on hospital policy. That would be a rare event—but an available option.

Systems Problems

Early on, it became apparent that barriers to optimal care were often systems problems and not the fault of the individual physicians. For example, if a laboratory sample or tissue specimen was lost or if a report was not generated, the physician managing the patient could hardly be blamed for not addressing it except against an unreasonable standard of responsibility given the available time and resources available to manage individual patients. Peer judgments are important because only peers in the same medical environment who are subject to the same time and resource limitations can make fair judgments against individuals, but they do have the responsibility through the QA process to spotlight resource deficiencies that could compromise patient care.

Specimen-handling problems were actually identified as part of the QA program early on. They were corrected by making changes to the standard operating procedure for handling specimens and the reporting of results. This became a system-wide benefit for all practitioners, and it was the direct result of a well-functioning QA program. The QA program has been, and remains, a powerful physician ally when making the case for clinical resources. Systems problems have been the cause of many more quality issues than individual performance.

No-Blame Culture

The purpose of any QA program should be to identify problems early and correct them. It is not to assign blame or to politically disadvantage an individual or department. Systems problems are best corrected by establishing policies and standard operating procedures that address the problem.

Addressing the quality of individual physician performance is more complicated. If doctors are held to an unreasonably high—arguably even impossible—standard of perfection, if a QA program is designed to be punitive, passive resistance or even sabotage can be expected. In any system composed of human beings, mistakes will occur. It is inevitable. QA-based discipline should never be employed to set an example. The purpose of the QA program is to detect problems and then analyze them for the purpose of preventing them in the future. If this involves the individual physician, discussion of questionable outcomes provides a valuable clinical learning experience for everyone in the department. For sporadic problems, that is often enough for the doctor involved.

Bad trends may highlight a system problem or a performance deficiency by an individual physician. In the latter case, the chief needs to get involved. The chief may prescribe a problem-focused medical education effort, mentoring, close department supervision of that kind of case, or even loss of privileges. Loss of privileges is a hospital executive committee function. The latter could result in HPMG-determined (not hospital) compensation penalties if other department physicians have to pick up that physician's workload. It should be noted that compensation and even termination are not quality assurance functions; they are HPMG functions initiated by the department chief at the HPMG executive committee and board of directors level.

It is rare for a physician to be terminated for quality reasons because the QA program focuses upon re-education. Negative clinical outcome trends are identified early so that improvement efforts can begin promptly.

While often not seen as a benefit by physicians subject to performance improvement actions, these actions, if successful, have and will save careers. The usual reason for quality assurance-related termination is physical impairment (stroke, neuromuscular disease etc.)—in which case, the generous HPMG disability program provides support. An uncommon reason for termination for cause would be the willful refusal to accept the QA judgment of peers—a key value of HPMG.

Confidentiality

While a successful QA program must be based upon a no-blame culture to function, this is not the culture of tort law, at least not in the United States. Blame must be established for a malpractice tort to be successful. The more blame that can be assigned, the higher the award for the plaintiff and the attorney presenting the case who is usually paid on a contingency basis (a significant percentage of the award). There is near-universal agreement by physicians that US tort law is heavily biased against them. For a QA program to function, QA data must be kept strictly confidential. Otherwise, there will be a physician conspiracy of silence—the "white wall"—and physician nonparticipation. No physician participation means no effective peer review of cases. Peer review participation is essential for any QA program to be perceived as fair and therefore legitimate. Fortunately, at the time of this writing, there are robust legal protections for the confidentiality of peer review activities.

KP Hawaii's QA Contribution to the Program

By mid-1986, the program was working so well that Dr. Craddock (CEO of Medical Management Associates) and Jim Vohs (CEO of KP) came to Hawaii to see the program in person. In 1987, it was presented to the KP National board of directors. Subsequently, the Hawaii program had a major influence on the development of QA elsewhere in the program.

Soon, retrospective disease audits were out, and prospective screening was in. The principles of the Hawaii QA program have continued virtually unchanged to this day. It is but one example of the Hawaii region making program contributions well out of proportion to its size. It is likely due to the medium size of the Hawaii region that such a comprehensive QA program could be developed. It is small enough for most of the doctors to know each other and key Health Plan partners, yet it is large enough to internalize almost all of the medical services and have the resources to fund an innovation.

As important, HPMG has a flat chain of command with only four levels or fewer between the president of HPMG and the practicing physician. In addition, almost all physician administrators have at least a 70 percent full-time practice so they are on the front line of care-delivery.

In HPMG, one physician—or a small group of physicians—can potentially initiate important care innovations with a reasonable chance of success. The tremendous professional satisfaction attained by doing so is a rarely recognized HPMG career benefit.

CHAPTER 9

HOW MUCH IS A DOCTOR WORTH?

What is a well-trained, capable, efficient, honest, personable, and ethical doctor worth? The short, cold answer is the *cost of replacement*. Determining that cost is the hard part. In most free societies, occupational compensation is determined by the length of training, competitiveness, the difficulty of the work, hours worked, responsibility, and personal risk. In the last chapter, the required competitiveness, performance, and extensive training necessary to become a doctor were described. Physicians are expected to work long hours at very high levels of consistency, accuracy, and complex decision-making. Few careers have the same levels of responsibility—literally life and death. Finally, the personal risk of physicians from occupational exposure to blood and airborne contagious disease, anesthesia gases, radiation, suicide (two to three times), and lawsuits (two to three times) is much greater than that of the general population. Most societies recognize this. Indeed, doctors are compensated at a rate of two to six times the average of other occupations around the world. The US and other prosperous developed countries are at the higher end of the scale, and socialist or less developed countries tend to be at the lower end.

Arguments about the relative value of physicians to society between Kaiser Health Plan and HPMG—and within HPMG regarding the relative value of the different specialties—are potentially endless and pointless.

Indeed, that was the experience of HPMG during the first thirty years of its existence. In the end, no one really cares what KP or HPMG thinks about the value of physicians. The market determines that value, and bucking the validity of market value almost destroyed HPMG at least three times—in 1960, 1975, and 1988. It took thirty years of learning things the hard way to achieve a working formula.

The History of Compensation Policy

In the beginning, there were the five partners of the Pacific Medical Associates who were handpicked by Henry Kaiser on the basis of their social standing. They maintained their existing fee-for-service practice while providing token professional services to the new Kaiser program, which they regarded as more of a management contract than as a professional contract. Between their fee-for-service practice, the payments from Kaiser Health Plan, and the use of free facilities, staff, and supplies, the five partners were compensated at about two times the top 1 percentile of contemporary US incomes. To service the growing Kaiser Health Plan membership, they hired salaried doctors at about one-quarter of their own income. This created an unfair, two-tiered system of compensation that was resented by the hired physicians. When it came time to end the Pacific Medical Associates contract, Health Plan officials, working in partnership with other Permanente Medical Groups, were able to exploit this resentment to organize the new Hawaii Permanente Medical Group partnership from the PMA-hired doctors.

In the early years of HPMG, the program was struggling to survive. It did so by maintaining low membership dues. As a result, care resources were scarce, and doctor salaries were very low compared to the earning potential of comparable fee-for-service practice. Salaries were determined based upon ad hoc recruiting needs. There was little reliable external data regarding physician salaries; thus, they were based upon guesswork, and they were very low. As long as the program was small and on Oahu, this more or less worked, but there was high physician turnover, and the service and care reputation of the program was average or below.

By the end of the 1960s, the program was well established, in the black, and with both geographic expansion and membership growth. Because of the internal political instability during the first five years of Bill Dung's administration, after the unexpected death of Phil Chu in 1970, HPMG was distracted by internal conflict, and a poor Health Plan partnership impaired salary negotiations.

Outside of KP, specialty salaries were outpacing primary care salaries at an accelerating speed, and HPMG was falling behind. By the mid-1970s it became apparent that competitive specialty salary levels were well above HPMG specialty salaries. The result was that the primary care specialties were relatively well staffed with able physicians, while specialty departments had a steadily worsening ability to recruit. This led to unstable specialty departments and unfilled specialty staff vacancies. This, in turn, led to an increase in outside referrals to maintain service levels. Since specialty outside referral care was three to five times more costly than the cost of internalized care, program-wide financial problems resulted. KP had a growing reputation for not being able to handle complex specialty problems, and worse, the community specialty care competition was being subsidized by KP at the expense of the entire program, including the specialty departments that could have solved the problem if salaries had been competitive.

Without an external "gold" standard, salary scales were left to internal political processes, which had a leveling effect. Understandably, it was not obvious to a pediatrician that the market value of an orthopedic surgeon could be (and was) two to three times more than pediatrics. In a large multi-specialized medical group serving a general population, there are always more primary care physicians than specialists. HPMG is, after all, a democracy.

While specialty salary scales were slowly adjusted upward, they did not keep pace with market-based salaries. Within HPMG, specialty salary scales really didn't begin to differentiate until the mid-1970s. Progress was very slow. By 1981, the difference between the highest-paid specialty ($90,000 maximum) and the lowest-paid specialty ($60,000 maximum) was still only 50 percent. Outside, the highest-paid specialties were 250 percent or more than that of the lowest-paid specialties.

As the salary discrepancy worsened, even aggressive recruiting became an exercise in futility. Fortunately, the temptation to fill vacant positions with incompetent or impaired doctors was avoided. There were always plenty of them looking for a position and willing to work at a discount. Some departments made the decision to stop actively recruiting. They rationally, if somewhat cynically, decided to let departments shrink to crisis levels of staffing, which would make a better case for salary correction. In the meantime they would put their administrative energy into managing the increased load of outside referrals. That was of course terribly destructive to the program.

At one point, the cost of orthopedic outside referrals, despite strenuous efforts to internalize the most expensive cases, would have paid the corrected full market value salary of an orthopedic surgeon every three to four weeks. The HPMG board of directors continued to be unable to agree on competitive orthopedic salaries. At one point, the HPMG orthopedic surgeons offered a plan to shut down the Orthopedics Department, resign from HPMG, and organize an independent outside medical group that would provide all KP orthopedic services at a favorable, contracted, discounted rate compared to what was being paid for fee-for-service outside orthopedic care. This was narrowly avoided only because shortly thereafter HPMG leadership realized that the problem of orthopedic salary discrepancies needed a solution for purely financial reasons if nothing else.

In the late eighties and early nineties, with new leadership, better recognition of the problem, and a well-validated, external, market-based salary benchmark, the problem was aggressively addressed. While there were many external standards for physician salaries, most were poorly validated. For a time, HPMG utilized benchmarks from the magazine *Medical Economics*. While these benchmarks demonstrated clearly the inadequacy of HPMG specialty salaries, they were too imprecise to be used as the basis of a salary scale.

After studying dozens of purported salary scales, HPMG settled upon the Medical Group Management Associates (MGMA) scale, which was based upon the detailed compensation packages compiled by the business managers of large multispecialty urban practices similar to HPMG. These reports included overhead and benefit costs as well as salary levels. This well-validated scale correlated well with what potential candidates were telling chiefs about the competing salaries that they were being offered.

The MGMA scale was adopted as policy and then rapidly implemented in the early 1990s as soon as the expanding KP budget allowed.

By 1995, HPMG salaries reflected market value at the fiftieth percentile for all specialties. This enabled HPMG to quickly become very selective in its recruiting. Voluntary staff turnover became very low (~2 percent), and morale soared. The program was getting seventy-fifth to ninety-fifth percentile physicians at fiftieth percentile salaries because along with the competitive specialty-based salaries HPMG could also leverage the practice and lifestyle advantages of being in a large, prepaid group practice and a generous benefit package.

Health Plan could afford the increased compensation because the KP program was more efficient than the competition. Because of the advantages of prepaid versus fee-for-service practice, HPMG was able to employ one-third fewer doctors than the fee-for-service competition while delivering an equal or higher level of service and quality. HPMG leveraged the lifestyle advantage of a large group practice, including less call, better support, and better vacation and educational opportunities. This plus a fair salary, an excellent retirement program, and full medical and disability coverage made for a very appealing recruiting package. This attracted many outstanding doctors who, in turn, attracted other outstanding doctors. Program patient care and service provided by HPMG grew at an accelerating pace. By the end of the 1990s, more than 98 percent of patient care was provided internally. Documented physician and patient satisfaction was significantly better.

The Advantages of Market-Based Salaries

Market-based salaries addressed several major problems. Once the market-based fiftieth percentile salary standard was established, conflict among departments over compensation nearly disappeared. If every specialty was at the same relative market value (fiftieth percentile), the lofty burden of proof to break scale—have a salary greater than the fiftieth percentile— was on the department trying to make the case. Since every department could come up with dozens of reasons for why it should get an above the average salary, such arguments were met with gimlet-eyed skepticism from other departments. Most understood that if the scale was broken even once, it would soon be meaningless since every department would then try to break scale. Alternative measures were found to avoid this; the most popular of which was to recruit a physician at a higher step on the longevity scale.

The acrimonious board salary discussions of the previous thirty years, which could last for hours and generate long-lasting rancor, almost immediately disappeared. Once HPMG consensus was reached that an external market-based standard was fair, salary compensation discussions were quick and easy. The board would pass the scale for the coming year with little or no debate, standardized mathematics formulas would be applied, and the salaries were set. It was to the eternal credit of the lower-paid specialties, already at market value, to allow, on principle, their salaries to stay at market value so that the higher market value specialties could catch up. They understood that improved specialty services would benefit their patients.

Alignment of Recruiting Incentives

Once fiftieth percentile salaries were established, given the security of a generous benefit program and the lifestyle advantages of being in a large medical group, recruiting was rarely a problem. In the Surgery Department, by the early 2000s, there were typically dozens of applicants for every open position.

Before the fiftieth percentile salary standard was adopted, with no reliable salary standard, it was not known whether a department's difficulty recruiting was due to poor recruiting or noncompetitive salaries. Indeed, poor recruiting resulting in unfilled vacancies would reinforce the argument for increasing a department's salary scale. Conversely, an aggressive, successful recruiting effort by a chief could actually hurt a department's case for a more competitive departmental salary scale. Doctors, being smart, soon learned that the best argument to get a department salary increase was to have multiple vacant positions despite the increased clinical stress caused by understaffing. In the long run, this was very destructive to physician morale, patient care, and the global program budget as medical care needed to be sent outside at three to five times the internal cost to maintain service levels until new staff were recruited.

With an accepted external salary standard that applied to everyone, using the failed recruiting argument to increase departmental salaries became a bad plan. If one department was unsuccessful in recruiting when almost all the other departments—usually the case—were successful at the fiftieth percentile standard, the burden was on that department's leadership to explain why they couldn't recruit when the other departments could. By aligning recruiting incentives, this behavior largely disappeared. Recruiting efforts improved across the board, and this directly led to an era of steadily improving HPMG stability, prosperity, and improved performance.

Care and Service Improvement

The ability to implement and maintain care and service improvement programs is directly proportional to the desirability of a position in HPMG. The author vividly recalls a separation discussion at the height of the late eighties salary crisis with a poorly performing surgeon. He essentially said that we couldn't discharge him because we would not be able to replace him with our compensation package.

The author replied, "We will figure something out." Patient care and service was not going to be compromised. What that something was going to be was not clear to the author at the time.

The surgeon to be discharged was right. We couldn't recruit a replacement for more than a year, and that was only after the department salary scale had been raised significantly because the department had withered to 40 percent of approved staffing levels.

By the mid-1990s, HPMG positions were highly sought after. Quality and service efforts in HPMG could proceed realistically because there was little need to be concerned about being able to replace a poorly performing doctor.

Internalization of Care

By 1990, the outside services budget was greater than 15 percent of the Hawaii region budget and accelerating as specialty departments collapsed because of recruiting difficulties. It approximated that of the entire HPMG budget. To internalize care, departments needed to be fully staffed, and that required a competitive compensation package.

Ideally, HPMG wanted to be able to honestly say that if it couldn't be done by HPMG, it couldn't be done in Hawaii. With only 16 percent of the doctors in Hawaii, HPMG would need to sub-specialize. Sub-specialization allowed fellowship-trained physicians to concentrate upon certain sub-specialties within the traditional specialties. A subspecialist usually had a sub-specialty fellowship training for a year or two after standard residency training. For example, orthopedics was eventually subspecialized into hand, shoulder, foot and ankle, total joint, and sports subspecialties. There will be more on this in a following chapter. By the end of the nineties, because of the ability to recruit sub-specialists, HPMG had internalized 98 percent of KP membership care.

Principles of HPMG Salary Policy

These are the policies that have worked for HPMG. They evolved over decades, but they have provided political and staffing stability since the early 1990s.

Fairness

Salaries are maintained as close as possible to the national fiftieth percentile for every specialty. From a societal and Health Plan negotiation standpoint, this is quite defensible. Recruiting had to be at the national level because the pool of available local doctors was too small – especially among specialists. Hawaii is a small state. Most reasonable people would concede that if compensation is systematically too low, there will be difficulty recruiting anyone – especially high-quality doctors. An excellent case can be made that the difference between a high-quality doctor and an average-to-low-quality doctor to the survival of a health program is much greater than just about any other employee classification. The product of KP is health care, and the doctors lead it.

KP Hawaii is unionized, and this has maintained very competitive employee salaries. The doctors are not unionized, and they can be left behind in the budget process as they were for most of the first thirty years unless HPMG is effectively negotiating for their fair share of program resources. This requires HPMG to balance the responsibilities of maintaining medical professionalism and union-like advocacy within the same organization. It is a difficult tightrope to walk.

This argument applies to the Health Plan negotiations. Health Plan can defend the fiftieth percentile doctor salaries to its customers who might try to complain that Health Plan is paying the doctors too much. Even though doctor salaries are high on an individual basis, physician compensation is a relatively small piece of the health care pie. Nationally, it is about 18–20 percent of the total medical budget, and well over half of that 18–20 percent is overhead. Paying physician salaries at half of their market value would save only about 5–6 percent of the KP Hawaii regional budget. This is what was essentially done during the first thirty years of the program with the resultant recruiting, reputation, and outside service costs.

The missionary spirit of the founding doctors inspired by the ideals of Kaiser Permanente should not be forgotten. It kept the fledgling program alive in the early years, but eventually KP had to expand or die—and die it nearly did in 1960, 1975, and 1988 as a direct result of noncompetitive salaries. There simply aren't enough quality doctors to be found who will work for half of their market value to treat the one sixth of the population of Hawaii that KP serves.

For HPMG and Kaiser Foundation Health Plan, when defending doctor salaries to its critics, a useful analogy would that if you are running an airline, you don't save the money on pilot salaries—even if they are among the highest-paid employees.

Benefit Structure

By the end of the 1970s, HPMG had funded a generous benefit structure. With excellent retirement, health insurance, disability, vacation, and medical education benefits, physicians did not have to worry about their security and that of their family. They could concentrate on the quality of their patient medical care and service.

Lifestyle

Almost from the beginning, the HPMG physician leaders learned that they could exploit the advantages of being in a large medical group to improve their work-life balance. Because of the large size of most clinical departments, vacation and educational leave was easy to arrange with automatic, competent, and noncompetitive coverage by partners. Your job and your patients would be waiting for you when you returned.

For some doctors, especially those who joined HPMG after being in private practice, it was worth a significant proportion of their salary. With reasonable performance, a HPMG physician had job security rarely found in other practice situations. Once salaries reached the fiftieth percentile, the turnover rate dropped to 2–4 percent per year, and most of that was due to retirements, doctors leaving distant Hawaii for family reasons, or less commonly inadequate performance. Very few doctors left HPMG for what they perceived to be better positions. Of those who did, many later tried to rejoin HPMG—usually unsuccessfully. The ability to work with other highly skilled physicians was a major draw—as was the ability to subspecialize in clinical areas of interest.

Finally, a doctor fresh from training, joining HPMG, had a full practice and the mentoring of physician colleagues from day one—just when they needed it the most to become seasoned doctors. In contrast, when starting out in private practice, it usually takes three to five years to build a practice and often it is done alone since colleagues are competitors.

Divisible Surplus

During the history of HPMG, during most years, there was what was called a *divisible surplus*. It ranged from 0–10 percent of the yearly salary. HPMG is *capitated*, which means that it is paid on a per-member, per-month basis, which is the source of the HPMG budget. If, at the end of the year, HPMG comes in under budget, the surplus is distributed to all doctors equally—without regard to specialty. The admirable rationale is that the surplus was due to the efforts of everyone in HPMG working together. Over the years, it went a long way to promote group solidary.

The Problem of Incentive Payment

On a regular basis, all through the history of HPMG, the issue of merit bonuses has been raised. The core principle behind HPMG compensation policy is that it should be competitive so that HPMG can recruit and retain exceptional doctors. In return for the fair compensation package, career security, and a sustainable lifestyle, the physician is expected to practice at a uniformly high level of professionalism. The compensation policy is intended to isolate compensation issues from medical decision-making, and it does.

With everyone in the same specialty paid essentially the same shortly after beginning a career with HPMG, the self-centered cynic could conclude: "Since we are all paid the same, the harder I work, the less I get paid." Human nature, being what it is, always produces at least a few of these characters. Some of these slackers are able to translate this work versus pay equation into a high art form. They do just enough work to keep from getting fired. As a response, HPMG leadership recognized early on that outstanding work needed to be rewarded. Anything else would be unfair. It took more than forty years to figure out how.

Doctors, like most people, will usually do what you pay them to do. Incentives are a two-edged sword. Thoughtlessly applied, they can lead to a number of unintended consequences that are at cross-purposes with the success of the program. Almost all HPMG compensation is fair and fixed for which is expected a high level of professionalism. The incentive problem is that even a small incentive program can disproportionly shift effort away from overall professionalism to specific incentivized behaviors. In this compensation setting, adding incentive payments to the fixed base salary would be the only way to raise salary.

Caveat: Partners or Competitors

Doctors are naturally competitive. Medical training selects for competitive, perfectionist, individualists. It is demanding, complex, high-level, intellectual work. Barring individuals with exceptional intellectual brilliance and personality, noncompetitive people do not get selected for, or fare well, in medical school and the subsequent competitive training programs. There is little room for easygoing when delivering health care at the physician level.

Physicians working together as a team, without the noise and friction of intradepartmental economic competition is one of the major strategic and lifestyle advantages of practicing within HPMG. At what point does the percentage of incentive salary convert department partners to competitors? Given the naturally competitive nature of most physicians, that incentive percentage is not likely to be very high.

Caveat: Behavioral Distortion

The base salary is based upon the expectation of highly professional behavior, but it is fixed. Marginal increases in salary above that base can only come from incentive bonuses. At what point does a physician decide that if it there is no incentive payment for some desirable activity, then it needn't be performed because it detracts from the incentive efforts? The risk of distorted professional behavior can only be avoided if the actual incentive payments are so low that the risk of putting disproportionate effort into bonus activity at the expense of overall professional behavior threatens the base salary. Thus, incentive payments must be kept very low relative to the base salary scale to prevent incentive-driven, unintended, undesirable behaviors. These behaviors are often difficult to detect. It would be best to avoid such behaviors to begin with.

A clinical example comes from another KP region long ago. As told to the author by doctors from that region, there came from high-level PMG leadership, a drive to increase the number of colonoscopies. This was in response to suddenly increased publicity about the need for colon cancer screening. A significant portion of the base salary was placed at risk and could be earned back or even exceeded by doing more colonoscopies. As expected, there was a boom in the number of colonoscopies performed. Little noticed was a concurrent increased difficulty scheduling more complex, time-consuming, but necessary, procedures from that specialty as effort was shifted to colonoscopy production.

Incentives are not a good way to allocate clinical resources. Professionalism coupled with evidence-based medical resource allocation by dedicated, informed, physician PMG leadership at the department level is much better.

The Solution

In the beginning, HPMG salaries were based upon history, guesswork, immediate need, and politics. There was a deeply felt need for the recognition of meritorious behavior, which resulted in sporadic bonus awards. Some early salary proposals were based entirely on a merit system. The problem was defining merit.

As specialty market-based salary formulas evolved in the late 1970s, the clamor for bonus recognition continued. By the early 1980s, there was a yearly bonus award structure of $1,000, $5,000, and $10,000 based upon chief recommendations for specific program-wide improvement programs initiated by individuals. These, however, were only awarded to a small percentage of physicians.

There is a management saying that good managers catch employees "doing something right." Unfortunately, chiefs are more commonly expected to catch employees "doing something wrong." In the late eighties and early nineties, chiefs were encouraged to issue "mahalograms." Mahalo means thank you in Hawaiian. These were notes to individuals from chiefs acknowledging specific meritorious behavior. While generally appreciated for the thoughtfulness of the chief, there was no associated financial reward. As a result, many chiefs didn't bother. This was in contrast to the chiefs addressing bad behavior, which was usually associated with a financial penalty if it persisted. Bad behavior got a pay cut, and good behavior got a mahalogram. This didn't do much to support a chief's standing among department members. By the mid-1990s, the mahalogram program had pretty much died out from disuse.

By mid-1994, everything changed with the addition of a small financial bonus to an individual recognition program. The new recognition bonus program was quickly accepted by the chiefs and the PMG doctors. The rules were clear. Each chief was given a certain number of "chits" (budgeted at three per doctor) based upon the number of doctors in their department. A chit consisted of a hundred-dollar American Express check and a note card in a matching envelope. To issue the recognition, a handwritten note acknowledging a specific meritorious action was required. An individual could get more than their allotment during the year or none at all depending upon their behavior. Chiefs were specifically not allowed to issue equal bonuses to everyone in their department, and a chit was not valid without the note. Chits not issued by the chief were returned to the HPMG general fund at the end of the year on a use-it-or-lose-it basis. Putting department award money back into the general fund at the end of the year would be an unpopular option for chiefs. There were many benefits:

- It powerfully reinforced the value of good behavior well out of proportion to the cost of the program to HPMG. The total cost of the program was 0.2–0.3 percent of the HPMG budget. Once fair compensation is achieved, for most doctors, personal satisfaction for a job well done and professional recognition by superiors and colleagues are more important than money. If they are not, HPMG isn't a good fit for them anyway.
- It is at most a fraction of 1 percent of salary which discourages unintended behavior just to boost the chit score.
- Almost every doctor does at least one right thing per year that can be recognized, so almost all doctors benefit from the program. It powerfully reinforced good works.
- It is worth the extra effort for a chief to think about and acknowledge good behavior. Too often, only the very best and very worst

doctors get the attention of the chief's—while the rest of the doctors go unrecognized. This program encourages chiefs to give concrete recognition to the vast majority of the doctors who, after all, do most of the work. A program moves forward by moving forward the rank and file more so than the outliers.

- It greatly improves the standing of the chiefs. They not only are the initiators of the relatively uncommon, unpopular, disciplinary salary cuts, but they are also the initiators of the much more common, and popular, recognition bonuses. As of this writing, more than twenty years later the program is more popular and stronger than ever. It has become one of the more pleasant aspects of the HPMG culture.

Staffing

Without a proper staffing model, a salary scale is meaningless. Consider this simplified model. If there are one hundred HPMG doctors, and the HPMG budget is one thousand units of pay/year, then there is available for each doctor ten units of pay/year. On the other hand, if there are fifty doctors doing the same amount of work, there is available twenty units of pay per year. Conversely, if there are two hundred doctors doing the same amount of work, there would be available five units of pay/year. Why is this? It is because HPMG is capitated—paid on a fixed amount per member per month.

HPMG is paid by the number of patients that it cares for—not by fee-for-service, which is the number of medical interventions that each doctor performs. In turn, the upper limit of the capitation amount is itself fixed by societal and market forces. If the HPMG yearly budget is fixed by capitation—the number of patients it serves—then it needs a clear, prospective staffing model to fairly distribute resources. With a fixed budget based upon capitation, there is little room for the "if we build it, they will come rationalizations" that might apply to an expensive piece of equipment, overbuilding, or overstaffing, which might be true in a fee-for-service setting. If there is a fixed budget determined by capitation, giving disproportionate resources to one area means taking them from another area. Human nature almost dictates that the managers of all patient services will have many reasons why they should get a disproportionate share. In a fair model, no one can. Again, like the salary scale model, to avoid a "squeaky wheel" staffing model, an outside gold standard is again required. What is that gold standard?

For purposes of illustration, urology, a surgical specialty, will be used as an example. In urban areas of the United States like Boston or San Francisco, the patient-doctor ratio of urologic surgical specialists might be as low as 1:20,000, but 1:40,000 or more in rural areas with generally similar outcomes. In the Republic of Ireland, due to government policy that favored primary care doing nonsurgical specialty care, the ratio was 1:184,000. While urologic outcomes and the availability of services might be less than in the US, the overall health statistics are similar or even superior to those of the US. In some developing countries, there are few or no urologic surgeons. The economy simply cannot support that level of medical care. The medical care statistics may not be as good as developed countries, but to have the maximum impact upon health, the resources that are available are better spent on clean water supplies, immunization, condoms, and mosquito nets.

A urologic surgeon is about twice as expensive to maintain as a primary care doctor. In a planned economy, that would be the rationale for using primary care doctors for nonsurgical urologic problems. Such nonsurgical problems include primary urinary tract infections, prostatitis, nonsurgical medical bladder problems, and urologic cancer follow-up. The cost savings might be worth it, but only if the primary care doctors have the same interest and training in these specialized problems as a fully trained urologist. They rarely do. Indeed, in Germany, urologic care is not provided by primary care but by surgical urologists (~30 percent) and clinic urologists (~70 percent). In a free economy, such as the United States, patients prefer to see a urologist for urologic medical problems. In relatively non-planned economy of the US, training programs are not limited by the government but by the market economy. Based upon market forces, many more urologists can be trained and supported by patient demand. A sixty-five-year-old man with aggressive prostate cancer is not likely to be consoled about the absence of urologic care by knowing that the immunization rate of the population is very high. Fortunately, the economy of the United States of America can support both.

KP has the freedom to vary somewhat from a free market model, but that is sharply restricted by patient demand and evidence-based medicine. Indeed, KP planning could sharply restrict specialty departments and more generously staff primary care, but it would still face the competition of a medical community that reflects a patient demand for unrestricted access to specialists.

It is always risky not to give the customer (patient) what they want. Excessive specialty restriction can and has been used against KP marketing efforts in the past. KP Hawaii historically has solved the problem by being more generous with primary care staffing and less generous with specialty staffing. As a result there was not wide-open access to specialty care, barriers to specialty care were set low enough so that the specialists were still used efficiently, but at the same time, patients felt that they were getting good specialty service. In 2012, when a staffing analysis was performed, the primary care doctor-patient ratio was 70–80 percent of that of the community, and the specialty staffing ratio was 40–50 percent. This was essentially unchanged from a previous similar study from twelve years earlier.

Model Modification 1

While there is flexibility for innovative staffing models within KP, periodically, radically different staffing models are proposed by one KP region to other regions at interregional meetings. These models generally propose that specialty department staffing be radically reduced with the resources diverted to increased primary care staffing. The response by the specialty chief audience is skeptical: "Your region first." Their experience with similar past experiments is that typically primary care doesn't have the same interest or training in the specialty problems, the specialty department ends up seeing the problems anyway with reduced staffing, and after failed primary care trials and long specialty wait times, which delay care, the cost of care is ultimately higher. Historically, after a few years, these models are not heard from again. On the other hand, many specialty chiefs have enthusiastically supported primary care and physician assistant staffing along the lines of the German model within and under the control of the specialty department to increase the efficiency of care-delivery.

Model Modification II: Physician Extenders

Another alternative model is to use more ancillary care providers as doctor extenders. From the beginning of its history, HPMG has employed such ancillary providers with considerable success. Ancillary care providers are medically trained professionals who are quite capable of competently performing some physician duties under the supervision of physicians. They can include physician assistants, advanced practice nurses, nurse anesthetists, midwives, podiatrists, optometrists, audiologists, and psychologists, but there are caveats.

Caveat 1: Supervision

Ancillary care providers are neither physicians nor physician substitutes. Ancillary care providers have two to five years of additional training after college. In contrast, a physician has four years of medical school, one year of internship, and then a residency of two to five years—and often an additional one to two years of subspecialized fellowship training—for a total of seven to twelve years of medical training after college. Along the lines of "with responsibility must come authority" since physicians are held responsible for medical and liability outcomes of a department, it is HPMG policy that physicians are the supervisors of care delivered by ancillary care providers.

Attempts in the past by ancillary care providers in KP Hawaii to have complete independent practice with little or no accountability to the departmental supervising physicians have not been successful. A historical example from the early 1990s was a nurse anesthetist demand by a minority of the nurse anesthetists that they have their own quality assurance program independent of the anesthesiologists and accountable only to hospital nursing and administration. HPMG administration made clear to hospital administration and Health Plan that this was unacceptable to the anesthesiologists and the surgeons. The involved nurse anesthetists threatened a strike, which resulted in emergency contingency arrangements by HPMG to move to a permanent all doctor anesthesiologist service within a month's time at no additional expense. The crisis was quietly averted when a few of the most militant nurse anesthetists did not report for duty, abandoning their scheduled cases. They were promptly and permanently replaced by their own nurse anesthetist leadership. After this crisis, the close coordination between the anesthesiologists, surgeons, and nurse anesthetists resumed and has continued.

Caveat 2: Cost Savings

While ancillary care providers may have less than half the postgraduate training of a doctor, their compensation and benefits, at least in KP, are not typically less than half of a doctor's, especially when compared to primary care physicians. Even if they were, productivity must be also taken into consideration. Most ancillary care providers are unionized, which can bring mandatory break times, lunch hours, overtime, and more complex disciplinary procedures. While of proven value to our form of care-delivery, physician extenders are not necessarily more cost effective than doctors. Proposals to replace doctors with physician extenders for economic reasons need to be examined critically, taking into account salaries, benefits, and productivity.

Caveat 3: Market Competition

HPMG embraced ancillary care providers earlier and more extensively than our market competition. Most patients still want to see a doctor or at least know that a doctor is closely supervising the practitioner. This is especially true in primary care where there is patient resistance to independent practice by non-physician practitioners.

The KP use of non-physician providers has often been distorted by KP critics. "You don't see a doctor at Kaiser" has been and is used against KP marketing efforts. It is another reason why HPMG maintains a close and visible supervisory role over the employment of ancillary care providers.

Caveat 4: Physician Burnout

For most doctors, the most difficult part of the job is "call." Call is a clearly defined period of availability where the on-call physician covers the entire department for all problems related to that specialty from nursing questions to all night medical and surgical emergencies. During the workweek, the call physician is usually expected to put in a full day of clinic work the next day. Call periods are the times of greatest risk and stress for physicians. Most ancillary care providers cannot take call. Consequently, if ancillary care providers replace doctors, then there are fewer doctors to rotate call, increasing the frequency of these high-stress, high-risk call periods.

If the non-physician ancillary providers manage the routine cases, the management of difficult cases is concentrated in the hands of fewer doctors. At the same time, these doctors have the additional responsibility and liability burden of the supervision of the work of the non-physician providers. This may appear to be more efficient in the short run, but excessive stress is likely to lead to physician burnout and the resultant medical errors and disruption of the continuity of care caused by physician turnover.

Solution

The use of lower-cost nonphysician providers to replace high-cost physicians is often attractive to high-level administrators. They should not be making these operational decisions. Administrators should provide financial data to support such decision-making at the operational level. As stated many times in this book, "With the responsibility must come authority." The department physicians have the operational responsibility for the clinical and liability outcomes of their department. Therefore, they should make the decisions about the provider mix for their department.

In the early 2000s, this actually occurred in one of the primary care departments. During a rare staff downsizing, due to an unexpected and sudden membership loss, the department was presented with a difficult decision. It needed to decide whether to downsize either three physicians or five nurse practitioners. With the financial tradeoff equalized, the department members decided to keep the physicians. The deciding factors were call and difficult caseload burdens. Why was the decision allowed to be made by only the department physicians? Because the clinical and liability "buck" stops with them.

Physicians deciding to keep physicians—what is so surprising about that? The decision could be and has been different under different circumstances. There have been cases of departments delaying or forgoing increased physician staffing to increase non-physician providers, especially in the surgery specialties where physician assistants are widely incorporated into the care-delivery team. The important point is that staffing mix should be made at the department level by those immediately responsible for the clinical and liability outcomes. The only role of administration should be to provide the data necessary to make rational decisions about tradeoffs.

The Development of the HPMG Staffing Model

Starting in the early 1980s, HPMG worked hard to develop a prospective staffing model. Doctor-patient ratios were initially calculated from other KP regions. These were imprecise, did not reflect the local Hawaii competition, and did not account for contracted outside services provided by non-PMG doctors, which falsely raised the patient-to-PMG doctor ratios. Because of this, PMG nationwide ratios represented only the upper limit of acceptable patient-doctor ratios.

Another patient-to-doctor ratio standard was obtained from within Hawaii. Being a small state, it was not difficult to calculate accurate, non-HPMG patient-to-doctor ratios. These were much lower than the HPMG internal ratios, but they did represent the local service competition. They could be used as the lower-limit patient-to-doctor ratios. The actual historical HPMG patient-doctor ratios turned out to be the best ratio for the final model in that they accounted for internal workload-distribution agreements that had evolved over the years. For example, who treats pyelonephritis (a serious kidney infection)? Is it internal medicine, urology, or infectious disease? Actually, all three departments treated pyelonephritis cooperatively. Informal interdepartmental agreements set up the workflow. Uncomplicated cases are treated initially by primary care, usually with success. When necessary, they call in urology if there is an anatomic problem such as a stone, which might need surgery or infectious disease if there is a complicated bacterial-resistance problem. It is of interest is that these internal doctor-patient ratios have changed little over the years, probably because they reflect the totality of these – usually informal - clinical agreements.

Let's use urology again as a model. When the first ratio was set up in 1992 for the specialty care model, the KP National ratio was calculated first. It was one urologist per forty thousand patients. The HPMG Urology Department actually knew all of the practicing urologists within Hawaii. Dividing the number of practicing private urologists into the non-KP civilian population gave a doctor-patient Hawaii ratio of one to twenty-three thousand. The HPMG historical ratio for the previous ten years had hovered around one to thirty-five thousand members. When the ratio exceeded to thirty-five thousand, urology patient access suffered.

Because it takes two to three years to recruit a good candidate, these ratios help predict staffing needs. This avoids "panic hires" because of staffing crises due to unexpected retirements, resignations, and illness. The department was given the go-ahead to begin recruiting at a 1:32,000 ratio and could consider bridging mechanisms to maintain service levels when the ratio got to 1:37,000. Bridging mechanisms were approvals by the HPMG executive committee to authorize and pay for extra clinics at salary rates. Thus, long-term service levels can be maintained—and recruiting is orderly.

By 1995, there was a staffing scale based upon specialty patient-to-doctor ratios to accompany the salary scale. A quick study of the staffing scale combined with an estimate of KP membership growth could provide HPMG management with an accurate recruiting plan for the next several years in a matter of minutes. Together they provided a rational basis for an attractive compensation benefit funded by an efficient and rational staffing ratio. The staffing scale fit on a single page. There were seven columns: the current HPMG staffing, the KP National doctor-patient ratio, the Hawaii doctor-patient ratio, the HPMG historical staffing ratio, the agreed ratio to begin recruiting, the ratio qualifying for "bridging mechanisms" to maintain service, and the cost of outside services generated by services that could not be provided internally by the department. The outside services budget acted as a "fudge factor." Again using urology, if urology sent out

$200,000 of urologic oncology cases a year, and the ratio was approaching the recruiting threshold, the department might be told that they could begin recruiting early—but only if they were recruiting a urologic oncologist. Thus, the staffing scale was also an incentive for departments to sub-specialize, enabling the internalization of more and more care.

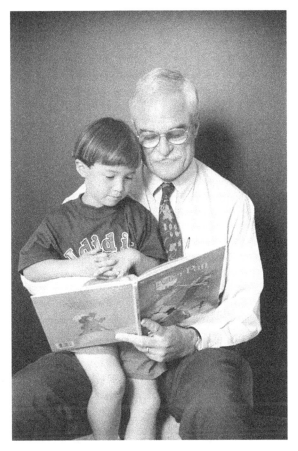

Michael Chaffin, MD, the third HPMG medical
director from 1992 until 2007.

CHAPTER 10

MICHAEL CHAFFIN, MD: THE THIRD PRESIDENT OF HPMG

When Dr. Michael (Mike) Chaffin became the third medical director of HPMG on January 1, 1992, things were looking up for HPMG. The toxic election of 1989 was now more than two years in the past, and the rancor it had generated was now a distant memory. Since the departure of Dan Wagster in early 1991, Cora Tellez, regional president of the Kaiser Foundation Health Plan, had organized a capable Health Plan administration now working in true partnership with HPMG. During his two-year partnership with Bill Dung—first as executive vice president and then in his second year as president-elect and acting president working in partnership with Cora—Mike was ready from the first day in office. His first year in 1992 was a year of recovery, progress, and optimism.

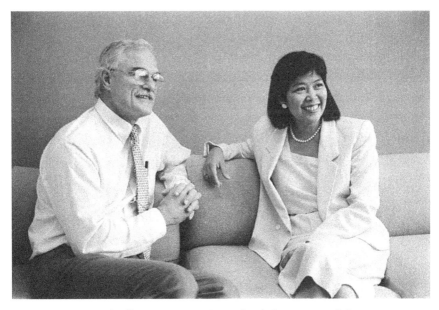

Mike Chaffin, MD, HPMG medical director, and Cora
Tellez, regional president of Kaiser Health Plan and
Hospitals Hawaii. It was partnership at its best.

Among Mike's first acts was to appoint his vice presidents. He made it clear that they would report directly to him and that their role was to be content experts rather than supervisory over other physicians. The chiefs and PICs would remain supervisory and continue to report directly to him. Steve Miller, MD, was appointed vice president of finance and was named his successor if Mike was incapacitated. Karl Pregitzer, MD, was appointed vice president of outside services and later special projects. Geoffrey Galbraith, MD, a rising star in HPMG and the quality assurance director, was appointed vice president of quality.

Except for one, he then reappointed the existing chiefs and PICs over the next several board meetings for three-year terms as specified in the bylaws. The second presidential succession had occurred with a minimum of fuss. The year was spent rebuilding HPMG by tracking the rising market-based salaries. The recruiting effect was immediate. By the end of the year, most of the vacancies had been filled by high-quality physicians who for the most part remained with HPMG until the end of their careers.

May 14, 1992, marked the passing of an era. On that date, the board of directors honored the retiring executive secretary of HPMG, Sumi Croydon. Sumi had served Drs. Chu, Dung, and Chaffin for thirty-two years since the founding of the HPMG. She was the living corporate memory of HPMG, deeply loyal to ideals of Kaiser Permanente, and a mothering figure to many of the new doctors after they joined HPMG, including the author. Without the system of archive preservation that she established, this story would not have been possible. She had carefully trained her equally dedicated successor, Shelly Young, who served as executive secretary for Drs. Chaffin and Sewell for an additional twenty years until 2012. Shelly continued the archive preservation policies of Sumi. For the first fifty-two years of HPMG, there were only two executive secretaries.

Call and Comp Time

Since 1992 was an era of good feeling for HPMG, at the October 1, 1992, board meeting, an update of the 1993 "comp" time policy was quickly ratified. It had rarely been so easy before or after. Most PMG physicians would agree that call is the most difficult of their duties. After hours on call, emergencies occur when most of the support staff is off duty and often in the middle of the night when a person's mental and physical resources are at their lowest. As such, it is a period of high stress, career risk, and quality of life disruption. Being the largest medical group in Hawaii allows the sharing of call so that when the doctor is "off" call, the doctor is truly "off." While this greatly improves the overall quality of life for all HPMG physicians, when the doctor is on call, the intensity of call is increased because the on-call doctor is typically covering all KP patients for that specialty. Backed up by a fully staffed and capable emergency department, this call system is fair, safe, and maximizes physician overall quality of life.

As the Medical Group grew and differentiated, a compensation program was instituted in the 1970s to offset the risk and inconvenience of call. As a result of this program, getting doctors to come in at night or off hours was rarely an issue. Depending upon the time and duration of the call-in episode, the call doctors could be compensated in salary or "comp time" hours, which were used like vacation hours. To avoid piling up call time to increase compensation and to allow for needed rest, in time, it became an hours-only program. Since the hours were covered by the other members of the department, all of whom benefitted from the policy, it promoted dependence and cooperation within a department. It had no overall financial consequences on the HPMG budget because the departments were expected to manage schedules to cover their own call without extra staffing. Patient service should not be impacted because all departments are expected to maintain preset patient and physician service levels. Departments were expected to and did enact department efficiencies to cover their own call.

With the salaries most of the way toward the goal of the fiftieth percentile of MGMA by the end of 1992, most of the vacancies had been filled with high performing doctors. Mike Chaffin's administration was well established, and 1992 was to be the beginning of more than a decade of peace, growth, and prosperity for HPMG and the Hawaii KP program.

The HPMG Values Statement

While 1992 was a year of rebuilding, 1993 was a year of positive progress. One such event was the passage and promulgation of the HPMG values statement. Kaiser Permanente nationally was structured around a group of semiautonomous regions. The leaders of each region met regularly at national meetings where ideas were exchanged and national policies were discussed and endorsed. These meetings were called the "Kai-Perm" meetings. At one of these meetings, Simi Lisse, MD, the medical director of the Northeast Permanente Medical Group presented the Northeast PMG Values Statement. It was an explicit statement of the values of that medical group. Mike Chaffin brought this idea back to the HPMG board of directors.

On June 10, 1993, the board of directors established a committee of voting board members chaired by Drs. Nathan Fujimoto and David Waters to develop a HPMG values statement. The committee went about its work, diligently studying the values statements of other groups. The committee developed the HPMG values statement based upon these and locally evolved values. To validate their work, the proposed values statement was vetted in a series of stakeholder meetings. On November 18,

1993, the values statement was approved unanimously by the HPMG board of directors.

Unchanged since that time, it reads:

> The Hawaii Permanente Medical Group seeks associate physicians who support and promote Kaiser Permanente's mission of providing quality of care and comprehensive medical services in an accessible, cost-effective manner for members. In addition, the HPMG board of directors has identified the professional and personal values that enhance individual and collective medical practice. These are our core values:
>
> The characteristics of professional competency, reliability, compassionate caring, and a striving for excellence are core values necessary for our associates. Furthermore, we value good-natured team players who are approachable by colleagues and staff. We expect our associates to be hardworking professionals capable of an innovative approach to solving problems, who make efficient use of time and resources. We expect our colleagues to maintain a professionally appropriate appearance. We expect a professionally appropriate attitude toward patients and staff that excludes bigotry and prejudice.
>
> We value individuals who are responsive to constructive criticism and who demonstrate courtesy and respect to fellow workers as well as patients. We place value on quality work with consistent standards. It is important for us to recognize professional limitations in forming the boundaries of work, matching competence with confidence.
>
> We seek associates who will actively assist the organization to function efficiently and effectively. Our strength comes from a shared sense of responsibility for the Medical Group and from our collective talents as medical professionals. Finally, we believe that along with hard work, we

seek to achieve a balance between a satisfying career and a fulfilling personal life.

This statement was not mere sloganeering. Along with the approval of the values statement, the board required that it be the basis for HPMG associateship. The board enacted a sixteen-point survey based upon the values statement, which was to be given to every prospective HPMG associate during orientation if not during recruiting. Each candidate was made to understand that this survey would be distributed to all HPMG doctors after the associate candidate's first year of service and again prior to the voting on associateship. Poor performance on the survey would be grounds for delaying or denying associateship. This gave the policy teeth. Over the years, a small but significant number of associate candidates were denied associateship as a result of poor performance on this values statement survey.

Because at least two value statement questionnaires were distributed for each new candidate to every HPMG doctor, dozens of surveys were distributed to every HPMG doctor every year. In subsequent years, as "wrongful termination" became a growth industry for tort attorneys, this policy provided a robust defense for HPMG. No HPMG physician could reasonably claim that they were unaware of the HPMG values—the "house rules" of HPMG.

Board Certification

By the 1970s specialty board certification was widely established. The specialty boards were made up of specialty program directors who would come together to examine candidates for board certification after these candidates completed their specialty residencies. This was an important validation to be obtained. It certified by experts that the candidate physician was competent to practice the specialty in the eyes of the specialty's training experts.

Previous HPMG policy had established that board certification was required to become a HPMG associate. On the September 2, 1993 the board passed a board certification policy for associates who had already become associates or "grandfathered" prior to the board certification requirement for new associates. It stated that current associates without boards had three years to obtain board certification; otherwise, there would be a 5 percent reduction in salary until board certification was obtained. Physicians with term-limited board certification would have two years to renew their board certification after expiration; otherwise, they too would be subject to the 5 percent pay reduction until their certification was reestablished. Board-certification expenses and time away from the practice to take the test would be covered by the Medical Group as an extra educational leave package. The importance of board certification, and eighteen years of HPMG controversy about the need for specialty board certification had finally been settled firmly in favor of board certification for all associates.

Point-of-Service

With the 1992 succession of Jim Vohs by David Lawrence, MD, the program changed sharply away from the genetic code of KP, to that of a health care corporation. There were even leadership comments overheard that were interpreted to be favorable to a for-profit business model. A for-profit business model would have the advantage of being able to quickly generate very large amounts of capital from the sale of stock to fund rapid expansion.

Lawrence enthusiastically proclaimed the need for drastic change at the national Kai-Perm meetings of the regional executive leadership. At one of these meetings, Mike Chaffin, who observed that the genetic code of KP had been increasingly successful in Hawaii for more than three decades, skeptically asked, "Change to what?"

For this, he was asked to lead the "Change to What?" committee by his equally skeptical colleagues. Some of the newly proposed changes were a direct threat to the traditional exclusive partnership between the Permanente Medical Groups and Kaiser Foundation Health Plan, which would later lead to "Tahoe II."

One such change was the introduction by Health Plan leadership of a "point-of-service" (POS) plan. The idea was that an employer wishing to offer KP was provided the option to employees of the traditional program restricted to the PMG doctors or Kaiser Health Plan-affiliated non-PMG community doctors for some of their care. The PMG doctors would be paid by traditional capitation, and the community doctors would be paid by fee for service. Mike Chaffin announced this proposal to the HPMG board of directors on October 21, 1993. He pointed out that it would be acceptable to the Permanente Medical Groups only if they controlled it. He announced that Dr. Karl Pregitzer, his vice president of outside services and one of the chief skeptics of the point-of-service program, would represent HPMG interests in a newly formed Health Plan point-of-service task force. "Point-of-service had some pros and many cons.

The rationale that Health Plan used for the point-of-service program was that many potential members rejected the idea of trying Kaiser Permanente because patients would be restricted to Permanente doctors. With a point-of-service option, these patients, especially company executives, would no longer be restricted to Permanente physicians. Health Plan proponents of point-of-service buoyantly explained that once they tried KP point-of-service, they would convert completely to the traditional KP program.

The PMG leadership was quick to point out the point-of-service flaws. They noted that restricted choice of physicians was not a problem for the Mayo and Cleveland Clinics. They postulated that if the clinical services of the PMG Medical Groups were resourced at the same levels as these world-class institutions, restricted choice would similarly not be a problem. KP initially survived because of its cheap prices due to its widely recognized frugality and tight clinical resourcing. It was the overly tight clinical resourcing that had resulted in poor compensation and overly tight staffing, which blighted the service and sometimes even quality reputation of the program. It was this mediocre service and quality reputation that the KP Hawaii was trying to get out from under in the 1990s. The PMG Medical Groups, saddled with this unenviable legacy, were now expected to compete within their own Kaiser health plans with private medical community physicians. Historically, these private community doctors had been better resourced.

To participate in Kaiser Health Plan, the community physicians would expect the same fee-for-service-based reimbursement that they had been receiving from the KP competition. Kaiser Health Plan would have to pay these higher fees to make the program acceptable to these community physicians. Furthermore, these physicians would be practicing at competing hospitals for which Kaiser Health Plan would be required to reimburse at rates multiples higher than those paid to the Kaiser Hospital. Like outside service contracts, the program could be subsidizing the competing doctors and hospitals with already scarce clinical resources from the core product. Finally, Health Plan would have to build an expensive infrastructure to manage fee-for-service billing, which it hadn't needed in the past. Since all resources would come from the same Kaiser Health Plan budget, any point-of-service budget deficit would further divert already scarce resources away from the KP core product and toward the community competition. Thus, point-of-service had the potential to divert resources from the core program while subsidizing the competition since the point-of-service program usually ran at a loss.

Another real risk was that if pricing and sales incentives were not carefully managed, the point-of-service program would cannibalize members from the KP core program rather than from the community competitors. This would also happen if the POS plans were priced at or close to the core plan. It initially was, and it did.

The greatest risk of all to the program was the risk to the partnership. Medical Group skeptics were convinced that this was a ploy by Health Plan to gradually break the exclusivity contract between the Permanente Medical Groups and Health Plan. If community doctors were competing within the Kaiser Health Plan with Permanente Medical Groups, once there were enough community physicians in the program, Health Plan would no longer need the Permanente Medical Groups and would use this leverage against them at the time of the medical services agreement negotiations. Of course, this could work both ways.

Not unreasonably, some Permanente leaders argued that if Kaiser Health Plan could partner with the Permanente Medical Group's community competitors, there should be no reason why the Permanente Medical Groups shouldn't partner with the community competitors of Kaiser Health Plan. Either way, the loss of the partnership would end Kaiser Permanente's role as the potential "third way" model for health care-delivery between government control and for-profit business health care models—if not Kaiser Permanente itself. Point-of-service was just one issue that led to a "Tahoe II" confrontation later in the decade between the Permanente Medical Groups and Kaiser Health Plan.

The point-of-service task force addressed the potential problems. It was agreed that the point-of-service program could not operate at a loss so as not to take resources from the core product. It was also agreed that the point-of-service program must be bringing in new members into the core program and not cannibalizing the KP core membership. Both deficit funding and cannibalization of the core KP membership did occur at times during the following decades and only close, time-consuming scrutiny by HPMG partially controlled these concerns.

The traditional KP program itself has major cost advantages over fee-for-service medicine as previously described. To avoid subsidies to the POS program from the core program, it had to be priced at a premium compared to the traditional program. As such, it remained small. As a result, the point-of-service program never grew very large and may have actually added to the core membership. Point-of-service remains a potential threat to the core program if administered badly. It bears close scrutiny for as long as it exists.

By the end of 1993, steady membership growth despite the recent rate increases increased membership to 190,500. This membership growth, plus the stanching of the outside services cost hemorrhage due to internalization of services, and the improved contracting by Dr. Pregitzer's Outside Services Department, fueled continuing progress toward the median of MGMA salaries.

1994

This was the year that important HPMG policies were established. It was also the year when the changes in the national medical economy began to impact the Hawaii region.

Virtual Offices

An example of the dialogue between Medical Group and Health Plan was the presentation of virtual doctor's offices in February as a significant program cost savings idea. It was true that multiple doctors sharing offices and examination rooms would have resulted in some facilities savings. Not surprisingly, the concept was very unpopular among the clinical staff and doctors who would be expected to deliver efficient and confidential clinical care without a "home base." Patients expect doctors, who direct essentially all of their health care, to have an office. The lack of an office would have been a clear mark of the low status in which doctors were held by the program—a program that existed to deliver medical health care driven by physicians. HPMG representatives on the committee, somewhat tongue in cheek, suggested that they could further explore the concept but that it should be broadened to include virtual offices for everyone, including managers and executives. The initiative quickly lost momentum. While there are a few hospital service physicians that share offices, a quarter of a century later most HPMG doctors still have offices.

Medicare Risk Contract

In April 1994, HPMG ratified the first KP Hawaii Medicare risk contract. Previously, Medicare paid for services using a fee-for-service model. The idea behind a Medicare risk contract was that Medicare would pay a fixed fee per patient. It was intended to encourage cost-effective, coordinated, preventive care for Medicare patients. Since KP was already doing these things, it was an excellent line of business until 2016 when the federal government demanded rebates, claiming that KP patients were healthier than the average Medicare risk patients. How much was due to cherry-picking and how much was due to conservative disease coding and the better management and resultant better health of KP Medicare risk patients is, at the time of this writing, being challenged by the program in the courts.

Cora Tellez Leaves Hawaii

A harbinger of problems to come with Central Office in Oakland was the resignation of Cora Tellez as regional president as of June 1, 1994. Cora had arrived as the associate regional president in 1989 and then became regional president in 1991. She saw the Health Plan-Medical Group partnership as the key to regional success. In close partnership with Mike Chaffin, Medical Group leaders, and her own capable management team, a faltering partnership and program had been turned around. She had been personally recruited to KP from the Oakland city government by Jim Vohs who had mentored her. She believed in the ideals of Kaiser Permanente that Vohs had championed during his twenty-two-year administration. She saw early on that David Lawrence intended to change the organization away from the ideals of the founders toward a more commercial, corporate entity, and she wanted no part of it. She went on to a highly successful career as a health care executive and entrepreneur. She successfully positioned DeeJay Mailer, her capable hospital administrator, to be her successor. DeeJay successfully carried on Cora's partnership policies with HPMG for another five years. As Kaiser Health Plan continued to change, for similar reasons, she resigned. She followed Cora first as a successful health care executive in California and then as the successful chief executive officer of the Hawaii Kamehameha Schools between 2004 and 2014.

Board Certification Defined

The policies and procedures that were formulated in 1994, a busy year, have persisted unchanged to the present. In January, because of the proliferation of competing board certifications, board certification was defined as only those boards that were accredited by the American Board of Medical Specialties. In February, 1994 the board certification requirements were placed in the HPMG employment contract. There were some HPMG doctors who were boarded in more than one specialty. There were other doctors providing specialty services who did not qualify for board certification because they had not completed a residency in that specialty and thus were not even eligible to take boards. This caused specialty salary confusion. In March, the board of directors resolved the confusion by restricting specialty pay scales only to physicians practicing in that specialty and who were board certified or board eligible.

In March, it was announced that KP Hawaii had the highest patient satisfaction of any KP region on the STAR patient-satisfaction survey. In May, to promote more physician accountability, the board passed an amendment to the bylaws allowing dismissal of an associate by a vote of seven out of nine members of the board. Prior to that, dismissal of an associate required a nearly impossible to achieve unanimous vote of the board. In June, the board passed the family leave policy and in August the leave without pay policy. In August, funds were appropriated for the first hundred-dollar bonus chit program, which had successfully solved the "incentive bonus" issue. In December, the Psychiatry Department announced a department name change to the Department of Mental Health.

1995

In February, the disciplinary hearing policy was ratified. It defined in detail due process for denial of privileges, suspension, and termination, including the appeals process. In May, a disability policy was ratified. In July, a Kaiser wide email system became operational. In October, further expansion occurred on the Big Island of Hawaii as the Waimea (Kamuela) and Hilo Clinics were opened.

Membership Losses

While membership stood at 190,500 at the end of 1993, in 1994 and early 1995, there was a slow but steady loss of membership. By the end of 1994, it stood at 187,000 members. This was due to the proliferation of mostly for-profit HMOs, which were not averse to buying market share. In Hawaii, both the Queens and Kapiolani Medical Centers attempted to establish their own health plans to get out from under the near Health Care non-Kaiser monopoly held by HMSA. As this put downward pressure on rates and membership, KP Hawaii had to adapt by increasing efficiency. It did so successfully.

1996

At the February 1 board meeting, it was announced that the Computerized Medical Record Task Force had made the decision to partner with a small

Silicon Valley computerized medical records startup called Oceana. The intent of the partnership was to develop a medical records platform called the WAVE.

Thriving in a Busy Practice

At the March 21, 1996, board meeting, "Thriving in a Busy Practice" was introduced. This was a Southern California PMG program designed to help doctors cope with the increasing stress and demands of a rapidly changing medical environment. This idea was to evolve into an important local program that eventually was integrated into the HPMG quality-of-service and peer-to-peer programs. It became an effective resource for those HPMG physicians who were identified by these programs as falling behind.

At the June 6 meeting, Yi Ching, MD, who joined HPMG in 1967, the long-term, respected chief of pediatrics and a forward-looking pioneer of HPMG, announced his retirement at year's end.

Kaiser Permanente National Product Council

Further evidence of KP centralization was the presentation of the National Product Council and the National Purchasing Office, which were supposed to leverage the purchasing power of the whole program, but they were to take away some of the regional autonomy of the Regional (Hawaii) Product Council. While lower supply prices were usually negotiated, there were situations where locally negotiated prices could actually be lower. Frequent changes of medical suppliers, such as surgical sutures, could be clinically disruptive. Fortunately, there was usually a 20 percent escape clause to accommodate local clinical needs.

Clinical Retraining of HPMG Managers

In August, the board ratified a policy for the retraining of HPMG physician managers returning to full-time practice. Doctors who had served more than two years in a half-time or greater position would be given paid leave for retraining calculated on the basis of percent of administrative time times years of service.

Divergence from the Genetic Code

Under David Lawrence's administration, national Kaiser Health Plan policy continued to diverge radically from the KP "genetic code." The "change to what" committee failed for lack of agreement on the basic principles of partnership between the Heath Plan and the Permanente Medical Group participants. Later in 1996, in a bid to weaken the regional partnerships between medical directors and Health Plan regional managers, the Kai-Perm committee, which had met at least annually for decades to coordinate policy, was dissolved.

As the leadership of the PMG Medical Groups saw the partnership being weakened, in response, they reorganized the "Permanente Medical Groups Interregional Services Office" to become the "Permanente Federation." The new Federation was organized to more forcefully represent the interests of the Medical Groups in Central Office, which was now called "Program Office." The articles of Federation required the ratification of all of the Permanente Medical Groups. They were ratified by the HPMG board of directors on December 15, 1996. The political unification of the Permanente Medical Groups was to lead directly to the "Tahoe II" agreements of the next year, which are detailed later.

Financially, 1996 had been a good year for HPMG. Membership growth recovery, a higher marketable dues rate, combined with cost efficiencies, financed a salary scale that approached the MGMA mean. Nineteen ninety seven was to be an even better year.

Kaiser Permanente, Queens, and Kapiolani Health Plans

Influenced by McKinsey's recommendations to seek partnership with non-HMSA plans, starting in January 1997, talks were initiated between KP and the Kapiolani Health Care Program and later with the Queens Health

Care Program to seek out areas of mutual benefit. Both health plans were having difficulty competing with HMSA. The talks didn't amount to much as the interests of the three competitors were too divergent. Both the Kapiolani and Queens Health plans shut down within a year. That was just as well because true partnership with the Kapiolani Health Plan and the Queens Health Plan would have ended the integrated facilities KP strategy as well as the exclusive partnership of Health Plan with HPMG. The strategy of integrating the financially sound KP with the failing Queens and Kapiolani Health Plans while giving up the KP principles of integrated facilities and the Health Plan HPMG partnership was a bad one and likely would have led to the demise of the region.

Mike Chaffin Ratified for a Second Term

At the June 5 board meeting, Mike Chaffin's ratification for a second term was announced. He had been ratified by a comfortable margin with 82 percent approval. The vote was 174 yes, thirty-six no, and one abstention, with 117 necessary for ratification.

Permanente Medical Group Federation Ratified

In July, the Federation leadership, responding to attempts by Kaiser Health Plan to offer only non-exclusive contracts (Health Plan could contract with non- PMG community doctors) to some of the smaller, weaker, Permanente Medical Groups, proposed an amendment to the articles of federation. That amendment stated that any Permanente Medical Group that signed a medical services agreement—without an exclusivity contract with Health Plan and the consent of the Federation—would no longer be a member of the Permanente Federation. This was ratified by the HPMG board of directors at the August 11 meeting and by all twelve Permanente Medical Groups by the end of the year. The stage was set for Tahoe II.

Physician Sudden Impairment Policy

HPMG had established a very comprehensive disciplinary and appeals process, but such a process would necessarily take time. This protected the physicians and HPMG, but what about the patients during that interval? The question was raised by chiefs about what could be done about a sudden physician impairment that could not wait for full due process. The board ratified the following proposal to the bylaws in November:

> The medical director or the physician's chief may summarily suspend any physician with pay upon determination that immediate action must be taken to protect the health, safety or welfare of any patient or if there is a question of substandard professional care. Oral or written notice of the suspension to the physician shall constitute sufficient notice provided that any physician who is suspended for fourteen (14) days or more under this section shall be provided with the notice and the hearing rights in effect at the same time as the suspension.

Before long, it would be used.

Ben Tamura, MD, Chief of Medicine

At the December 18 board meeting, Dr. Benjamin Tamura was appointed the chief of medicine to replace Martin Leftik, MD, who had served since 1985 in this position but was not re-ratified by the board. Ben was to serve first as a revered clinician and chief of medicine and then as associate medical director (AMD) of primary care for twenty years. Ben resigned as AMD of primary care at the end of 2017 to develop important clinical projects prior to his eventual retirement. Dr. Leftik was reassigned to concentrate on the eventually successful implementation of the computerized medical record.

From a financial standpoint, 1997 was even better than 1996. The Hawaii region was accumulating a surplus, which was intended to finance the expansion and renovation of the Moanalua Medical Center.

The MGMA scale increased to 91 percent of the fiftieth percentile—up from 88 percent. At year's end, membership had more than recovered and stood at 210,000 members.

The KP Open-Heart Program

In 2017, the KP Hawaii region celebrated the twentieth anniversary of the first open-heart procedure at the Kaiser Permanente Moanalua Medical Center. The open heart program had a difficult birth.

Expect Resistance to the Internalization of Medical Services

Except when the capital outlay is too much, medical services should be internalized within the KP program whenever possible. It allows direct control of quality, and it is almost always much less costly than when delivered by competitors. This loss of income to the community doctors is almost always the source of the resistance. The internalization of cardiac surgery was the most difficult administrative challenge that the author experienced in a long administrative career.

Open-heart surgery was developed and refined in the fifties and sixties at large academic centers. Hawaii was not too far behind. The first open-heart surgery in Hawaii was performed at the Queens Hospital in 1959. The first coronary bypass surgery in Hawaii was also performed at Queens in 1970. It was performed by Dr. Richard Mamiya, a nationally respected, gifted, and innovative cardiovascular surgeon. While the surgeries were performed at the Queens Medical Center, they were referred from the other Hawaii hospitals, including Kaiser.

By the mid-1970s, cardiac heart surgery had become standardized, more common, and had developed cardiovascular specialty training programs. Academic centers were training cardiovascular surgeons in good numbers, and some established themselves in Honolulu.

In 1975, the largest cardiovascular surgery group in Honolulu was approached by Mike Linderman, the HPMG business manager, about a discounted contract for all KP Hawaii cases. Up to that time, the HPMG cardiologists were free to refer to any cardiac surgeon, and they usually preferred the established Dr. Mamiya. Dr. Mamiya was very busy and had no need to discount his services. A contract with the cardiovascular surgery group for the KP Hawaii heart cases would have provided a considerable savings to KP – but only if the outcomes are equal or superior. The HPMG partnership contract with Health Plan gives HPMG the exclusive right to arrange for care that cannot be internalized by the Medical Group. Dr. Straehley was the HPMG-respected HPMG thoracic (chest) and vascular (blood vessel) surgeon, but he had not trained in cardiac surgery. He was involved with the group's quality assurance program and coordinated with the cardiologists and the cardiovascular surgical group to study the outcomes of cardiac surgery group making the offer and Dr. Mamiya. No significant outcome differences were noted. The cardiologists were, from then on, much more comfortable with the contract.

This arrangement worked well for about a decade, although it was noted in early 1977 that the Hawaii region was doing about five times more cardiac surgery cases per 100,000 than the other KP regions. The issue was never resolved and was probably related to the rapidly evolving and loosening indications for heart surgery. In 1982, Dr. Straehley, anticipating his retirement, invited Philip W. Wright, MD, to look over HPMG with the idea that he might take his place. After visiting the program in November 1982, Dr. Wright was interested. Dr. Wright had obtained his BS at Occidental College, his MD at Northwestern University, and his internship and residency at UCLA. He was in midcareer, and a well-recommended Southern California cardiovascular surgeon. Dr. Straehley had met him through activities of the prestigious Western Thoracic Society. The plan was for Dr. Wright to perform thoracic surgery and some vascular surgery at the Kaiser Moanalua Medical Center, and once established, to partner with the cardiovascular surgery group to do some of the KP heart cases at Queens Hospial. The cardiovascular surgery group had agreed to this.

Dr. Wright arrived in November 1985. Things were going well for about a year as he assumed the vascular and thoracic surgical caseload of the now retired Dr. Straehley with apparently no problems. Problems started in early 1987 when he began his partnership with the cardiovascular surgical group at Queens as per the understanding. While that group cordially welcomed him and introduced him to the Queens cardiovascular community, problems surfaced within a few months.

The cardiovascular surgery group was spreading rumors at Queens that he was a technically poor cardiac surgeon with too many surgical complications. They were not communicating these concerns to him, and they certainly weren't helping him correct any perceived deficiencies. In late 1987, they finally communicated their dissatisfaction to the author as chief of surgical services and Bill Dung, MD, medical director. They stated that they would no longer operate with Dr. Wright on heart cases at Queens. This was something of a surprise. The plan had been from the beginning that Dr. Wright was going to lead the effort to internalize cardiovascular surgery at the Kaiser Moanalua Medical Center, partnering with the Queens cardiovascular group. By the late 1980s, the Kaiser Moanalua Medical Center was the only major private hospital on Oahu without a cardiovascular service, and its reputation suffered accordingly. It was the only high-expense major specialty not internalized by the program.

This was a major problem. If Dr. Wright could not do heart surgery at Queens, he would quickly lose his cardiac surgical skills, and there would be no near-term prospect of internalizing cardiac surgery. On the other hand, heart surgery is not aromatherapy. It must be done right. It was imperative to quickly assess the accuracy of the accusations. It would be wrong to put patients in the hands of an inadequate cardiac surgeon, and such a person could not possibly establish and lead a heart program.

Internal inquiries of our vascular surgeon and pulmonologists surfaced no problems regarding Dr. Wright's competence, but there were no other cardiac surgeons on staff to assess his heart surgery competence. The partnering cardiac surgeons weren't exactly dispassionate bystanders. If the program successfully internalized cardiac surgery, their lucrative contracts could be threatened. Since all of the KP heart cases were being performed at Queens, their base hospital, the shift to doing cases at the Kaiser hospital would be inconvenient. Suspiciously the partners didn't have any problems with Dr. Wright doing chest and vascular surgery at the Kaiser Hospital, including their willingness to assist him with surgery there. Dr. Wright's references were rechecked. New calls were made to Southern California. No issues surfaced.

Preliminary arrangements were quietly made for Dr. Wright to be checked out by the KP Northern California cardiovascular surgery program, which was located at the Kaiser Permanente Hospital in San Francisco. Here was centralized the cardiac surgery care for the two and a half million northern California KP members. The *Los Angeles Times* had rated it as one of the top three cardiac surgery programs in the state of California both in quality and size. It was roughly twice the size of the Queens program.

Dr. Wright was subjected to a harsh test. He was offered the opportunity to forget about cardiac surgery and to continue on with HPMG as a thoracic (chest) and vascular surgeon. Other thoracic surgeons had elected this option in other hospitals in Honolulu. If he had chosen this safe option, then maybe there was something to the partners complaints. At the very least, it would suggest that he didn't have the confidence necessary to start up and lead a new cardiac surgery program against what was now clearly going to be prolonged, major opposition.

As an alternative, he was offered a paid six-month leave of absence to be "checked out" by the KP Northern California cardiac surgery program starting January 1, 1987. Without hesitation, he elected the far riskier "checkout" in San Francisco. For the next six months, he was a full participant in the Northern California cardiac surgery program. About a month before the completion of the "tour of duty" in San Francisco, the author had a half-day meeting with the cardiac surgery chairman to assess Dr. Wright's performance. The chairman was fully supportive of Dr. Wright. He noted that when Wright first got there, his surgical technique was a bit rusty, but that this was to be expected as he had been away from full-time cardiac surgery for over a year except for the cases he did with the uncooperative partners in Honolulu. In San Francisco, he very quickly got up to speed as would be expected for an experienced cardiac surgeon. The chairman noted that he had an exceptional fund of clinical knowledge and the maturity to successfully establish and lead a cardiac surgery program. In summary, he didn't detect any problems.

Shortly after, the partners independently contacted the chair of the San Francisco KP cardiac surgery program. He gave them the same favorable report regarding Dr. Wright's performance. A few days later, the cardiac surgery partners called a midweek dinner at an elegant, even intimidating, private dining room at Alfred's fine dining restaurant in the imposing

Honolulu Century Center building. In attendance were the cardiovascular surgery partners, Mike Linderman, the HPMG business manager, and the HPMG cardiologists. After dinner, they announced that despite the favorable report from San Francisco, they were planning to discontinue their clinical association with Dr. Wright and that if he was allowed to perform cardiac surgery cases by KP, they would refuse to do any KP cardiac surgery cases, including those cases scheduled for the following Monday. Dr. Wright would not be able to do cardiac cases without backup at Queens. They thought they had the program over a barrel.

It was now apparent that quality had not been the real issue with Dr. Wright. He had opted for the high-risk option and had completed a successful checkout in San Francisco. As chief of the surgery services, the partners were told that fairness absolutely dictated that Dr. Wright be given a chance and that they should consider this decision carefully. KP even then covered one-sixth of the population of Hawaii and had experienced more than a quarter century of steady growth. If they carried out this decision, their partnership with KP would be canceled immediately, completely, and more important - permanently.

The partners turned to Mike Linderman and asked if the chief of surgical services spoke for the program. Mike had worked closely with them over the years on the original and subsequent contracts. Nevertheless, without hesitation, Mike supported the stated KP position. They then turned to the cardiologists who were responsible for patients who were already scheduled for surgery and asked them. Rescheduling scheduled heart surgery patients and establishing new relationships with the remaining community cardiac surgeons would be a lot of work and potentially disruptive to patient care. With the exception of one cardiologist, who was at the time making covert preparations to leave HPMG for a community position, they replied that they would proceed to make alternative arrangements for their patients if the partners carried out their threat. Some of the cardiologists' defiance came from their perception of being treated as second-class citizens when they participated in the care of KP patients at Queens—a lingering effect of the long-standing bias against KP by the local medical establishment. Two days later, on the following Friday afternoon, each of the partners called each cardiologist with whom they had worked most closely in the past and informed them that they would no longer be doing cardiac cases for Kaiser Permanente patients. This included the cases scheduled for the following Monday, which they had canceled. As promised, this was the end of a decade of partnership, which was indeed to be immediate, complete, and permanent.

Even though he was in San Francisco, Dr. Wright saved the day. Once he realized that the relationship with the CV partners was souring, he had taken the precaution of making a detailed study of the history of cardiac surgery in Hawaii. In 1987, one of the most respected cardiac surgeons in Hawaii was Dr. Michael Dang. Mike Dang had been born and raised in Hawaii. He had graduated from the locally respected St. Louis High School and then obtained his BS degree at the University of Hawaii. He went on to obtain his MD at the University of Colorado and then did his internship and residency in general surgery at Baylor University in Houston. There, he was selected to do a fellowship in cardiovascular surgery. After completing his training, he was recruited to the faculty of the Baylor heart program. Baylor was considered one of the best and most innovative cardiac surgery programs in the world under the leadership of Dr. Michael Debakey.

In 1979, Dr. Dang decided to return home to Hawaii. Despite his impeccable credentials, the same CV surgery group, now well established at Queens, had resisted Dr. Dang's establishment there. He survived in Hawaii largely because he had been recruited by the Honolulu Medical Group, which was one of the largest medical groups in Hawaii with five cardiologists who would refer all their cases to him.

By 1987, his innate skill and training had refuted any resistance, and he was well respected at Queens. Just before Dr. Wright left for San Francisco, the partners attempted to deny him future cardiac surgical privileges at Queens. Dr. Mike Dang, who chaired the cardiovascular credentials committee, pointed out that if they denied Dr. Wright cardiovascular surgery privileges, his career would be destroyed because Wright would have to report the denial of privileges in any future hospital privilege application. Dr. Dang proposed a period of observation if they wanted to postpone the approval of privileges. This passed by a five (all the non-partner community cardiac surgeons) to four (all the partners) vote. If the partners had been successful with this action, Dr. Wright wouldn't have been able to operate at Queens even if he did check out in San Francisco. Dr. Wright had identified a natural ally. Dr. Dang indicated his willingness to help before Dr. Wright set off for his checkout.

The partners had apparently timed their ultimatum prior to Dr. Wright's return so that he wouldn't be in town to provide damage control. Working the telephones from San Francisco with the full cooperation of Dr. Mike Dang, he arranged for the smooth transition of Kaiser Permanente cardiovascular surgical care from the previous partners to himself and Dr. Dang over the weekend. The cases that had been suddenly canceled by the partners were quickly assumed by Dr. Dang and rescheduled. Upon Dr. Wright's return, he began a partnership and friendship with Dr. Dang that continued on at Queens up to and beyond the internalization of cardiac surgery at the Kaiser Moanalua Medical Center a decade later in 1997.

The partnership with Dr. Mike Dang went well. In 1992, Dr. Jean Leduc was recruited as the second HPMG cardiovascular surgeon. He was a well-trained cardiac surgeon with an exceptional fund of knowledge. Sadly, Jean later developed Parkinson's disease that precluded his continuing as a cardiac surgeon. He had the option to go on full disability, but instead, he took a pay cut to organize and establish an exceptional surgical intensive care unit during his last five years before retirement.

Attention now turned to the long-term goal of cardiac surgery internalization at the Kaiser Moanalua Medical Center. The reasons for the internalization of cardiac surgery were quality of care, reputation, and cost. As financial analyses subsequently demonstrated, the cost of doing cardiac surgery outside of the program was two to three times higher than internalization. Being the largest hospital in the islands without a cardiac surgery program supported the subtle community bias that KP wasn't clinically up to it. Most important, the acuity of cardiac surgery would force an upgrade of all supporting services. There was no place for "Hawaiian time" in any program with a well-functioning cardiac surgery service. All KP patients would benefit.

The program could not just set up a cardiovascular surgery program. It needed state approval through a Hawaii certificate of need (CON) process. In 1974, a certificate of need process had been passed into law. It was intended to control the overbuilding of medical facilities and thus to control the cost of medical care. For marketing reasons, no hospital wants to be left behind regarding access to new medical technology, but such technology is usually costly. A potential exists to have expensive duplicative services that would raise the overall cost of health care in the state. The idea was that any additional services would have to be approved by the Hawaii State Health Planning and Development Agency (SHPDA) to prevent such duplication.

The CON process, which was tried in many states, is controversial. Fifteen states have repealed their certificate of need laws. On one hand, it can prevent the building of expensive duplicative services. On the other hand, it is a bureaucratic, expensive process that could hold back the implementation of worthwhile new medical technologies. It also has the real potential to suppress competition by establishing a government-supported monopoly for a given service, the owner of which service can then charge monopolistically high prices for that service. The CON is also a political process potentially favoring politically well-connected institutions.

In Hawaii, connections matter—and the best connected hospital was Queens. Queens stood to lose a significant portion of its cardiac surgery caseload if it was internalized by KP to the Kaiser Moanalua Medical Center.

With full HPMG and Health Plan backing, the program applied for a cardiac surgery CON. The effort was coordinated by Dr. Wright. Dr. Wright was socially active in the Hawaii community, well-spoken, and strategic. Three public meetings to solicit community comment were part of the CON process. It was no surprise when Queens led what community opposition there was, maintaining that there was no need for another cardiac surgery program in Hawaii.

Among those supporting the KP CON application at public hearings were patients who had been operated upon by the KP cardiac team at Queens. Queens could not, however, overcome the KP argument that internalized costs would be approximately one-third of the current Queens charges. If the CON application was rejected, these charges would have to be passed on to the membership, increasing the overall cost of health care in Hawaii. Since the rationale for the CON process was to reduce the cost of health care in the first place, the CON was approved.

Preparation by the medical center for the new cardiac surgery internalization required an enormous amount of operational work that was successfully completed. Special recognition goes to Alison Miyasaki, can, the only cardiovascular certified clinical nurse specialist who organized and led the exceptional cardiac surgical support team staff during its foundational years.

A few weeks before the scheduled start of the new cardiovascular surgery internalization at the KP Moanalua Medical Center, Queens made an offer to Health Plan to continue to perform KP cases for half the cost they had been charging. This transparent action to derail the internalization of cardiac surgery was declined. The offered discount would still be a third more than the cost of an internalized cardiac surgery program.

On February 10, 1997 the first open-heart case—a two-vessel coronary artery bypass graft—was performed at the Kaiser Medical Center by Drs. Wright and Leduc with Dr. Peter Schneider assisting, and it went well. It was featured on page 3 in the afternoon *Star Bulletin*. In a favorable article, the patient, Taue'etia Taulillili, said, "I praise all the nurses and doctors who helped me. It was the most wonderful thing in my life … It is a miracle." The article noted that 230 to 250 open-heart cases per year were being performed by the HPMG cardiac surgery team.

The KP cardiac surgery outcomes equaled or surpassed those in the community as measured against a rigorous observed to expected mortality standard. In 2000, the Cardiac Surgery Department and cardiology were reorganized into the Kaiser Permanente Heart Program to coordinate all cardiac care. The Cardiology Department was subspecialized with an emphasis on interventional cardiology to minimally invasively treat coronary artery disease and cardiac rhythm disorders. With frequent firsts often publicized in the local newspapers, the heart program earned the respect of the community.

After retirement from HPMG in June 1999, Dr. Wright extended his career for several years going on to follow Dr. Mike Dang as the chief of thoracic and cardiovascular surgery at Queens Hospital. Within a year of the fateful dinner meeting at Alfred's, with no KP business, the partners' group fell apart. Is business war? Not really, but it can get very nasty.

1998: Call Centers

At the January 22 board meeting, Jay Post of clinic engineering presented two approaches to the telephone appointment-making process. Offered was the highly centralized California approach where appointments were scheduled in large call centers remote from the clinics that they served. They were cheaper, but there was little or no accountability or communication between the actual clinics being served. The alternative was a refinement of the decentralized, clinic-based process being used in Hawaii. There was a strong preference for the Hawaii decentralized program. It was noted that the satisfaction with telephone appointment access in the Hawaii region was far higher than in the regions that used call centers. The call center idea was put on hold.

Drugs and Alcohol—Zero Tolerance

At the April 2 board meeting, a strict zero-tolerance drug and alcohol policy was passed.

Neighbor Islands Management

On July 2, it was announced that there was to be a change in the clinic administration of the neighbor islands. Instead of one PIC there would be two—one for Maui and one for the Big Island of Hawaii. Donna McCleary, MD, who had been the physician in charge of the neighbor islands since 1981 and had presided over the membership growth and then expansion to the Big Island, was appointed a HPMG vice president assigned to concentrate on the state and federal Medicaid and Medicare programs.

KP National Financial Crisis

At the September 17 board meeting, the echoes of the worst national KP financial crisis in modern times were being heard in Hawaii. It was announced that the Texas Permanente Medical Group was to be dissolved along with the Texas region. Also announced by DeeJay Mailer, regional president, was an eighteen-to-twenty-four-month KP National freeze on all capital expenditure.

Year-End Financial Results

As of December 31, 1998, membership stood at 215,000, but there was no significant regional or HPMG surplus. Despite the highest membership of all time, it included six thousand point-of-service members who were proving to be a very high-cost, unprofitable population and were difficult to service or please.

1999

On January 17, 1999, DeeJay Mailer announced her resignation as regional president to the board of directors. She had been recruited to the position of chief of operations of Health Net by Cora Tellez, who was now chief executive officer of that company, which numbered more than two million members—ten times the size of KP Hawaii. Bruce Behnke was appointed the new regional president. Bruce had been the capable hospital administrator during DeeJay's administration. He had excellent credentials, having served in hospital administrative roles at the Mayo Clinic's Rochester Methodist Hospital and then in the Southern California region.

At the April 15 board meeting, Dr. Wright's retirement was announced to take effect at the end of the month. Dr. Francis Duhay took his place as department chief. At the May 6 meeting, there was a discussion about whether alternative medicine should be a Health Plan benefit. There was a spirited discussion, the upshot of which was that if we were going to be forced to offer alternative medicine as a covered benefit by the market, then it should be offered as a rider outside of the program by outside practitioners in a carefully monitored environment. It was financed by a 10 percent elective program rider that was expected to pay for itself to avoid diverting resources from the internalized, scientifically based medical care of the core program. There was a strong feeling expressed during the discussion that there is medicine that works and medicine that does not. The scientific method—based on statistically valid, blinded, well-designed, placebo-controlled studies—is the only thing that separates the two. To avoid harm or interference with evidence-based (scientific) medical treatment, what was to be covered and who would be credentialed needed to

ALBERT J. MARIANI, M.D.

be carefully controlled. At the same meeting, the importance of board certification was again emphasized.

Other Events in 1999

Between 1958 and 1985, the Kaiser Medical Center had been located in Waikiki, and there was a significant amount of Waikiki tourist medical emergency business contributing to the bottom line. This was lost when KP moved out of Waikiki. On August 1, 1999, the New Ventures Department, led by Dr. Pregitzer, opened a fee-for-service emergency clinic in the heart of Waikiki, hoping to reconstitute the tourist business that had been lost when the hospital moved out of Waikiki. While a promising idea, like many freestanding acute care clinics, it eventually proved to be unprofitable. Since the rationale was to provide additional resources for the core program, when it did not, it was appropriately shut down.

By the mid-1990s, Queens and Kapiolani were the two largest health systems in the state outside of KP. Their leadership was increasingly worried about the non-KP HMSA health plan monopoly, which controlled their income. Like KP, they attempted to establish their own health plans. While they possessed clinical expertise, they did not have the Health Plan marketing or budget control expertise of HMSA. Nevertheless, their plans grew quickly. At one point, the Queens Health Plan, with more than 150,000 members and growing, threatened KP's status as the largest HMO in the state. Unfortunately for them, a large membership did not guarantee profits—both programs operated at a loss. It was announced at the August 5 board meeting that the Queens Health Program was to cease operations. Shortly thereafter, at the October 7 board meeting, it was announced that the Kapiolani Health Plan was to close. The provider attempt by the state's two largest hospital systems to establish financial independence from HMSA had failed.

At the October 21 board meeting, Stacey Honda, MD, was selected to be the chief of pathology. Thus, another clinically sharp, administratively capable, multi-decade chief began her administrative career.

For two years, the Information Technology Department had been preparing for Y2K. Y2K referred to various Armageddon-like scenarios that were supposed to happen on January 1, 2000. Early computer programs often used only the last two digits of a date to save two bytes at a time when memory was expensive—for example 1999 encoded as 99—was supposed to be the cause. At midnight on December 31, high-level program executives were on hand at the Moanalua Hospital to manage unanticipated disasters. Nothing much happened.

2000

At the January 6 board meeting, the Mental Health Department (formerly Psychiatry) announced another name change to the Department of Behavioral Health. On January 26, the board passed the fair hearing protocol. In March, a contract was to be offered to Geoffrey Sewell, MD, as a hospitalist. He had been president of his class in medical school and had set up the hospitalist program at Emmanuel Hospital in California and had an interest in electronic medical records. Geoff was to go on to be the fourth president of HPMG six years later.

Also in March, it was announced that Leighton Hasegawa was chosen as the chief financial officer; he was to replace Mike Linderman who was to retire later in the year. Mike had served as the first CFO of HPMG for a quarter of a century and deserved much of the credit for putting HPMG on a sound financial footing. Leighton went on to a multi-decade career with HPMG, continuing and improving upon Mike's legacy of financial accountability. Universally admired and clearly recognizing the need for competitive compensation to maintain a quality medical group, he was and is distinguished for his kindness, fairness, personal discipline, and most important, capability.

In June, the board passed the HPMG Family Leave Program providing for up to twelve weeks leave of absence without pay for family illness. At the June 15 board meeting, Cal James, the chief executive officer of the PMG Federation Ventures program, presented a new investment program being offered by the Federation to the Permanente Medical Groups. He proposed that HPMG invest $120,000 in a Federation offering, which was to invest in emerging medical technologies and services. At the July 7 board meeting, the offer was turned down. The arguments against participation were: (1) HPMG is not a venture capitalist firm—it doesn't have the expertise to judge good or bad investments. (2) Such ventures would divert attention from the main mission of delivering patient care. (3) It would be diverting funds from individual HPMG physician compensation that could be invested, or not, by individual HPMG physician's as they saw fit.

Electronic Medical Record

Envisioned by Sidney Garfield and proposed for exploration by Dr. Yi Ching in the early 1960's. The computerized medical record was seriously explored in the Hawaii region since the early 1980s. By the early 1990s, the program had committed to a unified electronic (computerized) medical record. Earlier development had been impractical because of inadequate and expensive computer power, memory capacity, wide-area digital communications systems, and workable software. By the mid-1990s, the very rapid development of both hardware and software had lowered the barriers to implementation.

Hawaii had decided by the mid-1990s to become a pioneering region for an electronic medical record. The rationale was based upon the lead that it would give the region both in implementation and influence. At the March 20, 1997, board meeting, it was announced that the Hawaii region would partner with the small startup software company called Oceana and its nascent WAVE electronic medical record software. This was done with the blessing of Program Office. At the same time, the national program was considering programs being developed by IBM, Oasis, Oceana, and Epic. At this point, the technology wasn't mature enough to support a unified KP National system.

One of the most powerful medical advances in the history of medicine has been the implementation of an electronic medical record. The electronic medical record provides three communication innovations that had never been reliably achieved before:

1. The medical record can be available in real time twenty-four hours a day and at any clinic location. There is no longer and need to store bulky paper records or to maintain the large staff infrastructure to

transport the paper records to where they were needed. KP Hawaii was one of the best for record availability, but despite enormous effort, at no time did clinic and hospital record availability get better than 80 percent. That availability was even less in emergency situations where the records were needed the most.

2. The records are filed by the program in a standardized way and easily searchable through data filters. Importantly, they are 100 percent legible. It eliminates the need to make jokes about physician handwriting.

3. Most important is the potential to link data and provide information for real-time medical decision support.

In early 1998, Mike Chaffin appointed Peggy Latare, MD, to lead the implementation of an electronic medical record. Also important to the effort were Drs. Martin Leftik and Howard Landa. In mid-August 1998, the national program announced that it had decided to partner with IBM to build a proprietary, program-wide electronic medical record system called CIS (Clinical Information System). Hawaii had been pioneering the Oceana startup. Central Office had concluded that Oceana did not have the size to scale up a national program of millions of patients in multiple regions, so the Oceana effort was terminated at a national KP cost of about $18 million. Oceana was later bought out by Cerner, another large medical software company and the chief competitor to Epic.

The original KP National rationale was along the lines of "no one ever got fired for choosing IBM." Someone should have. After two years of expensive development, the IBM product, CIS, was a complete failure. It would have been nearly impossible to use in a clinical setting, it was expensive, it was crash prone, which would be a clinical care disaster, and couldn't be scaled up to a medical care organization the size of Kaiser Permanente in any reasonable time frame. Taking a $400 million loss in 2002 the KP under its new CEO George Halvorson abandoned the CIS initiative. The organization fell back on the Epic program still being developed in the Northwest region with good success. Once this was decided, progress was rapid.

In Hawaii, the Epic-based Health Connect was fully implemented in the clinics by 2005 and in the hospital by 2009. It cost $4 billion to implement the Health Connect Electronic Medical Record program-wide, but it was worth it. From then on, for the first time in program history, medical records were 100 percent available region wide and eventually nationally twenty-four hours a day, they were always legible, and the structure was in place for unlimited, online, decision support. Peggy Latare described the process as akin to pushing a large stone up a steep hill.

Dale Crandall CFO

At the September 7 board meeting, it was announced that Dale Crandall was appointed president of Kaiser Permanente nationally. He was an established turnaround executive who took over most of the CEO duties from David Lawrence. He was largely successful at extricating KP National from the 1998 budget crisis by reversing some of the failed policies and by applying strict financial discipline.

Chief's Approval for Extra Educational Leave

At the September 21 board meeting, the executive committee policy of requiring chief's approval for extra educational leaves prior to executive committee approval was endorsed. Also endorsed was a policy of not crediting back vacation days for sickness during vacations.

Supplemental Employee Retirement Program (SERP)

At the November 20 board meeting, a major retirement policy modification was passed. The retirement amount had traditionally been based upon salary. The IRS passed a ruling limiting the amount of income that could be placed in a retirement account. This amount was less than the amount necessary to fund the retirement of some of the higher-paid specialties. For these physicians, to maintain this policy, it was necessary to separate the retirement into the standard Permanente Physician Retirement Plan (PPRP), and for those physicians exceeding the IRS limits, the remainder was deposited into a Supplemental Employee Retirement Program (SERP).

At the December 31 board meeting, it was announced that the program had reached 217,000 members. Despite the membership growth, the financial performance was not as good as it had been in the past, but it was good enough to provide a program surplus.

2001

At the July 19 meeting, standards for associateship were ratified by the board. Over the prior decade, HPMG standards for conferring associateship had gradually become stricter as more competitive compensation packages led to more candidates for each open position. Not all chiefs adhered to the newer, stricter, but informal expectations when presenting candidates to the board for associateship. Therefore, the board formalized these standards. All candidates presented were required to have current board certification. No candidate would be presented who was in the bottom tenth percentile of the peer-to-peer or quality-of-service surveys. Indeed, it was expected that any candidate presented would be at a higher average percentile than that of the department. Finally, there should be no negative quality assurance or risk-management trends. New candidates were expected to be strengthening and not weakening departments.

At the October 18 board meeting, it was announced that HPMG physicians on the neighbor islands would be compensated at par by HMSA for medical services. HMSA maintained its near health care monopoly outside of KP in Hawaii by offering doctors two options: par and non-par. Non-par physicians had to bill and collect directly from the patients. HMSA would then make a small payment directly to the patients. This payment was typically much lower than the doctor's fees. Not surprisingly, many patients just kept the payment and didn't pay the doctor's bill. To be a par physician, the physician had to accept the HMSA fee schedule, which was low relative to the mainland USA. HMSA would pay the physician minus any co-pay that the doctor was expected to collect at the time of service. Balance billing—additional fees to make up for HMSA low-fee schedule—was prohibited. Because KP was HMSA's only real competitor in Hawaii, prior to this time, HMSA had not allowed KP doctors to participate as par providers. The reason for the change of heart was that because of high overhead, small populations, and low HMSA reimbursements, the specialty care infrastructure on the neighbor islands was collapsing and only KP was maintaining such an infrastructure for its own patients. HMSA still did not allow PAR reimbursement for KP physicians on Oahu.

In October and November, the board ratified a leave of absence policy and a workplace harassment policy. Despite continued growth, the divisible surplus at year end was only five hundred dollars. The good news was that HPMG had doubled its size in fifteen years with 260 associates. Additionally, there were dozens of doctors on associate track who had not been with the program long enough to become associates. HPMG was by far the largest medical group in the state of Hawaii.

2002

At the March 7 board meeting, it was announced that the hospital bed days for Medicare patients was the best in the program. This was due to the internalized Skilled Nursing Facility (SNF) and the efficient management of the Community (Outside) Services Department led by Geoff Sewell. It was also announced that George Halvorson, an HMO executive from Minnesota, had been selected as the acting CEO of KP as of May 1 and CEO upon the retirement of David Lawrence at the end of 2002. At the May 16 board meeting, the sick leave and temporary disability policies were updated as was the board of directors' election process at the October 3 board meeting.

At the November 21 board meeting, Bruce Behnke announced his retirement on January 3, 2003. He had served for three years. He was frustrated with national KP centralization policies, which were progressively limiting regional autonomy, and the mysterious disappearance of the Hawaii surplus, which was tapped by Program Office to fund the failed region shutdowns. That surplus had been earmarked for the Kaiser Moanalua Medical Center expansion.

The years 2000 to 2002 were years of stability, growth, standardization of policy, and prosperity for HPMG. Similar to a previous time of prosperity and stability—1977 to 1980—many of the next generation of doctor leaders were recruited. They included such notables as Geoffrey

Sewell, David Bell, Michael Caps, John Chen, Karen Ching, Tarquin Collis, James Griffith, Dean Hu, Todd Kuwaye, Keith Ogasawara, Samir Patel, Kathryn Shon, and Mark Yamamura.

At the end of the year came the retirement of Steve Miller. Steve had joined HPMG in 1978 and had served as chief of surgery from 1979 until 1983. Subsequently, he served as HPMG vice president of finance under Bill Dung and Mike Chaffin and had been instrumental in the development of the rational staffing and compensation policy. As a clinician he was the only retina specialist in the Ophthalmology Department. He was asked to stay on as a consultant, and he did so until 2007.

2003

At the beginning of 2003, the future of the Hawaii region appeared very bright. There was a new regional president, Janice Head, who came highly recommended based upon her work managing the Central California service areas. The Hawaii region was setting KP National standards for quality of service and care. Independent sources rated it in the top five nationally for Medicaid and top twenty for Medicare quality of care. There were matching high overall national rankings in news magazines. Locally, it was winning corporate awards. Other regions were sending delegations to Hawaii to learn how to duplicate this performance. The region was continuing to grow in membership as the dissolution of the Queens and Kapiolani Health plans released tens of thousands of patients who were forced to find a new local health plan - many tried KP. Membership continued to grow and was to peak in 2005 at 225,000. HPMG had experienced more than a decade of accelerating growth, improved compensation and quality of life, the peaceful establishment of wide-ranging policies and procedures, and steady quality of care and service progress.

At the February 6 meeting, a formula to determine the medical director's salary was ratified. It would consist of the average of the medical directors of the regions outside of California and would be adjusted every two years. At the March 6 board meeting, the "disruptive physician policy" was ratified. In May, the moving allowance was adjusted for inflation. In September, the National Committee for Quality Assurance (NCQA) rated KP Hawaii as second in the Pacific and the top KP region for Healthcare Effectiveness Data and Information (HEDIS) care measures. At the November 6 board meeting, the HPMG pension policy was revised to include domestic partners.

2004

In May, the Nanaikeola Clinic on leeward Oahu and the Obstetrics and Gynecology Department went live with Health Connect. At the August 31 board meeting, teeth were put into the board-certification policy. For the first three years of un-boarded status, there would be a $1,000 pay reduction. At three years, it would increase to 10 percent of salary, at four years, 15 percent of salary, and at five years, 20 percent of salary. Already passed had been a policy that board certification was required for associateship. With this new policy, HPMG indicated that it really wanted a board-certified doctors group. In September, a revised family leave policy was ratified, allowing up to three months of unpaid family leave. Also in September, Program Office announced the "Thrive" ads would replace all local advertising programs. In Hawaii, that meant the end of the "Treating Patients Like Family" advertising program that had resonated with the Hawaii market. Nationally, the $40 million "Thrive" advertising program emphasizing preventive care was generally considered successful.

2005

Alas, a perfect storm broke in 2005 that threatened the very existence of the KP Hawaii region.

Adverse Market Trends

The oldest funding principle of KP is prepayment. It had saved Sidney Garfield's Desert Center contractor's hospital from bankruptcy and had been a core program principle ever since. By having population-based, fixed prepayment, finances were stabilized and facilities and staff planning and investment could occur, preventive care was incentivized, and fee-for-service billing overhead would be largely eliminated. By the early 2000s, with more than 95 percent of the income from prepaid dues, KP billing departments were small and unsophisticated.

Most Americans were insured through their employers. This began as a way to recruit employees during the labor shortages brought on by World War II. Health care costs had remained modest throughout the fifties and early sixties, and medical coverage had become a standard benefit. With improved, but increasingly expensive, technology, drugs, government-subsidized health care and increasing benefits, the cost of health care began to grow much faster than the consumer price index. It had become a serious and worsening overhead burden for business. Businesses were naturally looking to minimize this unsustainable and growing expense that hurt their competitive standing in an increasingly free trade international environment.

Fee-for-service health plans tried to control health care costs in the early nineties by closely regulating services with aggressive pre-authorization policies which, when abused, resulted in a downright unethical denial of care. While initially lowering the rate of health care inflation, it was increasingly unpopular. Individual and class action lawsuits as well as legislation addressed the worst of the abuses, limiting the ability of health plans to further lower rates by these methods. Nevertheless, business continued to demand lower rates. Some eliminated health care benefits entirely. The remaining option was to offer "skinny" health plans with high deductibles paid by the patient and low monthly premiums paid by the employers. Health plans obliged. Since most were fee-for-service indemnity plans, they already had a fee-for-service billing infrastructure in place. It was just a matter of changing the way that services were billed: lower payments from employers and higher co-pays from patients.

This was not the KP model, which was based upon comprehensive prepaid coverage with few and low deductibles to lower the barriers to early treatment of disease. Since employers wanted low-cost, high-deductible plans, any health plan that did not offer matching low-cost, high-deductible plans would be eliminated from consideration.

The KP National response in the early 2000s was the "New Generation Products," which attempted through high-deductible fee-for-service-like plans to match the low monthly rates of competitors. While there was little choice but to offer skinny plans if KP was to survive, the lack of a billing infrastructure prior to the "New Generation Product" launch in the Hawaii region proved to be a marketing disaster. Patients had preferred KP precisely because they didn't have to deal with medical bills once the dues had been prepaid—usually by their employers. Now they did—and the billing system wasn't ready. The medical staff was unused to charging for services beyond nominal, simple co-pays. Now there were complicated, unresourced, co-payment procedures that were required but not in place. Often the charges were missed. Even if the charges were filed, they often were not collected because there was little or no infrastructure in place to collect. Thus, KP was delivering comprehensive care at sharply discounted rates because the new, substantial co-payments were either not being charged or collected. This began to show in 2003 when records were being set for increased membership while at the same time there was poor financial performance. This worsened with each passing year. Ill-fated attempts to rapidly build the required billing system were fraught with problems. KP Plans had maximum yearly deductibles built into the contracts, but the billing department had no way of knowing when the maximum deductible payments were exceeded, so patients continued to get billed. When patients complained about the overbilling, they were given a large manila envelope and told to put their receipts into the envelope, and when they exceeded their maximum deductible, they were supposed to contact the billing office so that billing could be stopped. This kludge of a workaround was obviously not acceptable. A low point was reached in 2005 at a meeting of upper-level Health Plan and HPMG executives at which the billing department was presenting their solutions. They stated that the worst had passed. Simultaneously, a recent charge statement for two cents with two shiny pennies taped to it recently received by one of the audience was being passed around the room.

As membership peaked at 225,000, members were expressing real dissatisfaction with the billing process as they received multiple bills for the same service and were not being credited for payments made. That and the inflexibility of the Marketing Department to design competitive plans were simply too much. A membership slide began late in the year and accelerated until 2009. Eventually more than 15,000 members were lost largely due to billing problems. With the program hemorrhaging membership and co-pays not being collected to make up for artificially low prepaid dues rates, the program was descending into a serious financial crisis.

Compliance

Another consequence of the inadequate billing infrastructure led to a federal investigation of the region by the Office of the Inspector General of the Department of Health and Human Services. The consequences of a bad review had the potential to shut down the region.

The first incident was a due to a confusing credentialing issue. A physician assistant in the Dermatology Department had started his practice long before the initiation of a 2001 physician assistant licensing requirement by the state of Hawaii. He had a certificate from the navy credentialing him as a PA. He also had a certification given him for his work as a PA by Hawaii Governor George Ariyoshi (1974–1986). He had checked with the state after the PA licensing law was passed and was reassured by the response that he was grandfathered as a PA, and there was language in the law that seemed to cover his practice. A whistleblower turned him in, maintaining that he was practicing without a license. It looked like an amicable settlement with the state could be reached and friendly but desultory discussions were ongoing.

Shortly thereafter, the chief of anesthesia noticed that nurse anesthetist services were being billed improperly by the billing department. He brought it to the attention of the HPMG leadership, which brought it to the attention of the appropriate civil authorities. Again, after it was reported to the authorities, desultory but generally cooperative discussions ensued. Unexpectedly, the state, spurred on by an aggressive assistant attorney general who was later discredited, suddenly turned hostile. At about this time, an anesthesiologist who was being discharged for cause decided that this would be a good time to declare herself a whistleblower and claim that nurse anesthetists were not being properly supervised. One of the causes of the discharge had been that individual's difficulty with working with nurse anesthetists. Nurse anesthetists had been an integral and successful component of the Anesthesia Department for decades.

Local leadership wanted to challenge the charges, but Program Office insisted upon settlement.

The investigation uncovered billing discrepancies but no patient care issues or evidence of intentional fraud. The settlement included a $1.9 million payment and a five-year stern corporate integrity agreement. The corporate integrity agreement subjected the region to annual billing and coding audits and also mandatory time-consuming corporate integrity training for all providers. More than a quarter of the award was awarded to the Medicaid Investigation Division and hundreds of thousands of dollars were awarded to the whistleblowers. Many questioned the self interest of both. It could have been much worse—bad enough to close the region. To the credit of the HPMG administration, the corporate integrity agreement was strictly adhered to with no further issues. This incident was embarrassing and discouraging, especially to a leadership that had worked so hard for decades to continually improve the quality, service, and reputation of the program. In subsequent years, several other large health care entities in Hawaii had fines levied by the same Medicaid investigation agency.

Botched Hospital Expansion

The hospital, now twenty years old, was overdue for expansion and renovation. In the early eighties, during the planning and construction of the new Kaiser Moanalua Medical Center, there was extensive cooperation between HPMG and Health Plan. Clinical Department leaders were sought out to offer planning suggestions to improve clinical and workflow outcomes. For example the Emergency Department was placed next to the Diagnostic Imaging Department. Most of them were adopted. Central Office, with Jim Vohs as CEO, saw the regions outside of California as Kaiser Permanente "missions" that could spread KP ideals to eventually becoming a nationwide—even worldwide—health care movement. The financial backing by the national organization had been essential to the construction of the new Hawaii hospital. Their contributions to planning were helpful based upon extensive construction experience elsewhere in KP. There was little interference with the local, detailed planning. The hospital came in on time and under budget. It received architectural awards and served the region very well.

The situation in 2005 was very different. The attitude of Program Office toward the regions was now appeared to be centered upon the corporate bottom line—not spreading the ideals of Kaiser Permanente. Regions were expected not only to support themselves but also various Program Office-Health Plan centralization services supported by a mandatory, burdensome, corporate tax levied against the KP regions.

Since 1998, regions had been shut down in Texas, North Carolina, New England, and Kansas City because they couldn't. At the January 4, 2001, board meeting, the master plan for the Kaiser Medical Center was presented. Program growth coupled with the restricted expansion potential of the Moanalua site required that some services be moved off-site. It was decided to keep the procedural (operating room) specialties at the Moanalua hospital and move most primary care off-site to the clinic hubs of Mapunapuna, Honolulu, and Waipio. Stakeholders were then invited to participate in the renovation design, which they did. The product was two three-inch binders documenting this work.

"Value engineers" were then brought in by KP National facilities to reduce costs. There was little local input into the final building contracts—nor was such input welcomed. The final result was that there were a number of serious problems that required redoing much of the work, long delays, and increased (doubled) rather than decreased costs. There is a lesson to be learned. The lesson is that when outside consultants are being brought in on a building project, local leadership should make sure that there is relentless, close, local involvement, whether it is welcomed or not, so that everything of value is not engineered out of the project by value engineers.

Breakdown of Partnership Communication

With Bruce Behnke's retirement on January 2, 2003, Janice L. Head was announced as the new president and regional manager of the Hawaii region. She came well recommended. Her career began as a registered nurse with a BS and MS in nursing from the University of Colorado and a MBA from Northern Illinois University. She had spent eleven years in various administrative positions at Intermountain Health Care in Salt Lake City, Utah. She joined KP in 1996 and served successfully in in various management and executive positions. A KP public relations release stated:

> "Jan Head earned her promotion to president of the Hawaii region with her excellent work as head of our TriCentral Service Area," said George Halvorson chairman and chief executive officer of Kaiser Foundation Health Plan and Hospitals. "Her commitment to service, quality care, and staff development all made her the best candidate for the job."

The Tri-Central service area encompassed 700,000 central California KP members. Unfortunately, managing a California service area was not the same as managing an autonomous region 2,400 miles away from the Oakland Program Office. Most of the executive functions, such a marketing, government relations, and regional facilities planning, were performed in the California regional offices and not by service area managers.

Jan, a pleasant person, had a hands-off style not previously experienced by the regional leadership. This was especially true for HPMG leaders who had been accustomed to close communication with previous Health Plan regional presidents. It was this communication that fostered coordination and cooperation between Health Plan and HPMG. It was typical for major chiefs to have had fewer than two meetings with her during her entire four-year tenure. Some chiefs and HPMG vice presidents had none. Coordination with leadership partner Mike Chaffin was also minimal.

For the first two years, things went relatively well. Jan had an experienced team in place when she arrived, and most routine issues were handled by them. When the perfect storm of inflexible Health Plan offerings, billing problems, and dysfunctional hospital construction came in the second half of 2005, requiring decisive executive action, things came apart fast. By early 2006, her leadership team was dissolving. By mid-2006, the vice president of business development (formerly known as the Health Plan manager-sales) since 1998 had resigned due to falling membership, the vice president of finance had resigned because of declining financial performance and the "New Generation Product" billing issues, and the director of facilities resigned because of worsening problems with the hospital renovation. The very well-respected, long-serving, vice president of human resources, Kaki Jennings, decided that this would be a good time to tender her resignation to care for her two young grandchildren.

At a Health Plan all-hands meeting in the fall, Jan's presentation clearly indicated that she was overwhelmed. By then, Mike Chaffin had already announced his early retirement, and HPMG was in the process of choosing his successor. In early November, harsh belt-tightening measures were announced along with newspaper headlines featuring the layoff of fifty KP employees. Even these measures would only temporarily stave off financial failure if the dire membership and financial trends continued.

A delegation from Program Office, led by Greg Adams, a rising national KP executive, visited the region with preliminary plans for a Program Office takeover of local Health Plan management. Bad ideas surfaced during those meetings, including aggressive recruiting of loss-generating Medicaid members to raise membership, expensive outsourcing the most advanced specialty services, and separate Health Plan contracts for non-HPMG providers. These proposed policies did not bode well for the future of the region. Indeed, when Program Office previously took over the troubled Texas, Northeast, North Carolina, and Kansas City regions with similar recommendations, they all failed within two years. On November 3, Janice Head announced her resignation at the end of the year. The Hawaii region was in serious trouble.

Succession Planning

By 2005, the author was seriously concerned about the lack of HPMG succession planning. The "middle" generation of leadership was approaching retirement. By 2009, when Mike Chaffin's third term would expire, the long-standing leadership team, including Mike, Gladys Ching, and the other leaders of the middle generation would be at or well past retirement age. The culture of excellence progressed during Mike's administration as a result of HPMG stability, a fair compensation package, and good leadership. The recruiting had become very selective. There were fifty-two candidates for the single open cardiac surgery position in 2002. Associateship required board certification as well as high patient satisfaction and peer performance. Associateship was no longer automatic—nor did associateship provide immunity from accountability. Mike had inherited a HPMG riven by strife and factionalism. Slow, careful process had brought about peace and stability and steady progress toward accountability and excellence. The HPMG of 2005 was very different from the HPMG of 1990.

The next generation of potential leaders were typically outstanding clinicians, popular, exhibiting an exemplary work ethic, and were of very good character. They were impatient with any residual mediocrity in HPMG and had no memory or knowledge of the intragroup conflict that had plagued HPMG during the first half of its existence. Without mentoring or leadership experience, this impatience could translate into zealotry, and zealotry quickly becomes unpopular. There was a real risk that this exceptional group would become disillusioned, and their talents would be lost to HPMG through resignation from HPMG or simply a loss of interest in leadership. There was a widening rift developing between them and Mike Chaffin's low-key, deliberate style of administration. This quickly widened when the perfect storm suddenly hit in mid-2005 and rapidly worsened.

Mike had wanted the author to become chief of specialties since 1996. Agreement could not be reached on the "with responsibility goes authority" part of it. Nine years later, things were much different. The author understood that if agreement could be reached with Mike, then it would provide an excellent opportunity to mentor the next generation of leaders, so the plan was resuscitated. As it stood, the author was chief of surgical services (seven surgery sections) and chief of the Heart Program (cardiovascular surgery and cardiology), and these departments were functioning well. The new position would be chief of specialty services. It would include the surgical specialties, including anesthesia, the medical specialties including the hospitalists, as well as the Pathology, Diagnostic Imaging, and Emergency Departments. Each of these chiefs would be appointed by the chief of specialty services with the concurrence of Dr. Chaffin and ratified by the board. Each would have chief rank, including chief administrative pay, administrative time, and advisory board status. The concept was subject to re-ratification in one year. Finally, the chief of specialty services position would cease to exist on the election of the next HPMG president—presumably in 2009. This was proposed by Mike Chaffin and ratified by the board of directors on July 21, 2005.

For chief of surgical specialty services, Dr. Mark Santi was chosen. Mark had taken the orthopedics section from one of the most difficult to manage surgery department sections to a model subspecialized surgery section. He had an exceptional sense of humor and a very pleasant personality, but this did not prevent him from having high performance expectations. He was an outstanding strategist. He was a respected clinician in his own right—perennially listed among *Honolulu Magazine*'s top doctors.

Dr. Christine Fukui was chosen for chief of medical specialties. Having joined HPMG in 1980 Chris was the model HPMG doctor. Hardworking, popular, and clinically exceptional, she had built the well-respected Pulmonary Medicine Department from scratch. She was also perennially listed among *Honolulu Magazine*'s top doctors.

The most controversial appointment was that of Dr. Geoffrey Sewell. Geoff was a smart, articulate, high-energy, personable problem-solver with previous leadership experience. Having an exemplary work ethic, he would legitimately and consistently confront mediocrity when he encountered it. He did so appropriately and carefully—but firmly. Those on the receiving end complained, and this put him out of favor with the administration, which placed a high premium on everyone getting along. This policy, however, was distancing the administration from a new generation of outstanding physicians who were far less forgiving of mediocrity. Geoff was a subsection leader in the Hospital Medical Services Department in the Department of Medicine so he was familiar with the issues that had plagued that department since its founding fifteen years earlier. He had bold solutions to these chronic problems, but no one was listening. He needed a chance to carry out these ideas by giving him the necessary authority, but in a relatively safe political and mentored environment.

With this new specialty restructuring, there was an organization in which to place the three dozen or so idealistic, accountably activist, next-generation doctors into mentored positions of authority such as section chiefs, committee chairs, and elected board positions. Apart from acquiring experience with day-to-day management issues, such as recruiting, discipline, schedules, and service, they needed region-wide accountability-reform experience. Their energy was focused on putting teeth into the now decade-old, validated, respected, peer-to-peer and patient-satisfaction surveys. The success of these efforts fundamentally changed the character of HPMG. That story gets its own chapter later. During what would prove to be an all-too-brief apprenticeship, these young, bright, reformers rapidly learned important lessons about the limits of human nature and the value of patience and compromise without sacrificing ideals.

Geoff Galbraith, vice president of quality improvement since the start of Mike Chaffin's administration, was a sponsor of the new Medicine and Management Program. This midlevel management course was organized and sponsored by the Colorado, Hawaii, and Northwest Permanente Medical Groups. There were three one-week sections held every four months in each of the sponsoring regions for all of the attendees. It was well organized and considered to be worthwhile. Dr. Galbraith had led the 2005 group from Hawaii that contained several of the "young activists." Responsible for mentoring a group of new and relatively inexperienced managers, the author received the endorsement of Mike Chaffin and Geoff Galbraith to lead the new managers, who had not attended the 2005 sessions, in the 2006 sessions. This was an immersive, intense, participatory management education experience that provided an invaluable opportunity to observe the performance of each of the future leaders. One stood out.

Since becoming chief of hospital specialties, Geoff Sewell had more than lived up to his promise. Within three months, he had resolved hospitalist staffing and work schedule issues that had plagued the department since its organization fifteen years earlier. The solutions were imaginative, innovative, and peacefully achieved.

In January 2006, during the one-week Colorado portion of the Medicine and Management training session, Geoff's energy, strategic thinking, engaging personality, and belief in excellence was on full display. On Friday evening, while the rest of the group was out celebrating after completing a successful first session, with the outside temperature at minus twenty to thirty degrees Fahrenheit, Geoff and the author had a casual dinner in the hotel restaurant that evolved into an interview.

The next day, while walking with him between meetings, the author opened the conversation by saying, "You need to run for president of HPMG." His name had not come up as a presidential candidate among those concerned about succession nor apparently in his own mind. He had been in HPMG for only six years and in a major management position for only six months. He immediately brought up these disadvantages. "Not important," was the reply.

During those six years, he had developed an excellent reputation, few if any respected enemies, and he had demonstrated the right stuff for executive leadership. Next, he said, "Suppose I don't want to do it" but not "I refuse to be considered."

The droll reply was, "It's not important what you want."

A recurring theme of Medicine and Management during the previous week had been that duty takes precedence over self-interest if one aspired to be an effective leader. He was the kind of person to take such concepts to heart. The discussion next turned to the scope and risks of such a responsible position. While the depth of the subsequent informed consent discussion about being a HPMG president may have been somewhat "abbreviated", clearly the fire was lit.

Back in balmy Hawaii the following week, with some respected HPMG opinion makers, the author individually discussed Geoff as a potential candidate for HPMG president. The response was, in every case, positive. It was like a light bulb going off in their minds when his name was proposed. The idea rapidly snowballed. The "young activists" and HPMG now had an outstanding candidate for its next president. The next HPMG presidential election was expected to be in 2009 when Mike Chaffin's third term as president of HPMG expired. The next election was not to happen in thirty-six months—but in six months.

By early 2006, Mike Chaffin was well past qualifying for full early retirement—the age at which there was no financial penalty for retiring. He had served successfully as president for fifteen years, and as such, he was the senior medical director of all of the Permanente Medical Groups by a wide margin. While he could take credit for peacefully leading HPMG to a new age of nationally recognized excellence and accountability, at the same time, he was increasingly frustrated with the erosion of the partnership both locally and nationally. More and more national meetings on the mainland were being convened with less and less to show for them.

Bruce Behnke, when he resigned as regional president at the end of 2002, noted that he was traveling more than one out of three days a month. At the same time, more and more Kaiser Health Plan authority was being taken away from regional control. Behnke's executive management team now also had to report to Program Office managers who, to justify their jobs, required more and more reports from the local managers. These time-consuming, detailed reports took valuable energy away from local competitive efforts.

The worst part, which ultimately caused Behnke to decide to resign, was the violation of the "with responsibility must go authority" principle. With his direct report executive managers now having to report to him and an often-conflicting Program Office boss, his ability to lead the region was seriously weakened. Even as he had less and less control over the management of the region, he was still held responsible for outcomes over which he had little or no control.

Behnke's successor, Jan Head, was far less engaged. Then, in 2005, the perfect storm happened. For all practical purposes, Mike had no regional Health Plan partner to push back against the national program to defend local program interests, while at home, the local Health Plan leadership was completely unable to cope with the perfect storm. Poor implementation of the "new products" coverage plans (high co-pays to offset "skinny" plan low monthly rates) resulted in poor collections and terrible billing problems for patients. This had caused the accelerating membership and financial losses. In late 2006, the low point was reached when local newspaper headlines featured the need for KP Hawaii to seriously downsize its workforce. This was the first time in history for KP Hawaii. Morale was at a nadir.

Within HPMG, there is an unspoken, traditional principle. When there is a choice between family responsibility and work responsibility, family must take precedence. If it doesn't, in the long run, both will suffer. Leadership was a small facet of Mike Chaffin's considerable character. By all accounts, Mike's behavior defined goodness. He was frequently but sincerely described as "saintly."

In the 1989 crisis year, he had reluctantly yielded to the pressure to become a candidate for president. He became president not from a desire for power or riches but for reasons of medical idealism. Mike and Rhonda

Chaffin have had a successful marriage of more than fifty years. As evidenced "by their deeds you shall know them" characterized by a lifetime of service together, they embodied the ideals of Christianity. When their three natural children were at school age, Mike and Rhonda wanted to do more. They did so by adopting children—eventually nine of them. Being raised in the Chaffin family was just about the best gift in life that one could receive. It meant that Mike and Rhonda were never going to be rich or have a lot of free time, but that was unimportant to them.

Things went well until the mid-2000s when serious illness struck the family. Mike's family responsibilities suddenly increased to overwhelming proportions. A turning point came on early Friday morning February 9, 2006, when HPMG senior leadership was called to inform them that Mike Chaffin was in coma and on the way to the intensive care unit. By midmorning, Mike was stabilized but still in coma and on a respirator. None of the senior medical staff in attendance could think of a recoverable diagnosis that would allow him to continue as HPMG president. This was a frightening surprise. There was an anxious weekend as the medical staff tried to establish the diagnosis, but on Monday, Mike woke up apparently without injury. Within the week, he resumed his presidential duties. Apparently, there had been a medication mix-up at home, and once the side effects of the medication wore off, he was back to normal. Nevertheless, this was a watershed event both for Mike and the leadership of HPMG. He and they were forced to think seriously about succession.

Politically, the gulf between Mike's effective but gradualist approach to management and reform, and the impatience of the young activists, was steadily widening. In the November 2005 board election, they further increased their majority on the elected board of directors. Since Mike was unwilling to confront them, communication had largely broken down. At the July 20 board meeting, in closed session, the board passed changes to the bylaws that imposed a two-term limit on the presidency. It was soon ratified by a wide majority of associates 203–5. Mike had quietly opposed this change. Within the month, he made the decision not to complete his third term. Twelve years later, the two-term limit was reversed.

Having served successfully and honorably for fifteen years, well past retirement age, with new serious family health issues that had to take precedence, facing a dysfunctional partnership with Health Plan and an expanding rift with the next generation of leadership, he decided that it was not in the interest of HPMG for him to complete his third term, which wouldn't finish until 2009. He was determined to make this the most peaceful and least disruptive succession in HPMG history. He succeeded.

He made individual calls to the HPMG leaders announcing his planned retirement and then facilitated the presidential search process. No time was lost. At the August 18 board meeting, the search committee was announced. The chiefs had elected Dr. Mark Santi the chief of surgical specialties. The elected board members had elected Dr. Tarquin Collis a very capable and well-liked infectious disease specialist. The associates had elected by popular vote Drs. Peggy Latare and Dave Bell both family practitioners and Dr. Craig Nakatsuka from Internal Medicine. Three internal candidates were carefully considered during a very deliberate interview and discussion process.

At the November 3 board meeting, Dr. Peggy Latare, chair of the search committee, announced Geoffrey Sewell as the unanimous choice of the committee. After making a presentation to the board, he was ratified unanimously with an 8–0 vote. At the December 7 meeting, he was ratified by the highest margin in HPMG history with 212 votes for and five against—a 98 percent majority. Geoff was to serve as executive vice president in 2007 with his six-year first term starting January 1, 2008. It was understood that Mike would turn over full executive responsibility to Geoff sometime during the first six months. Mike Chaffin presided over his last board meeting on May 11, 2007. His presidency ended on January 1, 2008, and Geoffrey Sewell's, the fourth president of HPMG, began.

During Mike's fifteen years as president, the program had grown by forty-three thousand members against fierce competition. It was now a statewide program with a presence on all of the islands. Peace, prosperity, and cooperation had characterized these years. Divisive factionalism was gone. It was replaced by recognition of the strategic value of cooperation. The gold standard of market based physician compensation had been achieved. This vastly improved the ability to recruit outstanding doctors in all specialties. That along with standardized, objectively measured, and enforced standards of physician performance had established a strengthened and accelerating culture of excellence. This progress was already being recognized within the program and nationally by quality and service awards recognition. The stable, balanced, and accountable governance structure established during Bill Dung's years was further strengthened. It proved able to peacefully and thoughtfully establish the policies and procedures that further contributed to a stable HPMG governance that would enable further progress. It also successfully navigated the stormy establishment of the first program-wide electronic medical record in Hawaii.

At HPMG, the policies established for governance, compensation, staffing, and performance were being handed off to the next generation. It was now well positioned to successfully scale up to any size. With the next leadership generation characterized by outstanding physicians of intelligence, character, energy, and idealism, HPMG's future was very bright indeed.

CHAPTER 11

WHY DO IT THEIR WAY WHEN WE SHOULD DO IT OUR WAY?

The Specialty Care Model: Aligning Incentives

Relieved of many regional administrative responsibilities after the 1989 presidential election, the author was free to concentrate on the Surgery Department. By 1992, aggressive recruiting made possible by the rapidly improving salaries had brought all of the surgery sections up to full staffing. Attention then turned to optimizing the efficiency and quality performance of the department.

Since the beginning, surgery department workflow was modeled after the fee-for-service medical care-delivery systems in the academic centers where most Permanente surgeons trained. Fee-for-service clinical incentives are often at cross-purposes with the capitation and preventive medicine incentives of KP. The clinical independence afforded by KP vertical integration—ownership of the hospital, clinic, and pharmaceutical services—as well as the security of an exclusive partnership between the Medical Group and Health Plan provided fertile ground for a complete rethinking of specialty care-delivery. This rethinking was intended to align the care incentives of the patients with those of the care providers and with the nonprofit KP program that funded these providers and their medical support systems.

New Patients versus Follow-Up Patients

The science is fairly clear about when initial medical treatment should be applied to a medical condition, but it is far less clear about when and how often a previously treated condition should be followed up. Fee-for-service payment models rewarded each care visit whether it was for the primary condition or for a follow-up visit. Little distinction was made. An original visit required the establishment of a new doctor-patient relationship, a detailed medical history and physical exam, the interpretation of test and diagnostic imaging studies, and the execution of a treatment plan, which often involved surgery. In a fee-for-service model, after a condition had been treated, it is disproportionally rewarding for a specialist to perform frequent follow-up visits. Follow-up visits could be done much more quickly and with much less effort than the original visit. As a result, regular, frequent, and often potentially unnecessary follow-up visits were incorporated into fee-for-service "standard" follow-up protocols. Most Permanente specialists uncritically followed these protocols learned during their training.

In the KP-capitated program, the fee-for-service-based financially driven model of frequent rechecks presented a perverse incentive to see easy, questionably necessary "rechecks" at the expense of harder to manage new patients. After a few years of practice, specialists could accumulate a sufficient number of patients "requiring" multiple rechecks that they would have little remaining space on their schedules for new patients. In a system where payment is by capitation, staffing must be by capitation: the number of patients served rather than the number of services rendered. If staffing is by capitation, as it should be, if resources are to be distributed fairly, staff numbers are fixed by the prepaid budget. Unnecessary follow-up visits would leave less space on schedules for the new patients with untreated disease. This would increase the wait time for the first visit to the specialist. Disease processes could worsen during this delay period and impact adversely the overall quality of care. This would also result in a disproportionate number of new "harder" patients being left for the newest and often least experienced doctors in a specialty department until they, in turn, had acquired enough follow-up patients to fill their schedules. Typically, that would take only a few years. Perversely, the new doctors and the doctors who were more careful about scheduling questionably neces-sary rechecks would end up with more harder to manage new patients i.e. more work. This even had a name internally, the "Kaiser reward," when one was rewarded for being efficient by having to work harder. There was even a name for overscheduling rechecks: "churning."

Various attempts by supervisors to control churning by measuring "new patient recheck ratios" or setting minimal numbers of new patients per day on rigid schedules failed because of their complexity. Naturally, specialty physicians perceived these attempts to control churning as a threat to their medical decision-making. If KP was to compete in an in-creasingly competitive market, it needed to address the cost of excessive staff and good access at the same time.

The solution was to remove the complex, rigid existing scheduling models, which threatened physician autonomy anyway, and start from scratch. Clinic managers would no longer be responsible for specialty access; departments and individual specialty physicians would be. "Productivity" was now defined by how many specialty problems were solved by the spe-cialist and not by how many "treatment things"—useful or not— they did. This aligned with the capitation model. After all, solving problems that other doctors can't solve is the economic basis for the existence of special-ists to begin with. In a series of contentious specialty physician meetings between 1989 and 1991, a number of agreements were reached:

Specialty Work Unit: Consultation

The economic basis for the existence of a specialty department is to diag-nose and treat specialty problems beyond the training of physicians not in that specialty. The work unit was no longer any intervention—consultation or follow-up—but the lifetime solution of a specialty problem. In other words, it was only a consultation (consult) for a new patient or problem. No special credit would be given for rechecks. The need for recheck visits was to be decided upon on the scientifically based clinical judgment of each specialist. Proper follow-up was the professional responsibility of the individual specialist.

In the well-established, comprehensive, and well-accepted HPMG quality assurance program, inadequate follow-up, if clinically significant, would be detected and flagged for action against the responsible specialist. This was subsequently demonstrated to be unusual. In the discussions, there was physician consensus that the risk of delayed treatment for follow-up care was much less than that for delayed care of patients waiting to be seen for the first time. Best yet, the specialist had complete freedom to decide when a follow-up visit was appropriate, but they still had to do their share of the department work by seeing their fair share of department work: new problems that were specific to that specialty.

Stable Doctor: Clinical Team

Schedule structure and content to optimize wait times (access) were now to be worked out by the physician with the assistance of a specifically assigned clinic assistant. This team—explicitly led by the physician who was responsible for the clinical outcome—now had the authority and the responsibility to structure a schedule that would optimize care and access. This authority and responsibility that had formerly been in the hands of clinic managers was completely now in the hands of the doctor responsible for clinical outcomes and access (wait time). Physician buy-in was likely to be better when they had control over their schedule—and it was.

To establish these work teams, clinic administration was made explicitly responsible to rigidly enforce the already established policy of assigning the same nurse or clinic assistant to the same specialist as often as possible. Every physician's style of practice is different—and necessarily so because every practice is different. Most clinic assistants, now saw their role as a member of a specific care team – not as an interchangeable part. They usually would quickly adapt to the physician's clinical style. If they couldn't, a transfer would be needed.

For clinic administrators, the most convenient scheduling is when clinic assistants and nurses function as interchangeable parts to cover vacations, sicknesses, and job changes. Clinic assistant scheduling to other than their assigned physician for the convenience of nursing administration was very unpopular with both physicians and clinic assistants. More important, it had a seriously negative effects upon clinic efficiency. A poll was taken of physicians and clinic assistants by surgery department administration. It asked, on a 200 percent scale, if 100 percent productivity was present when the doctor was working with the assigned clinic assistant, what was it when the doctor was working with an assistant from within the specialty department section versus outside of the specialty department section. Surprisingly, the results across departments for both doctors and clinic assistants were essentially the same. They felt that if 100 percent efficiency was present when the original doctor-clinic assistant team worked together, it was 75 percent if it was a clinic assistant from within the same department section, and only 50 percent if from outside of the same department section. The scale was set to 200 percent on the off chance that non-departmental staff might be more efficient than departmental staff. No one felt that way. If they had, it would have indicated that there was a doctor-staff mismatch that needed to be addressed. Physician-clinic assistant clinical partnerships often lasted for decades, and these partnerships often implemented innovative access solutions—far beyond what any clinic administrator could have imagined.

Fair Access Measurement

For this model to work, there needs to be an accurate outcome measurement. To measure the consultation wait times, the number of days that the patient waited for their consult was averaged. For example, if two consults were seen the same day and two others were seen ten days after the consult was generated, the average wait time would be 0+0+10+10=20 divided by the four consults for an average wait time of five days. The simplicity of this approach avoided the complexity of other formulas. One such calculation was to determine first three available appointments, which could be gamed and had the potential to interfere with the proper prioritization of patients by the doctor-assistant team. The average wait time for individuals and the department was fed back to the physician-assistant team and the supervising chiefs on a monthly basis. The chiefs had the responsibility to assess this data, identify both good and bad outliers, and then act on the findings.

Work Units Are Distributed Equally

With the work unit defined as the definitive solution of a specialty problem, fairness dictated that the work be evenly divided. The criteria for a work unit was a written consultation to include history, physical examination, review of tests, assessment, and treatment plan, and responsibility for a lifetime of follow-up visits for as long as the patient was in the program. "Curbside consults" didn't count. Formal hospital consults and consults sent to an individual doctor (termed "specials") did count—provided the documentation criteria were met. Specialty consultations were scheduled in such a way as to sequentially assign the consults to each member of a specialty department until all consults were assigned. It looked something like this:

- C= Standard consultation
- S=Specially assigned consults to an individual specialist who may have a specific subspecialty interest, skill, and training or by a patient request for a specific physician.
- H=Hospital consultation (usually urgent same day consultation

Doctor A	C1	C5	C8	C10	C14	C16
Doctor B	C2	C6	C9	C11	H	C17
Doctor C	C3	S	S	C12	C15	C18
Doctor D	C4	C7	H	C13	C16	Etc.

In response to the criticism that some consults would present far more work than others, Dr. Carlos Weber section chief of general surgery at the time responded to this objection by calling the sequential consult assignment scheduling the "wheel of fortune," implying that any inequities would eventually even out. The wheel of fortune concept, was later shortened to the "wheel" ("put the consult on the wheel") referring to the consult distribution system.

There was a provision for giving double or more credit for particularly difficult case types. To obtain double credit on the wheel, all that the concerned specialist needed to do was make the case for this adjustment to the other members of the department. Such presentations were met with appropriate skepticism. While double credit for certain difficult case categories was enacted by several departments, it eventually fell out of favor due to the complexity of implementation and subsequent sub-specialization of the specialty departments. This allowed pre-assignment of certain types of subspecialty consults to the appropriate subspecialist. The workload really did even out with time.

There was surprisingly little opposition to the new consult-distribution system. For those doctors who thought they were working harder than their colleagues—most of them as human nature would predict—by getting their "fair share" of the work, they thought that things would get easier. In reality, most doctors were working equally hard, but this apparent "equalization of workload" perception actually promoted the acceptance of this consult-distribution plan.

Lifetime Follow-Up

Lifetime follow-up is implied in the KP promise. The lifetime follow-up was established as a disincentive to superficial or inefficient care because the patient would keep coming back to the same specialist until the problem was successfully managed. Once established with a specialist, that same patient would generally be assigned to that specialist for other problems within the scope of that specialty. These specialists would, of course, get consult credit for managing a new problem, but it would be easier because the doctor-patient relationship had already been established. For example, if a urology patient had a bilateral vasectomy in 1983 and then came back in 2005 needing a transurethral resection of the prostate, they would see the same urologist, but the urologist would get credit for the new work unit. This was a real example.

Lifetime follow-up increased the "bonding" of patients to their KP doctors. It was good for the patient because the patient was known to the specialist. It was good for the specialist because it increased the therapeutic bond of the doctor-patient relationship. It was good for the program because this bonding vastly increased the resistance of patients to switch health plans, especially in Hawaii where relationships are especially important. Patients and specialists could always request a change. An unusual number of change requests would attract unwanted attention from physician supervisors and that physicians' partners who would now have to care for the disgruntled patient. The resultant negative feedback kept this under good control.

Sub-specialization

It was in the interest of the program, the specialists, and especially the patients to sub-subspecialize within the specialty departments. For the typical Kaiser Permanente patient, the specialist usually represented the end of the road for specialty care. As such, there was a responsibility to offer a level of care that was as good as or even better than that of the community. This could only be achieved by further sub-specialization of the specialty departments. The history of scientific medicine has been a history of increasing sub-specialization. The idea of the need to refer to specialists was not a new one. The Hippocratic Oath contains the sentence: "I will not use the knife, not even on sufferers of [bladder] stone, but I will give place to such craftsmen therein." In other words, get a urology consult.

At first, most doctors were general practitioners and then physicians and surgeons. As medical knowledge rapidly expanded in the late nineteenth and early twentieth century, physician and surgeon sub-specialization accelerated. By the 1930s, the major specialty organizations and their training programs were in place. By then, general surgeons were no longer general surgeons doing all types of surgery. Surgery on bony structures went to orthopedics, on the nervous system and brain to neurosurgery, head and neck to otolaryngology, pelvic and kidney surgery to urology, eye surgery to ophthalmology, reconstructive surgery to plastic surgery, blood vessel surgery to vascular surgeons, heart and lung surgery to cardiac and thoracic surgeons. General surgeons had become specialists in their own right as endocrine, gastrointestinal (gut) and trauma surgeons. Likewise, internal medicine physicians differentiated into endocrinologists (glands), cardiologists (heart), dermatologists (skin), gastrointestinal (digestive tract), pulmonology (lungs), and others. Gynecologists managed obstetric and other female conditions. Internists and family practitioners managed what was left, but their all-important role was to become the patient's advocate and care coordinator (quarterbacking) among the increasing number of different specialties.

As medical knowledge grew at a geometrically accelerating rate, by the 1970s, medical knowledge had advanced so far that the recognized specialties required further sub-specialization. The major specialties began to offer subspecialty fellowships beyond the standard residency and subspecialty certifications.

Sub-specialization Is Good for Patients, Specialists, and Kaiser Permanente

By the 1990s, the successful implementation of national average salaries coupled with HPMG practice lifestyle advantages, allowed the directed recruitment of fellowship-trained sub-specialists. Staffing models tracking outside service charges helped focus subspecialty needs. For example, if gynecologic surgery was spending $400,000 a year on gynecologic oncology surgery, then it was time to hire a gynecology oncologic surgeon. With outside services typically costing three to five times more than internalized services, it was cost-effective and strategically important for the program to internalize most subspecialty costs rather than subsidize community subspecialty capability of competitors.

With fellowship-trained subspecialist staffing instead of generalist staffing, for almost all cases, there was an HPMG specialist who was as trained and experienced or even more trained and experienced than the community subspecialists. The old complaint against KP of a lack of physician choice would be negated if HPMG doctors were equal to or even better than the community competitors. Hawaii is a small place. The word spread quickly. The reputation of the program rapidly improved. KP became an attractive health care option for comprehensive care, reasonable cost, and state-of-the-art specialty care. As stated earlier, restricted choice of specialists is not a marketing problem for the Mayo Clinic. Sub-specialization is good for the specialists. While HPMG often did refer to community specialists, the community almost never referred to HPMG specialists – no matter their training or experience.

By the end of the 1990s, it was apparent that a single specialist could not master all the subspecialties of a traditional specialty. General specialists fell further and further behind because the KP service population (~200,000) did not provide enough of the relatively rare advanced surgical specialty cases to distribute among all the specialists to maintain proficiency. By focusing subspecialty cases on designated fellowship-trained subspecialists within a department, subspecialty expertise and proficiency was maintained and expanded. With sub-specialization as department policy and subspecialty-focused recruiting, by 2000, most of the intradepartmental surgical subspecialties were in place. For example, in orthopedic surgery, there were subspecialist orthopedic surgeons focused on hand surgery, sports medicine and endoscopy, trauma, total joint, and foot and ankle surgery.

Fortunately, subspecialty cases typically make up only about 20 percent of the workload. The remaining workload consisted of "bread and butter" specialty cases that any well-trained specialist could handle as well as any other. This was necessary because the subspecialists in a department must share general call and therefore must all have proficiency managing all acute types of problems related to that specialty after hours.

Sub-specialization makes HPMG attractive to specialists. Subspecialists usually identified themselves with a subspecialty because they had a special interest in it. People do better work when they are interested in it. With increased interest and experience as a result of the focused caseload, the specialist becomes the go-to person for that type of case because they quickly become the most skilled at managing a particular condition. This reduces wasteful intra-department competition because everyone in the department is "best" at their skill. By having a subspecialist in the department to refer a difficult subspecialty case increases the experience and skill of the sub-specialist, reduces the stress of the referring physician who has their own sub-specialty to concentrate upon, and increases the co-operation within the department. Competitive behavior within a specialty makes no sense because it pays to be civil to a colleague who might tomorrow be taking off your hands a difficult sub-specialty case that you can't or don't want to manage. Similarly, you would be taking over cases from that person for the subspecialty that you had the greatest interest in. As such, sub-specialization fostered cooperation rather competition. Being among the best or the best in Hawaii for a particular subspecialty skill was not only possible within HPMG but a common source of professional pride.

Sub-specialization is good for patients. It is intuitive that in almost any activity a practitioner is interested—and has more training and experience performing a particular skill—outcomes will be better. This is as true in medicine as any other human endeavor. The medical scientific literature strongly supports this concept. In time, it was observed that as surgery departments subspecialized operating room times, hospital length of stays, blood loss, and complications rates all declined. This was observed across all specialties. Improved patient care is, of course, the most important reason to subspecialize.

Outcomes of the Specialty Care Model

By the end of 1991, after dozens of meetings to secure a reasonable consensus in each specialty department, the specialty care model had been implemented. Once implemented by redefining the work unit as a consult and then equally distributing the consults, new consult-measured wait times in the first three specialties which implemented the program dropped from six to eight weeks to two to three weeks within six months without increasing staffing. As subsequent specialty departments implemented the program, they noted a similarly improved consult access. Sub-specialization resulted in a 98 percent internalization of patient care by the end of the 1990s. The principles of the specialty care model have changed very little since its inception more than a quarter of a century ago. It was a significant cultural change.

CHAPTER 12

CHAOS THEORY AS APPLIED TO PHYSICIAN PERFORMANCE

C haos theory? Really? Chaos theory provides several useful conceptual constructs that may help understand the problem of managing physician performance, and more broadly, to promote a culture of excellence in a health care organization. The myriad imprecisely measurable initial conditions that contribute to a health care environment are too complex to predict a precise outcome. Small initial changes could result after a time in radically different outcomes: unpredictable chaos. Fortunately, there are patterns (attractors) that spontaneously occur in nature, and thus humanity, that can be used to understand, predict, and even be manipulated to achieve a general, although not precise, outcome.

The Butterfly Effect

At the end of the nineteenth century, most scientists believed in a "clockwork universe." They felt if sufficiently precise initial measurements were made and then if proven scientific principles were applied, precise future predictions could be made. In the early twentieth century, a new understanding of quantum physics demonstrated that only approximations of these initial states can be made. Thus, a precise future outcome prediction is not possible because of the necessary initial rounding errors that would amplify with time, resulting in a wide range of future possibilities. As a result, a limitless number of future possibilities could result from an initial state of necessarily imprecise measurements in complex systems. As one gets further and further away in time from the initial state, the possibilities rapidly proliferate: chaos. This explains why, despite a good understanding of the behavior of gases in the atmosphere and the availability of super-computers, even today, the best weather forecasting is inaccurate beyond ten to fourteen days. A conceptual tool used to understand this was "The Butterfly Effect" found in the title of a landmark chaos theory scientific paper. The provocative question to be answered was this: Could the at-mospheric disturbance of a butterfly flapping its wings in Brazil lead to a future hurricane in Texas? Chaos theory would predict an answer of yes as one of the innumerable future possibilities, but nature is not entirely random. There are observable repeating patterns. Chaos theory was de-veloped to reconcile chaos with these observable patterns. These patterns were called *attractors*.

Kaiser Permanente in Hawaii is composed of an immeasurable com-plex of hundreds of doctors, thousands of employees, and millions of patient encounters. Every individual, doctor, care provider, employee, and patient, at any given moment, has a vast array of changeable personality attributes that are influenced by genetics, past experience, values, mental and physical state, sense of security, etc., etc. These are just the human fac-tors. Add to these the external factors of changing physical, economic and political realities affecting health care policy and resourcing, the rapidly accelerating growth of scientific medical knowledge, and environmental physical effects such as weather and manmade and natural catastrophes. With all of these factors constantly changing from moment to moment, how does one begin to manage such a chaotic environment. Random, reactive actions to counter acute crises generated by the forces of chaos is another name for micromanagement, and micromanagement is not a formula for lasting success. Fortunately, chaos theory does predict a larger-scale order out of the chaos that could potentially be manipulated.

Attractors

In the first paragraph of Genesis, the writers recognized the presence of order in the universe organized from an initial state of chaos and attributed it to God. It was already an old idea.

Human beings have evolved to recognize patterns in nature. Pattern recognition and the ability to use this knowledge to predict events and manipulate the environment gave *Homo sapiens* an evolutionary advantage that allowed it to become the dominant species on earth. If the universe was completely chaotic, there would be no need for pattern recognition because patterns wouldn't exist. Indeed, the universe as we know it would not exist—never mind evolving life forms that could recognize patterns if they did exist.

Attractors are defined in chaos theory as repeatable patterns in nature. These patterns are not exact but work within a fairly tight range of values. Let's do a thought experiment. Let's say that we agree that most people want to help other people. There is good fossil evidence that even Neanderthal society believed this. This is an especially important attribute to understand if we are going to manage health care since health care is all about helping others. We found that HPMG's own validated patient-satisfaction data supports this human behavior.

Wanting to help others seems to be part of human nature. It is an essential characteristic of a good doctor, but this "attractor" has a range. There will be good and bad outliers. It is the responsibility of HPMG managers to reward good outliers to incentivize more of them, and to identify and, where reasonably possible, help those who are bad outliers. If the bad outliers cannot or will not improve, it is the responsibility of HPMG leadership to remove them from the Medical Group if they are going to live up to the HPMG value statement of patient service and satisfaction.

The history of Kaiser Permanente and the Hawaii Permanente Medical Group would suggest that there are a number of KP principles that could be achieved by proper employment of the attractors. Implementation of these principles have contributed to the success of the KP program for more than eighty years and HPMG for sixty. Ignorance or deviation from these principles is fraught with peril.

The Kaiser Permanente Genetic Code Principles

The KP program principles, formerly known as the genetic code to an earlier KP generation, has served KP well for eighty years. The following, based upon economic, political, and behavioral attractors, have applied: *Prepayment* gave KP the ability to allocate resources to give patients the greatest medical value for their money. An emphasis on *preventive care* and *comprehensive coverage* prevented, from a moral and financial, costly delayed treatment of disease. Earlier treatment of disease has better health outcomes for patients than late treatment. The resultant conservation of resources can then be applied to lower patient cost and provide more resources for better care—as long as KP remains *nonprofit*. The *exclusive Health Plan-Medical Group partnership* balances the realities of economics with the moral imperatives of medical care—both are necessary if the organization is to have the expertise to properly allocate resources. *Vertically integrated facilities*—control of the hospital, clinics, pharmacy, and ancillary services—permits the rational development of Permanente Medicine's way of practicing medicine without outside interference. It also avoids subsidizing the competition in an often hostile medical, political, and economic environment. Experiments in the 1990s, which left out components of the KP genetic code in new regions or turned away from them in established regions—usually the exclusive partnership, prepayment, and integrated facilities—failed. These regions are all closed or were taken over by regions that continued to observe the genetic code. The KP genetic code, where followed, has allowed KP to grow into the largest vertically integrated private health care organization in the world. Tampering with these principles (attractors) has not been successful.

HPMG Human Nature-Based Principles

The following policies grounded in human nature "attractors" have historically served HPMG well for the past sixty years. Within the traditional structure of the well-preserved KP genetic code in Hawaii, they have been associated with steady growth, increased prosperity, and the accelerated expansion of a culture of excellence.

Competitive compensation packages based on market benchmarks permitted recruiting from a wider base of physician candidates. *Careful recruiting* emphasizing competence, character, and caring from this wide base of candidates provided HPMG with the doctors who had the core values necessary to grow a culture of excellence. *Democracy with built-in checks and balances* afforded governance stability, which bought time to develop carefully, consensus-based, policies and procedures to define and implement these values of performance excellence. Once defined, the final step was to deliver on these defined values by *validly measuring outcomes and then acting upon them.*

Dynamic Equilibrium

To further the chaos theory analogy, let us consider some concepts of equilibrium. Interacting attractors suggest that a persistent equilibrium can emerge from the chaos, and it does seem to, but it is not static. It is dynamic. It is subject to change—sometimes rapid change—again because of the inability to exactly measure initial conditions and initial complexity as suggested by chaos theory.

Virtuous Cycle

The proper alignment of attractors rooted in human nature coupled with the economic and sociologic advantages of the KP Principles has, for HPMG, resulted in a positive feedback loop virtuous cycle of increased order, performance, and resultant prosperity. That is the theme of this history. Chaos theory, however, would suggest that slavish replication of HPMG policies by another startup KP region would not result in an identical history because the complex of initial conditions would always be different. Nevertheless, the dynamic equilibrium that would emerge would be more likely a virtuous rather than a vicious cycle. "History may not repeat itself. But it rhymes." This statement is often attributed to Mark Twain. Is it possible that chaos theory provides the explanation for it?

Punctuated Equilibrium

Random outlier changes in starting conditions can have vastly different subsequent effects (butterfly effect). Dinosaurs ruled the earth during the Mesozoic era for a 165 million-year ecological "dynamic equilibrium." A random asteroid struck the earth sixty-five million years ago, and they went extinct. The asteroid strike was an outlier event. While an asteroid is no butterfly, without it, non-avian dinosaurs may well have survived and dominated the earth to the present day. Instead, mammals, which had previously been small ratlike creatures, evolved to fill the ecological niches that the dinosaurs vacated to take their place as the dominant life forms. Like nature, human history is full of examples of punctuated equilibrium. Where are all the previous empires? When they went out of alignment with human nature, they became more susceptible to outside random events.

Vicious Cycle

Another outcome of punctuated equilibrium can be a vicious cycle. Misalignment of attractors can result in a negative feedback cycle in which things get worse and worse. For all of its serious faults, the thousand-year Roman Empire increased overall security, law, trade, technology, learning, and prosperity for its population. When the virtuous attractors of the founding Roman culture, discipline, responsible citizenship, and mutual reward fell from favor, the empire collapsed. The fall of the Roman Empire was followed by a "dark age" millennium of decreasing security, law, trade, technology, learning, and prosperity.

Imagine a real-world situation that could result in a HPMG vicious cycle that destroys the HPMG physician accountability program of service and care and then the entire program. Acting upon the results of the peer-to-peer surveys, patient-satisfaction surveys, and the quality assurance program results have been the bedrock of HPMG physician performance policy for decades. Important increases in patient satisfaction and doctor cooperation have been the result. Let's imagine that KP Hawaii has a series of bad financial years as a result of significant membership loss as happens periodically due to changes in market forces. Fewer members would mean less capitation income for the Medical Group. Less capitation income would mean lowering compensation packages, downsizing staff, or both. Performance data would be employed to provide a rational basis for selective downsizing based upon performance.

Hard times breed populist demagogues. For them, the physician accountability program used to downsize staff would be an attractive target. The demagogue, exploiting fear, proposes equal salary cuts rather than selective cuts based upon performance. In this way, no one is threatened with immediate job loss. Exploiting small imperfections in the performance measurements process and its expense, it is further proposed that the performance program be eliminated entirely. With salaries now below market value, outstanding doctors with options leave for better opportunities, while doctors without options stay. The vacant positions must now be filled, but relatively low HPMG compensation, makes recruiting outstanding physicians difficult or even impossible. Doctors would still be needed to service the remaining patients. The temptation would be great to hire mediocre or worse doctors to fill the emergent need for staff. Eventually, the culture of excellence gives way to toleration of mediocrity or worse. This, in turn, makes the program even less attractive to patients. Membership goes down further, lowering compensation setting up a vicious cycle that sends the program into a death spiral.

There Is Hope

There isn't much that HPMG management can do about an asteroid strike or a nuclear war, but these are unlikely events. Efforts must concentrate upon what can be managed. HPMG learned the hard way at least three times in its history that uncompetitive compensation for doctors threatens the existence of the entire program. Disregarding this principle again would likely have a similar effect. Any health care-delivery program, no matter how well thought out, is dependent upon human talent for survival. Careful recruiting and competitive fair compensation nearly guarantee the ability to recruit such talent. Over the years, HPMG developed a democratic but accountable form of government. The checks and balances incorporated into this government along with an accountable "strong chief" policy inhibits demagoguery. By the 1990s, HPMG was well positioned to establish a culture of performance excellence.

The health care market will always be presenting new threats to the existence of HPMG to which it must adapt or die. On the other hand, good health care is an essential commodity that will always command a priority allocation of society's resources. Health care programs will compete for these resources. This brings to mind the joke: "You don't have to run faster than the bear—you only have to run faster than the other guy." Historically, HPMG has demonstrated that, when motivated, it can run very fast.

Delivering on Physician Performance

Inherent to the medical profession is a general commitment to excellence and an intolerance of mediocrity. Undoubtedly, the gauntlet that an individual must traverse to become a doctor eliminates most of the mediocrities. Nevertheless, a few will slip through the net. Others may lose their commitment to excellence during the course of a medical career. The reasons include changing personal relationships, burnout, substance abuse, mental or physical disease, and financial stress. Those who may have joined the profession predominantly motivated by income potential will be disappointed, and it will show in their work. It is the responsibility of all physicians to protect patients from mediocre health care, especially those physicians in leadership positions.

HPMG was fortunate from the time of its founding to have had a disproportionate number of idealists who believed that the principles of KP were the way to ethically deliver health care. Many of them, stung by community opposition and criticism, rose to leadership positions and single-mindedly took on the task of developing of a culture of excellence. A careful reading of HPMG primary source documents shows that from the beginning, a disproportionate effort was dedicated to recruiting outstanding doctors and removing or improving doctors who were mediocre or had slipped into mediocrity.

Early on, the efforts were by individual leaders perilously relying upon the only information that was available: observation and anecdotal information. Nevertheless, HPMG made the effort, successfully avoiding wrongful discharge suits, and a quality medical group steadily grew. As the group became larger and geographically spread out, observation and anecdotal information became increasingly unreliable—and performance evaluation became a riskier business.

Early attempts at peer-to-peer evaluation for the purpose of awarding bonuses or adjusting salaries were unpopular and never implemented. Similarly, patient-satisfaction surveys were simplistic, sporadically implemented, and not tied to an outcome. Establishing objective measurement of physician performance turned out to be a long, complicated business. The failed previous attempts demonstrated that a number of issues had to be addressed before a physician performance program could be implemented.

Belief in Excellence

To implement a culture of excellence, there must be a critical mass of physicians who want to. The thirty-year effort by HPMG leadership to do just that through selective recruiting and the maintenance of performance standards was largely successful. That effort was very much facilitated by the improved compensation packages of the early nineties. They greatly expanded the potential candidate pool available to fill the many vacancies caused by the previous salary crisis and the concurrent rapid membership growth. By 1993, HPMG had a critical mass of physicians who were offended by any residual mediocrity and were ready to define excellence.

Defining Excellence

In the last half of 1993, there was a six-month effort by the board of directors to explicitly define excellence within an HPMG values statement. A board subcommittee developed the proposed definition. After developing this proposed definition, a successful consensus-building campaign directed at the entire doctor staff was mounted by the board members. The final values statement was then ratified unanimously by the full board of directors. It was intended to be more than a series of slogans.

HPMG now had an explicit definition of excellence that was to be immediately acted upon. This was done by distributing a values statement poll to each of the associate staff at the end of the first and again at the end of the second year for all staff who would be proposed as new associates. A bad result postponed or prevented new staff from being proposed for associateship. The frequent and widespread distribution of the values statement poll meant that no member of the group could reasonably claim that they didn't know what the HPMG values were. Prior to hire, all candidates were informed that they would be subject to at least two values statement polls and that they would have to perform satisfactorily to be made an associate. There was a consensus within HPMG leadership that if a candidate lost interest after being informed of this requirement, it would be best for HPMG and the candidate if they were not even offered employment.

Enforcing Excellence

The values statement polling applied only to new candidates. What about associates? Applying these expectations to existing staff would be politically much more difficult—but necessary. Thus, began a twelve-year process.

The cornerstone of Bill Dung's governing policy was that the elected board of directors was responsible for policy, and the advisory board of directors consisting of chiefs and clinic physicians in charge was responsible for operations. He insisted that they meet together to keep the elected board out of operations and to keep the chiefs out of policy. This changed during Mike Chaffin's administration. The elected board insisted upon separate meetings early in his administration, and this was consistent with the original articles of incorporation. They were scheduled usually at noon on the first Thursday board meeting day each month. In response, the chiefs started their own meeting on the first Thursday of each month to define their operational policy needs as a counterweight to the elected board meeting. Through informal agreement, since the mid-1980s, Thursdays had become the HPMG administrative meeting day. Although fraught with peril, these separate meetings actually worked out well for both groups and HPMG. At the elected board meetings, extreme proposals were moderated, and at the chief's meetings, operational needs were better defined. It was understood that no unilateral decisions were to be made at these meetings. Policy decisions could only be made at the combined elected and advisory board meetings.

The author, as senior chief, was chosen to preside over the chief meetings. Discussions initially covered a wide range of operational issues and were relatively unfocused. Eventually, a decision was made to dedicate the chiefs meeting to physician performance. The informal "chiefs meeting" title was formally changed to the Physicians Performance Review and Oversight Committee, thereafter known as the PPRO. Its long-term mission was focused upon standardizing performance based upon the HPMG values statement. These standards would apply not only for the new physicians but for all HPMG physicians, including associates.

For the HPMG associates hired before the formal establishment of the HPMG values statement, this would be a new expectation, and it needed to be implemented carefully. Fortunately, the vast majority of the associates already believed in, and acted out, the principles of values statement. For that reason, there was time to meticulously establish the process. It took more than a decade, but during that development process, performance excellence became an even more deeply embedded tenet of HPMG culture.

Defining Measurable Performance

The HPMG values statement had already defined and ratified sixteen behaviors that were expected of HPMG Associates. The task of the PPRO was to identify what could be reasonably measured to address these sixteen behaviors.

Quality Assurance

The quality assurance program had been in effect and largely unchanged for twenty years. There was wide consensus among the chiefs and physicians that it was working well and provided valid, easily interpreted, and actionable quality trend information. To recap: each quality concern was evaluated by department peers and given two determinations. The first determination was for three levels of culpability: below standard of care, equivocal standard of care, and meets standard of care. The other was the determination of severity. It ranged from 1 (minor), for example generously judged illegible handwriting, to the highest severity code of 6 (death). This data was already being recorded for each physician and could be easily incorporated into a chief's PPRO department performance report.

Medical Malpractice

Medical malpractice had been trended since the beginning of the program, but because of the perverse financial incentives of tort law results, it did not and does not correlate well with real malpractice. By the mid-1980s, each malpractice case was judged for validity by an involved internal process. The data for each summarized case included: the charge, the results of the internal review—since every case was automatically reviewed with a quality assurance review, the determination of the State of Hawaii Medical Claims Conciliation panel, and any award or settlement amount. Any case that expended program legal resources to defend a specific physician's care triggered a summary that was trended and reviewed. Information regarding past cases was also reviewed to spot any adverse malpractice claim trends. Since all this data was already being recorded, it was a simple matter to incorporate results into the PPRO performance report to the chief. The PPRO chiefs ratified the existing process.

Patient Satisfaction

After considerable discussion it became the position of the PPRO that *patient satisfaction is whatever the patient thinks it is.* It was the doctor's responsibility to accommodate as much as possible the special needs of each patient. Issues of languages services, illiteracy, lack of medical sophistication, and mental health, with patience and empathy, could almost always be accommodated with help from the support services where necessary. Where support services were lacking, it would be the physician's responsibility, with the assistance of the chief, to pressure the program to obtain adequate support.

What about the drug addict who tells that doctor that they will give a negative service rating if an unnecessary prescription for narcotics is denied? Another example would be a disability patient demanding an un-justifiably long disability approval. Often with understanding and careful explanation, these patients can be convinced to do what is right and best for them—but not always. Doctors being evaluated for their patient satis-faction would naturally worry about the impact of unreasonable patients on their results. While these incidents are not rare, they are uncommon enough that they are almost always fade into the data background noise as long as the doctors are all measured the same way. Patient satisfaction data, like all performance data, is subject to review by the chiefs. At that level, a special appeal is available. For example, successful consideration would be made for a physician who ran a depression clinic or drug addiction clinic. When support system problems were at fault, the patient-satisfaction program was a powerful corrective mechanism because it highlighted the patient-satisfaction impact of these deficiencies. Correction of legitimate support service deficiencies makes for better patient care.

Designing the Patient Satisfaction Evaluation

Several attempts had been made to measure patient satisfaction since the KP Hawaii began. They all eventually fell out of favor because they were too general, sampled too small a population, or were not randomized—and thus lacked statistical validity. Thus the data generated had limited legitimacy in the eyes of the medical staff.

Specificity

Previous patient-satisfaction surveys asked patients to rate the physician experience as very satisfied, satisfied, or unsatisfied. This was not very use-ful in that it did not demonstrate the problem areas. By the mid-1990s, a survey was introduced to Hawaii via the Colorado region called the "Art of Medicine Survey." The survey was short enough that patients would fill it out, yet it provided diagnostic information highlighting problems. It was demonstrated to have reproducibility and internal validity. As such, it was accepted as the regional measure of patient satisfaction. The final question of the survey: "Would you recommend this doctor to others?"

This was the key question that correlated best with the patient's overall service experience. This was compiled to make physician comparisons. When a physician had negative ratings, data from the other questions in the survey were available to give useful diagnostic information that the physician and mentoring chief could use to improve a physician's patient-satisfaction performance. Sometimes they had little or nothing to do with the physician's performance, such as parking, billing, receptionists, or nursing. This could be taken into consideration and sent to the proper program agency for correction.

Statistical Validity

Doctors have a better understanding of statistical significance than most. Such an understanding is required to evaluate the medical literature. Mark Twain said, "There are three kinds of lies: lies, damned lies, and statistics." Physicians were concerned that misapplied statistical analysis could be used against them. On the other hand, proper attention to statistical validity would reinforce the perceived fairness of the quality of service evaluation program. To do this, the patient sample size needs to be large enough to provide statistical significance. There also needs to be good sample randomization of the physician's patient population. After much discussion, the PPRO agreed that ideally 2 percent of a physician's visits needed to be surveyed. Independently randomized, return postage-paid surveys were mailed. If enough surveys—more than thirty—were not returned, then results would not be reported. Collecting valid, and therefore trusted, data is expensive. It includes the cost of printing, postage, compilation, and reporting. For patient satisfaction, tens of thousands of surveys need to be mailed every year. On the other hand, if it improves service to patients, it is worth it.

Peer-to-Peer Satisfaction

For most doctors, it is self-evident that doctor to patient service is an essential component of physician professionalism. Doctor-to-doctor service may be less evident. A major strategic HPMG advantage is that there are no financial barriers to cooperation and many incentives. The doctors within HPMG are not in economic competition. This is the rationale for a salary structure based upon national average salaries and a very modest bonus reward structure. There is no advantage to disparage the ability of a member of one's department.

While in fee-for-service practice, criticism of colleagues might provide more cases (business), all it does in HPMG is incite animosity. If there are more cases as a result of this disparagement, for the doctor doing the disparaging, it just means more work for the same pay. This is not in the interest of the doctor and especially the patient when it is three o'clock in the morning, a partner's help is needed, and there is preexisting animosity between the two doctors.

The doctor selection process is very competitive. The process favors confident, proud, independent, action-oriented, and intelligent individuals. Even though there are many disincentives to destructive, competitive behavior within HPMG, viciously toxic relationships, lasting for decades, have repeatedly occurred throughout HPMG history. The importance of cooperative teamwork and respect among HPMG physicians is explicitly stated in the HPMG values statement. The PPRO chiefs, who had the experience of managing the disruption caused by un-cooperative, disrespectful behavior, clearly agreed with these sentiments. The chiefs clearly saw that the competitive potential of a medical group of hundreds of doctors cooperating was much greater than the same number of independent practices acting in their own interests. The PPRO was highly motivated to support an evaluation that fostered such a culture of respect and teamwork.

This was easier said than done. Previous attempts at peer-to-peer measurement had failed miserably. Senior physicians in the group were interviewed to find out why. The reasons for the failure seemed to be the baseline compensation was too low for all the doctors, there was too much emphasis on tying the results to large bonuses that could increase economic competition within the group, there was no standardized disciplinary due process policies in place, and finally there were always technical flaws in the survey process—again centered around the data being non-randomized, nonspecific, and statistically invalid. All of these findings needed to be addressed. The first thing that opponents of performance reform attack is the validity of performance data.

After some discussion, it was decided by the PPRO to allow every doctor in HPMG to rate every other doctor. This raised the criticism of how one doctor would rate another doctor if they had no contact with them. It was made clear in the survey directions that if there had been no interactions with a particular physician for two years, then this physician should not be rated. While it was on an honor system, this restriction was apparently observed. At a time when HPMG had 350 doctors, any individual doctor would typically be rated by less than one-third of HPMG—and most doctors were rated by fewer than that. As with the patient-satisfaction data, because of statistical validity concerns, the results for doctors with fewer than thirty evaluations were not reported.

One concern raised was that every doctor's rating was equal despite wide differences of familiarity with the doctor to be rated. To correct this, various complex schemes were considered. In one such scheme, ratings would be restricted to thirty raters each chosen by the doctor, the chief, and random selection for a total of ninety potential ratings. After considerable discussion, the PPRO chiefs decided not to go this way. Such a program would be very complex, very time-consuming to administer, and very expensive. More important, it would be more vulnerable to manipulation, results would be less clear, and at any given time over three-quarters of the Medical Group would not be able to rate a given doctor.

The PPRO chiefs decided that the character of the Medical Group was such that they could trust an honor system enough that doctors who could not rate a doctor would not do so and that the ratings would be honest. It also sent a powerful message every time the survey was run—every one or two years—that cooperation and respect in addition to patient service and quality of care are values that are expected of all HPMG physicians.

The complexity of such a survey presented problems. Every doctor who participated in the survey would be evaluating hundreds of doctors—about six hundred by 2019. To get enough doctors to participate the survey, it would have to be simple. If too few doctors bothered to fill out the survey, it would lack statistical validity. It was designed with only four ratings: patient quality of care, patient quality of service, helpfulness, and contribution to the success of the HPMG mission. These were well aligned with the HPMG values statement. Rather than using a traditional ten-point scale, it was boiled down to a four-point scale 4 = A, 3 = B, 2 =

C, and D = 1—just like premed college grades. This was not coincidental. When applying to medical school, an individual with a GPA of less than 3.5 usually was rejected. The "grades" and the four values were qualitatively defined in the instructions. On average, any individual doctor would be evaluated by more than one hundred HPMG doctors.

The peer-to-peer survey was first run in the early nineties as part of the Surgery Department's specialty care model program. All HPMG doctors were asked to rate the surgeons. Almost immediately, other departments requested that they be included in the survey. By the time that the PPRO was organized, a majority of departments had joined the peer-to-peer survey. Several years of performance data had accumulated, and the process and the data generated were considered valid by most. The PPRO reviewed the peer-to-peer polling process. It decided that cooperation and respect were important behaviors within HPMG and were powerfully aligned with the HPMG values statement. It further concluded that the peer-to-peer survey was a valid process for measuring this aspect of physician performance.

The PPRO had completed its first task, practical measurement of physician performance, which broadly encompassed the aspirations of the HPMG values statement. Out of dozens of potential measures of physician performance, it had settled on the critical four that would encompass the aspirational goals of the HPMG values statement: *Patient satisfaction* as a core principle of the profession. It is whatever the patient thinks it is, and it was validly measured by the "Art of Medicine" survey. *Peer-to-peer satisfaction* promotes cooperation and respect essential for optimal patient care-delivery and is validly measured by the peer-to-peer survey. The prospective *quality assurance* process, in existence and well accepted since the mid-1980s, was adopted as the measure of the quality of the care delivered by a doctor. Finally, measuring *medical malpractice trends* and acting upon them, was felt to be essential for the financial health and reputation of the program. These four measures were not mutually exclusive but supportive of each other. There are usually high correlations among them.

Action Thresholds

Measurement of performance identifies problems, but it doesn't fix them. That is the job of the department chiefs working with the physicians in charge. When the process started, there was wide variation in chief response to identified problems. Among chiefs, no one wants to be the disciplinarian—and everyone wants to be popular. If one chief is a strict disciplinarian and another has a casual attitude toward performance, that would be unfair to all. As a result, the PPRO chiefs decided to identify a minimum mandatory response to identified performance lapses.

The PPRO decided that the best way to standardize the chiefs' response was to have a "mandatory performance action plan" for defined thresholds of performance. The committee then proceeded to define these thresholds. For medical malpractice cases, this was two per year—even if the physician was not judged at fault during internal review.

For quality assurance, the threshold was two cases per year judged to have equivocal or below standard of care. The patient-satisfaction and the peer-to-peer survey results were plotted on a distribution curve. Without knowing where individual doctors fell on the curve, the PPRO chiefs by consensus chose a threshold below which individuals would be subject to a mandatory improvement action plan. The line was approximately two standard deviations below the mean HPMG performance. Initially, it involved about 2 percent of the doctors—typically six to twelve doctors. It was of interest that the same doctors were often below both thresholds. With performance thresholds measured and then acted upon, there was now a consistent approach to physician performance. Between 2000 and 2005, the average patient-satisfaction score went from 84 percent highly satisfied to 88 percent highly satisfied. During the same period, peer-to-peer satisfaction went from a 3.1 to a 3.25 on the four-point scale. Considering that this data included thousands of data points, this was a highly significant improvement for both measures.

The Performance Curve Shifts to the Right: Significant Improvement

Once every doctor understood that they would have their quality assurance, peer-to-peer, and patient satisfaction measured by a valid measuring tool, most doctors eagerly benchmarked themselves against these widely accepted measures of professionalism. The performance distribution curve improved each time the survey was run. The distribution curve steadily shifted toward the right with improved scores.

By 2005, while most of the group was improving, a small core group of about fifteen to twenty out of almost four hundred doctors who were on the poor performance side of the curve (left side) stayed where they were or even worsened. This resulted in a small bump on the left side of the distribution curve as the poor performance of these doctors separated them further and further from the improving performance of the rest of HPMG. Several of these doctors had been subject to written mandatory action plans multiple times with little or no improvement—and some even worsened. Not a few were on the wrong end of both performance curves with problematic quality assurance and medico-legal trends to boot.

The sense of the chiefs, who were counseling the same doctors over and over without effect, was that this small minority of doctors didn't really accept the HPMG values statement or the authority of HPMG leadership to enforce it. By this time, the young activist doctors were a dominant majority on the board of directors, and they found this unacceptable.

Historically, once an HPMG doctor became an associate, typically after two years of probation, it was nearly impossible to remove that doctor from the group. It required a unanimous vote of the board of directors. This had been done in egregious cases, but it was rare. Similarly, significant salary reductions for performance reasons were unusual, but they had also been done. The bar to become an associate had risen steadily from the late seventies through the nineties at an accelerating pace. The vast majority of associates supported performance measurement and improvement, but performance had not been directly connected to salary or employment. The values statement survey had been effective in screening out weak candidates for associateship, but it did not apply to established associates. To avoid wrongful discharge suits and political turmoil, there would need to be a clearly defined progressive disciplinary process and a robust, objective performance evaluation on which to base performance judgments upon if compensation and employment were going to be directly tied to performance. By 2005, there was such a political consensus, a rational process for measuring performance, a process for evaluating this well-measured performance, a comprehensive appeals process, and a well-established remedial program. The time was right to tie performance directly to compensation and employment.

Test Case: Tying Performance to Compensation

In mid-2005 a test case was brought before the board. The individual involved had been in the Medical Group for twenty years. He had become an associate two years after joining at a time where associateship was almost automatic. In 2005, the peer-to-peer scores for this individual were in the bottom 1 percent (415 out of 420) at 2.45 on the four-point scale. The average for the department was 3.4, and for HPMG, it was 3.25. Patient satisfaction was 80 percent (seventeenth percentile). The average for the department was 88 percent, and for HPMG, it was 87 percent.

There was also a spotty malpractice and quality assurance record. Counseling had been attempted several times in the past with no apparent effect. Indeed, he claimed that the poor performance was all new news. Because of this, a mandatory meeting was arranged after office hours with the chief of surgery and the section chief. It was time to test whether associateship conferred permanent immunity from compliance with the HPMG values statement for associates.

The chief fashioned a board motion that had been reviewed and sharpened by discussion during a previous PPRO chiefs meeting. It was explained to this doctor in detail that a recommendation would be presented at the following voting board meeting. It outlined mandatory performance goals, which if not met, would result in a salary reduction of up to 20 percent on the next run of the PSAT and peer-to-peer surveys. This gave the individual twelve to eighteen months to improve and avoid any penalty. A salary reduction could be avoided by improving the peer-to-peer survey results to 3.0 and improving patient satisfaction to 85 percent.

Both of these performance measures were still below the average for the Medical Group and the department. Meeting this still-below-average performance bar would at least demonstrate an understanding of the gravity of the poor performance and meaningful efforts to improve. Mentoring by high-performing colleagues from the department was offered as well as the patient-satisfaction course of "Thriving in a Busy Practice." Other suggestions to improve the peer-to-peer image were also made.

The motion went before the board at the following meeting on June 16, 2005, and it was ratified. The recommendations were not embraced by the doctor in question. In the following years, things didn't really improve. Performance goals were not met, salary reductions persisted, and resignation from HPMG occurred within four years.

The Board Ties Performance to Compensation

With the ice broken by this successful test case, the movement to tie performance to compensation proceeded rapidly. On September 1, 2005, the board of directors ratified a restatement of the HPMG values statement from the 1993 HPMG code of conduct. On September 16, 2005, the PPRO chiefs were charged by the board with developing a HPMG performance policy. This came together quickly. On October 20, 2005, after two lively, extended PPRO meetings on that day, the professional chiefs were behind a HPMG-wide policy that was finalized for the board meeting that evening. The principles of the policy were as follows:

1. The purpose of tying performance to salaries is to improve the performance of HPMG doctors at the low end of the performance scale—not to save money. It is expected that most HPMG doctors will improve on their own for reasons of professionalism as a result of the validated performance data ("Hawthorne" or "report card" effect). This has been the HPMG experience prior to tying performance to compensation.

2. The purpose of tying salaries to performance is to give a wake-up call only to the seriously deficient. The purpose is not to establish performance-based competition within the Medical Group, which could have the unintended consequence of damaging cooperative

efforts within HPMG. Doctors who have been deficient in the past and who do not respond to counseling have often claimed that they didn't really understand the seriousness of the situation or even that they had not been counseled. By establishing a standardized protocol of an advance written notification of a potential salary reduction and a personal, documented interview (preferably with a witness), no doctor subject to such disciplinary action can reasonably claim that they do not understand the gravity of the situation.

3. The purpose of tying salaries to performance is to identify poor performers and to concentrate the chief's attention and performance improvement resources on these individuals. It is clear, however, that it is the sole responsibility of the individual to improve performance. It is not the responsibility of HPMG if rehabilitative efforts are unsuccessful. When an individual is hired by HPMG, by contract, they are expected to have a preexisting skill set, which is outlined during the recruiting process. HPMG is not a training program.

Opponents of the measure spoke before the board of directors meeting, which was held in closed session that evening. There were three lines of opposition. The first was skepticism that the program could be administered fairly. Each objection was answered in detail. It was pointed out that everyone would be measured the same way. Any doctor could dispute the data, which would then be subject to a hand count. Every effort had been made to maintain statistical credibility. Patient satisfaction data and peer-to-peer data was collected randomly and reported out by a third party. The chiefs judged the performance cutoffs without knowing who was where on the distribution graphs. Finally, it protected HPMG doctors from arbitrary chief judgments based on incomplete or flawed, unstandardized performance data. In this sense, solid patient satisfaction and peer-to-peer performance data would be protective for the individual doctor disliked by a chief.

The second objection was that these salary reductions would threaten traditional HPMG collegiality. This concern was raised in good faith, and tying performance to compensation in any way had the potential to do just that. In defense of the motion, it was pointed out that less than 2 percent of HPMG doctors were involved. These individuals had multiple opportunities to improve their scores, but they had not done so. Individuals would have twelve to eighteen months to improve before any salary reductions would take place. There would be no immediate salary reductions. These physicians were to be given one more chance with focused counseling before salary cuts would occur approximately a year later, after the next round of peer-to-peer and patient-satisfaction surveys. This fair and deliberate process and the honest intent of the chiefs to help physicians improve their performance went a long way to assuage this concern.

Who is hurt when a physician has poor quality assurance, patient satisfaction, and peer relationships? Most important is the patient who could be harmed physically or emotionally. Next are the physician's colleagues who have to repair the trail of damaged patient relationships and shirked responsibilities left in the wake of the poorly performing doctor. Everyone knows who they are. As a result, sympathy for these doctors is typically "a mile wide and an inch deep." The program is collectively hurt by a poorly performing doctor.

In Hawaii, when a private doctor performs poorly, it is not the health plan that is blamed, but the doctor. The situation is different for Kaiser Permanente. Because of the exclusive partnership, if a "Kaiser doctor" performs poorly, it reflects upon all of HPMG and the Kaiser Health Plan in addition to the individual doctor. Of course the converse is also true. Finally, it is the poorly performing doctor who is hurt if poor performance is not vigorously addressed. The doctor may persist in that behavior through self-delusion—or worse—apathy.

An attempt by the Medical Group to improve poor performance with monitoring and counseling is actually a gift that the doctor would not receive outside of HPMG. The performance policy gives every HPMG doctor the opportunity of an early warning of inadequate performance and the support and tools to improve that performance before it gets past the point of no return. No patient wants to see a doctor without empathy or skill. No other doctor really wants to work with them. For such a doctor outside of HPMG, feedback would likely be limited to a shrinking practice, no referrals, and consequent financial problems. Sadly, in such a situation,

271

if the poor performance worsens, it often ends badly with career-ending disciplinary and regulatory actions.

It was no surprise when the loudest objections came from those physicians who would be at risk financially if the policy was adopted. One claimed that this motion "weaponized" the physician performance process. The response by defenders of the motion was that it was indeed sad that it had come to this, but that it was sadder still that it had become necessary because of a core group who, even after years of effort by supervisors, were resistant to even low levels of improvement. The choice for HPMG was to enforce the HPMG values statement with concrete action or to leave it to be only an aspirational guideline. At this watershed moment in the performance history of HPMG, the board of directors supported tying performance to salary by a vote of four in favor, two abstentions, and zero no votes.

Out of the four hundred and fifty doctors in HPMG, seven doctors were at risk for 10 percent salary reductions for poor peer-to-peer evaluations (<2.5), eleven faced a 10 percent salary reduction for patient satisfaction of less than 70 percent (<3rd percentile), and an additional forty doctors faced a 5 percent salary reduction for a patient satisfaction of less than 77 percent (<10th percentile). All doctors at risk were counseled by the chiefs, and the counseling session was documented. The message travelled fast: HPMG leadership was serious about performance.

The First Survey after Performance Policy

After the performance policy was passed by the board, all of the doctors at risk were counseled, and the meetings were documented. The doctors at risk had more than a year to improve. The results of the first patient-satisfaction and peer-to-peer survey after implementation of the performance policy did not become available until early 2007. As the performance policy implementation date approached, the tempo of email and hallway scuttlebutt to overturn the policy increased.

At the beginning of 2007, Geoff Sewell, HPMG president-elect, assumed the role of executive vice president, partnering with Mike Chaffin. Mike presided over his last board meeting in May 2007, after which, Geoff was essentially in full control. A strongly supportive memo of the performance compensation policy signed by Mike Chaffin, Geoff Sewell, and the voting board of directors was sent to all HPMG physicians on March 1. It outlined the history and reasoning behind the performance policy with the promise that the policy would be reviewed at the subsequent March 15 board meeting.

At the March 15 board meeting, the performance compensation policy was again discussed at length. The board re-ratified the October 20, 2005, motion and the salary adjustments that were to occur as a consequence of continued poor performance. They went on to ratify adjusted performance standards for the following patient-satisfaction and peer-to-peer survey.

The board also ratified an important addition to the policy. What was to keep a doctor from making a rational decision to sacrifice 10–20 percent of their yearly salary so that they could ignore patient-satisfaction and peer-to-peer performance while continuing HPMG employment? The following addition was made to the policy: "Physicians who have had prior salary reductions due to failure to meet performance thresholds from the 2005 performance policy who again fail to meet the 2007 performance policy thresholds will in addition to the salary reduction, be referred to the HPMG executive committee for additional action." This action clarified that ignoring performance was not an option for continued HPMG employment.

Results

The effects of the 2005 performance-compensation policy were immediate and lasting. Staff relationships became much more cordial, and cooperation vastly improved, as did patient satisfaction.

The new policy radically changed the chief's role. Previously the chief had been responsible for gathering performance data from sometimes unreliable often anecdotal sources. They were then obliged to fashion a disciplinary action that would be subject to challenge because of poor data quality or political influences. Historically, successful challenges to such data had resulted in chief resignations. Since there was no standardized action threshold, chiefs were naturally reluctant to initiate disciplinary actions to begin with. Disciplining physicians was rarely popular. Who wants to be unpopular? Doctors being disciplined would often label the chief as a bully to anyone who would listen. This was especially true if a chief took performance seriously and initiated more disciplinary actions than average.

With the PPRO-designed performance program, everything changed. The chiefs were *required* to initiate disciplinary actions at a standard of performance that had been *collectively* determined by the chiefs on the basis of the *anonymous* peer-to-peer and patient-satisfaction performance graphs outside of the chief's influence or control. Thus, no case could reasonably be made that the chief was picking on an individual. Who was to be subject to disciplinary action was predetermined by the collective opinion of the chiefs. The chiefs' role had changed completely from policeman and judge to counselor and advocate.

With some overlap, the 2005 distribution graph thresholds had demonstrated eleven doctors at salary risk for poor peer-to-peer relationships and 55 for poor patient satisfaction—out of 450 doctors. By the next survey in 2007, nine doctors who would have been subject to penalty resigned (two) or retired (seven). Only six doctors had not improved sufficiently to avoid salary reductions ranging from 7.5 percent to 20 percent. Of these six, three embraced counseling and improved to mainstream performance and retired from HPMG many years after. Only three did not and resigned from HPMG within three years. Across HPMG, there was a significant improvement in both peer-to-peer and patient satisfaction, especially those who were at risk for salary reductions. Three of these at-risk physicians had a remarkable improvement in patient satisfaction—one by 20 percent and two by 11 percent.

Emergency Department Patient Satisfaction Immunity?

The group most opposed to the patient-satisfaction performance was the Emergency Department (ED). Emergency Department patient-satisfaction scores tended to be lower than average in the Hawaii region and all across the program. Admittedly, there were patient-satisfaction challenges unique to the Emergency Department. During a short emergency visit, there was not much time to develop a patient-doctor relationship. Visits were for an acute problem, and the patients were sick and often in pain when seen. Depending upon the seriousness of the problem, the patients often waited in uncomfortable surroundings for hours. Emergency Department visits by their very nature prevented scheduling and distributing the demand. Because the ED doctors worked in shifts, there was less of a chance to work out cooperative relationships between doctors and support staff. For the same reason, it was difficult to have department meetings where cooperative department policies and procedures could be established.

Immediately prior to the release of the first survey results under the new performance program, a representative of the Emergency Department made a presentation to the board of directors requesting that the Emergency Department physicians be held to a lower patient-satisfaction standard than the rest of HPMG for the above reasons. The board took no action on this request, and the policy stood.

As associate medical director of hospital and specialty services, the emergency Department was the author's responsibility. The author, decided to get directly involved and scheduled individual meetings with all of the Emergency Department physicians. There were Emergency Department physicians who had managed to achieve patient-satisfaction scores that were well within the mainstream of HPMG, proving that good scores were possible. These doctors were interviewed first and congratulated. They were asked about best practices that might have contributed to their good scores. They were asked if they would advise poorer performers. They agreed. They were then asked about the barriers to high patient satisfaction. They were frank. The lower-performing doctors were then interviewed. Without naming names, it was pointed out that some of their colleagues had managed to achieve good patient-satisfaction scores. The successful best practices were generically described. All who were interviewed were asked to work with their colleagues to improve the performance of the Emergency Department as a whole.

It was apparent that there was a widespread sense of fatalism within the department that assumed that high patient satisfaction could not be realistically achieved. Many felt the work environment mitigated against good patient satisfaction and that it couldn't be changed. Stark, uncomfortable waiting rooms, lack of timely information to patients who might have been waiting for hours, and lack of staff cooperation were given as examples. This fatalism was self-fulfilling and needed to be reversed. For a start, it was made clear to each individual that the board and the chief did not accept this fatalism as a reason to have a separate lower standard of patient satisfaction for the Emergency Department if for no other reason than some Emergency Department physicians had good scores. Fatalism was not an option. Each Emergency Department doctor was asked to take responsibility not just for their own performance but also that of the department. Regular and well-attended department meetings would now be an expectation. Support, and if necessary, resources from the highest levels of management were pledged to resolve environmental concerns and staff accountability, but the specifics needed to come from the department itself. A laissez faire shift worker mentality toward department management by individuals was to be no longer acceptable.

The new Emergency Department chief, Dr. Greg Strongosky, representing the interests of the department, was initially skeptical, but he was a problem-solver "driver". Working closely with the associate medical director and pointing out to the department members that there was little option but to improve, he began holding department meetings with better attendance. Staffing adjustments, increased accountability of support staff to the doctors, and improved policies and procedures included keeping waiting patients updated on their status, and an improved physical layout of the waiting area changed the attitude of the department—things could change for the better. By the time of the next survey, only one doctor out of the several who had been at risk was subject to a salary penalty. The department individuals' patient-satisfaction numbers had improved markedly—two by double digits. The department patient satisfaction continued to improve so that the Hawaii regional ED became a benchmark for the national program. This trend was reinforced over the next few years by the retirement or resignation of several of the doctors who had been under par on patient satisfaction. The performance culture of the ED department had changed.

Grading on a Curve

A universally despised feature of college premed was grading on a curve. This was a component of the premed winnowing process. It was employed by some professors to limit the number of mostly A and the few allowable B grades that were absolutely necessary to obtain admission to medical school. It entailed giving a test where the actual grades were marked on a distribution curve and then grade cutoffs that were based upon where one stood on the curve and not upon the actual number of correct answers. When being graded on a curve, one could have 90 percent of the answers correct and still get a D. A D in one or more courses would likely end all hopes of getting into medical school. Grading on a curve brought out the worst of student competitive behavior.

The intent of the performance policy was not to winnow out the Medical Group but to identify the worst performers who were resistant to improvement. Indeed, before performance was tied to compensation, simply reporting patient satisfaction and peer-to-peer satisfaction with counseling as needed had caused most of the performance improvement. The need to tie performance to compensation became apparent only when a core group of less than 2 percent at the low end of the performance curve separated out from the rest of HPMG. Most of these had willfully ignored poor results and resisted improvement efforts.

As both the patient-satisfaction and peer-to-peer data rapidly improved, the specter of grading on a curve emerged. After much debate, the PPRO decided that a patient satisfaction of above 80 percent highly satisfied and a peer-to-peer score of greater than 3.0 (above average) would not be subject to financial penalty. The reasons included:

1. Patient satisfaction and peer satisfaction were already part of the HPMG culture. Within a few years, the PPRO performance compensation policy, having withstood all political challenges intact, had become even more deeply embedded in the culture of HPMG. Within a few years, the core group of opposition, often those who would be subject to sanctions, had resigned or retired. The harsh reality was that, while friends of performance came and went, and enemies could accumulate, but this could only occur if those

ALBERT J. MARIANI, M.D.

enemies were still in HPMG. They were no longer. Peer pressure on mediocre performers to improve would now be even greater. In such a performance culture, deciding to stop performance effort at 80 percent patient satisfaction and 3.0 on peer-to-peer would be professionally very risky in a culture where performance was not overwhelmingly popular.

2. There was a recognition and bonus incentive program to reward those who did well on the surveys. As noted earlier, these modest rewards were not great enough to elicit destructive competitive behavior. Such behavior would in any case likely backfire, damaging the individual's peer-to-peer survey results. The bonus chits were distributed only for meritorious behavior. Mediocre performers would notice that they were getting very few or none. Such positive reinforcement further advanced the culture of performance excellence.

3. Within the program, there were wide variations in the practice environment that could put certain individuals at risk, such as under resourcing and uncooperative staff. These could put individual doctors at risk. Rare but possible data errors could also unfairly impact physician performance outcomes. If poor performance was due to forces outside of a physician's immediate control, it would be unfair to penalize them by marking on the curve.

This became long-term policy. With financial penalties limited to only the very worst performers, compensation and employment security were maintained. If there were environmental or data problems, there would be time to detect and repair these problems without inflicting unfair salary reductions. On the other hand, this policy helped avoid perfectionist, bizarre, destructively competitive performance (perfection is the enemy of good) behavior by establishing a baseline of reasonable performance environment for employment safety. Performance improvement beyond the baseline (80% patient satisfaction and 3.0 "better than average" peer to peer performance) would be accomplished with counseling, reward, and peer pressure.

Persistent Poor Performance Policy

On March 15, 2007, the board ratified a policy of HPMG executive committee review of physicians who failed to reach performance thresholds two times. The first failure would result in a standardized notification and counseling of the physician. If a certain performance threshold, set region wide by the PPRO and ratified by the board, was not met, the physician would be subject to a salary reduction. The physician was given until the next survey to meet this performance threshold to avoid the financial penalty. Region wide, yearly, a new performance threshold would be set for the next survey. If the physician did not meet the performance threshold by the third survey, they would be subject to the financial penalty and a review of their status as an employee of HPMG. This was serious. At this meeting, the doctor would be presented with a mandatory, strict action plan, involving formal, often off-site performance training, counseling, and mentoring. Failure to embrace the remedial course of action or persistent poor performance would result in the HPMG executive committee recommending to the elected board of directors that continued employment of this doctor should cease.

Improvement Resources

While it was within the right of HPMG to discharge physicians for poor performance, it was the culture of HPMG to help colleagues with problems, including performance. While it was made clear that performance was ultimately the responsibility of the individual, there is a long tradition going back at least to the Hippocratic Oath for physicians to help fellow physicians in need. This of course struck a chord with aloha-influenced HPMG.

For this reason, a robust improvement effort was incorporated alongside the sanction process. The intensity of this effort increased with the risk of sanctions. At the first level, the physician was at risk for a salary penalty if they did not improve to the threshold level by the next survey. Help consisted of mandatory chief counseling, mandated or voluntary focused medical education, participation in Thriving in a Busy Practice (now called

Communication Skills Intensive Course), focused medical education, and mentoring by a department physician with best practice performance. This was usually successful.

The second level of counseling was done at the level of the HPMG executive committee. This was mandated by previous board policy after the individual physician twice failed to meet minimum thresholds of performance. This was more serious. The typical performance-improvement program mandated by the HPMG executive committee included regular meetings with the chief to chart progress or the lack thereof and satisfactory completion of an intense, off-site residential performance course sponsored by the Southern California Permanente Medical Group. If there was a clinical issue-focused medical education, would be mandated.

The 2008 survey was the first opportunity to test the HPMG executive committee's review process. Only two doctors were involved. One of the doctors was a hardworking, clinically capable specialist who unfortunately had persistently low patient-satisfaction scores for decades and who refused to see it as a problem. This doctor chose to resign rather than attend the mandated Southern California residential patient-satisfaction program. This resignation was not perceived as a problem by the leadership. The second physician had weak overall performance but was eager to improve. Full cooperation with an intense program of chief monitoring, and participation in the local and Southern California patient-satisfaction programs as well as mentoring by colleagues enabled the individual to meet performance thresholds and continue HPMG employment until retirement. It would be a rare event for a doctor who had embraced the performance training to be forced to leave HPMG.

With a clear performance process of notification, the availability of rehabilitative resources, and a well-documented progressive discipline process followed by a clearly defined appeals process, it would be very hard to bring a successful wrongful discharge case against HPMG. This closed the performance loop for HPMG doctors.

Results

Within the first few years, especially after a spate of performance-related semi-voluntary resignations and retirements, opposition to the performance program completely died out. Quality of patient care, quality of patient service, and peer-to-peer cooperation were firmly established components of the culture of HPMG, and they improved steadily. Physicians at risk for salary reductions dropped to two or three per year. Usually these were new doctors who proved to be a poor fit with HPMG practice. By 2017, there were no physicians below the 80 percent highly satisfied patient satisfaction and none below 3.0 (above average) on the peer-to-peer survey. When the performance program started in the late 1990s, *highly satisfied* patient satisfaction averaged 84 percent. By 2017, it stood at 94 percent. During the same interval, the peer-to-peer survey results had risen from 3.25 to 3.7. Given that the surveys were unchanged and that there were tens of thousands of surveys during the interval, the improvement was unquestionable.

Back to Chaos Theory

It took twenty years—from 1985 to 2005—to evolve the performance standards that have been in place largely unchanged since then. The deliberate, well-vetted evaluation process did successfully change the HPMG culture to one of performance excellence. All this was made possible by the long-term economic and political stability of HPMG.

Economic Stability: The KP Genetic Code

The attractors, patterns of behavior reflected in program policies that provided the economic stability, were derived largely from the KP genetic code. These included the *exclusive Kaiser Health Plan—HPMG partnership,* which allowed both sides to develop in an environment of relative economic stability where both entities were in a mostly cooperative relationship and where each entity did what it did best. The economic stability permitted a *fair physician compensation* program, *enabling HPMG recruitment of high-performing doctors.* With predominantly high-performing physicians, the baseline culture of HPMG was already culturally sympathetic to a performance program. *Prepaid medical care incentivized preventive care,* which lowered the overall cost of care. *Salaried physicians isolated medical decision-making from reimbursement,* further lowering the cost of care. *Vertically integrated KP facilities* were present in the Hawaii region from the beginning. This self-contained environment permitted the innovations necessary to adapt the new prepaid concepts of medical care-delivery without outside interference. Prepaid care-delivery is a radical departure from fee-for-service-based care-delivery. Coexistence with fee for service is nearly impossible because the economic incentives of each are reversed. In non-KP hospitals, unless PMG doctors are a dominant majority, policies and procedures are made by and for predominantly fee-for-service competitors. In such an environment, Permanente physicians were forced into compliance with these fee-for-service-based policies or face career-risking sanctions. In such an environment, it is much easier to comply, which retards, possibly permanently, the adoption of Permanente Medicine.

Political Stability: HPMG Governance Principles

The political attractors that provided long-term governance stability were HPMG based. They included a *strong chief policy* necessary to have the persistence and authority to carry out important initiatives such as the performance policy. Executive overreach was prevented by a *democratically elected board.* Election to the board was open to any HPMG associate. It provided an opportunity for any associate to participate in HPMG governance, and it was a rich source of potential chiefs. This system of *checks and balances* prevented poorly thought out or poorly executed programs. The political stability of HPMG was such that there were only four medical directors during the first sixty years of HPMG's existence.

Professional Ethics

Arguably the most important attractors of an effective performance program are the baseline expectations of the profession itself. Quality of care, quality of service, teamwork, and respect for the others on the health care team and perfection are all expectations of the profession. Those who do not embrace these professional expectations can expect to do poorly in the profession. While a few bad apples get through the selection and training process or change after, most physicians are self-policing. That is the definition of a professional. This professionalism goes a long way to facilitate the implementation of any performance program.

Human beings are imperfect, but if there is any profession that demands perfection, it is medicine. Patient well-being and even lives depend upon it. A large medical group such as HPMG has the resources and expertise to establish a program that is valid, fair, legal, and directed toward improvement. For the rare HPMG physician who does not share these values, and doesn't want to, the only alternative for HPMG is the removal from patient care and separation from the group. *Who will protect the patients from poor physicians, if not good physicians?* There are many outside of the profession who would be happy to do so, but compared to peer physicians, their solutions would likely be crude, less fair, and in the long run, probably ineffective as physicians would react to perceived unfairness by building a "white coat wall."

Scam-Proof versus Scam-Resistant

With all of the safeguards that have been discussed, to some, the performance program could seem to be "scam-proof." Nothing is scam-proof. At best, a program can only be scam-resistant. Remember; most doctors are smart. For any reform program that can be thought up by the human mind, that same mind can develop a workaround that can be the source of unintended consequences.

In the author's experience, there were several examples of this. In one case, a relatively new physician was extraordinarily careful to provide a very high level of service to patients and referring physicians at the expense of essential departmental chores, such as availability to back up other department members, minor procedures, and test interpretation and documentation. The apparent motive was to replace a chief who had recently and successfully reorganized department. Higher peer-to-peer and patient-satisfaction scores were the justification offered to replace the chief. Further investigation demonstrated no wish to replace the chief from within the department, but there were concerns about this individual's contribution to the smooth functioning of the department. When told that the chief would not be replaced, the individual resigned. The judgment not to replace the chief was vindicated when it was learned that the individual was leaving behind more than 2,100 unfinished test interpretations. Only after the individual's medical license was threated were the test interpretations completed.

Because of examples such as this, any performance program will fail unless it is interpreted by intelligent, principled leaders of goodwill who will put all performance data into perspective. A successful performance program is all about quality leadership.

Culture Change

To build the HPMG performance program, many attractors needed to be skillfully aligned. With such careful design and vetting, it survived the necessary political challenges and successfully became an essential component of the HPMG culture of excellence. A dynamic equilibrium of excellence was established. A low tolerance of mediocrity was now at the core of the shared values of HPMG physicians. This was reflected in recruitment and orientation of new doctors, and it would be ongoing during a physician's HPMG career. As such, a mediocre doctor would be a poor fit. In turn, such a doctor would probably not be interested in joining HPMG. If by some recruiting accident, they did join, they would soon feel the uncomfortable cultural intolerance of mediocrity of their peers and leave. This self-renewing "virtuous cycle" continuously strengthens the culture of performance excellence.

Resistance to change must be successfully overcome to establish a high-performance culture. Likewise, once established, that same resistance to change will help preserve it. A positive dynamic equilibrium can be surprisingly resistant to change, especially when there is a built-in renewal processes. Indeed, the establishment of a true "positive dynamic equilibrium" is the only way to effect lasting change.

The persistence of the HPMG culture of performance excellence is now more likely than not. True cultural change characterized by shared values in a human society can last for hundreds or even thousands of years. Consider the foundational Greek contributions to Western civilization. They included rationalism, mathematics, science, democracy, philosophy, empiric medicine, literature, art, and architecture. They are still, 2,400 years later, accepted as good ideas. The loss of the HPMG culture of performance excellence would be a great loss to local society if the Kaiser Permanente program in Hawaii were ever to fail.

CHAPTER 13

CHANGE TO WHAT?
THE NINETIES

Kaiser Permanente

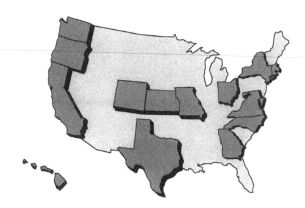

Expansion Study

February 1993

KAISER PERMANENTE

Kaiser Permanente at its maximum extent in 1993: Twelve regions.

After more than twenty years as de facto CEO of Kaiser Permanente, Jim Vohs announced his pending retirement in 1991. He expected that his successor would continue the principles, the genetic code of KP, that had been the governing doctrine under Cliff Keene and himself during the previous thirty-five years. They included prepayment, community rating, Health Plan-Medical Group partnership, integrated facilities, and high levels of regional autonomy. Both he and Cliff Keene continued the missionary spirit of the founders and promoted continued expansion into new regions to spread the ideology of Kaiser Permanente. This was not to be. The 1990s was to be a period of experimentation away from the KP core principles and this missionary spirit. This experimentation nearly bankrupted the program.

The frontrunner for the new chief executive officer to take Jim Vohs's place was Wayne Moon. Moon had started at KP in June of 1970 and steadily rose on the Health Plan side. Even though he was deeply imbued with the KP culture, he was not to be the chosen successor of Jim Vohs. After his unsuccessful candidacy, he was appointed by Vohs's successor, David Lawrence, to the position of executive vice president and manager of operations (COO) of the Kaiser Foundation Health Plan and Hospitals. In August 1993, about a year later, he left KP to become the CEO of Blue Shield—a KP competitor in California—and he served in that capacity until the end of the decade.

David Lawrence had joined KP in 1981 as the Northwest Permanente Bess Kaiser Area medical director. His background was in public health rather than clinical medicine. After his internship, he joined the Public Health Service and served in Peace Corps assignments in the Dominican Republic, Washington DC, and Chile. He obtained his masters of public health at the University of Washington where he ran the MEDEX physician assistant program for five years. He then returned to Portland where he was hired as the medical director of the Multnomah County Health Department before becoming the Multnomah County Director of the Department of Human Resources. Probably due to his public health, rather than clinical, background, his time as Bess Kaiser Area medical director in the Northwest region was rocky. He left this position when he was offered the position of Health Plan president of the Colorado region in March 1985. Now in an administrative role, he again did well.

In September 1988, he was promoted to the Northern California Health Plan senior vice president and manager and later, in 1990 and 1991, to California Health Plan vice chairman and chief operating officer. In August 1991, he was selected successor to Jim Vohs as the CEO of Kaiser Permanente. The deciding factor was the support of the medical directors. His charisma—no doubt honed by years of public service—and the fact that he was a doctor were the reasons for this support. The medical directors came to regret their decision.

Once the competitor corporate health plans, many of which were for-profit, figured out that there was a lot of money to be made in health care, they expanded rapidly. As the corporate big fish ate the little fish in the early nineties, there was rapid consolidation within the health care industry. Kaiser Permanente with its 6.5 million members, was by far the largest nonprofit health plan, but its number of "covered lives" was soon overtaken by larger and rapidly expanding national for-profit health plans. The for-profit health plans had the advantage of being able to generate large amounts of capital quickly by selling stock. Their initial profits came from leveraging provider costs down by pooling patients and by controlling the amount of medical care delivered with provider-annoying, hassle factor, preapproval policies. In the interests of speed and flexibility, they did not address the cottage industry: inefficient, fee-for-service delivery of health care. At the time, there was much unnecessary health care being delivered that was subject to denial, and there was a lot of money to be made by denying that care. Eventually, when the worst of the waste was driven from health care-delivery, the profits stalled. By the mid-nineties the most outrageous attempts to deny appropriate care to further increase profits had fortunately been constrained by bad publicity, lawsuits, and legislation.

The fundamental health care-delivery issues that the new for-profit health care corporations had sidestepped were the same issues that KP had struggled with since its inception. They included patient satisfaction, quality of care, and the provision of and then allocation of resources to deliver health care at a price that the average employed person could afford. For KP, balancing quality, service, and price had been a slow, difficult process. This was especially true when the relative strength of the regional health plans and the PMG Medical Groups were out of balance or not communicating. When this occurred, forward progress often stopped or even regressed.

The relatively stable heath care market of the sixties, seventies, and eighties had allowed KP to address these fundamental health care-delivery issues at a deliberate but casual pace. By the early nineties, market changes were moving so quickly that KP could no longer indulge in such a casual pace.

As the explosive growth of the large for-profit corporations surpassed and threatened the KP market position, Lawrence correctly saw that the pace of change within the organization needed to accelerate. What he apparently did not see was the fundamental value of the genetic code that embodied the core principles of Kaiser Permanente: partnership, integrated facilities, internalization of care, and prepayment. At high-level meetings, he constantly talked about the need to change and grow rapidly, but things suddenly became less clear when the question: "Change to what?" was raised by Dr. Chaffin at one of these meetings.

Political Shakeup in Health Plan

Within Health Plan, Lawrence began replacing many high-level KP veterans with outside executives from the fee-for-service, corporate health care world. When Jim Vohs retired, he retained a position on the KP board of directors. With Lawrence as chairman of the board and changes in the composition of the board, Vohs's efforts to retain the traditional genetic code doctrines were increasingly out of fashion. Vohs kept an office at KP for about five years after his retirement. Seeing that he was completely out of step with the current leadership, he gave it up.

Like many Health Plan executives before him, including Henry Kaiser, Lawrence was impatient with the slow, democratic process necessarily employed by the Medical Groups in their role of representing the medical expertise and ethic of the KP program. He felt that the Permanente Medical Groups were holding back the program from necessary, rapid expansion. He decided to hire McKinsey & Company as strategic consultants.

Consultants

The corporate consultant market is huge. As of 2017, it was a $250 billion per year business. There are four reasons why corporate executives hire consultants. The first is that they really don't know what to do to manage the changing economic environment. They can then tell their governing boards that they are doing something by hiring the consultants. A second reason is that they know what they want to do, but it would be politically or operationally difficult—so they find a consultant who agrees with them. Then they carry out the recommended policies—often involving "reorganization," otherwise known as downsizing. They are able to diffuse some of the political cost to the consultants in a "the devil made me do it" way.

Thirdly, if the policy doesn't work out when questioned by the governing board, they can blame the consultants—who are now long gone. Finally, consultants are not typically responsible for carrying out the recommended changes; that is left up to the corporate executives, who can choose to carry out the changes or not. Since consultants don't often have to deal with the human cost of their decisions, they can often be insensitive to it.

McKinsey & Company

In 1993, Lawrence retained the McKinsey & Company to develop the "change" strategy that he thought could best enable Kaiser Permanente to survive the rapid consolidation of the health care industry. McKinsey & Company was one of the top three consulting firms. It was founded in 1926, originally as a consulting agency, to apply accounting principles to management. As the company evolved, it broadened its scope until it had developed an outsized reputation and influence in American business. McKinsey is known for bringing in fresh ideas, encouraging self-examination, and disseminating an understanding of what other corporations have done to be successful.

McKinsey hires the best and the brightest from many disciplines, often outside of business, straight out of school. They work very hard, and there is an "up or out" company policy. If a McKinsey employee is not promoted, they are asked to leave. These young consultants are very smart, very hardworking, and they work cooperatively in teams. They do, however, often lack hands-on business experience. They develop a strong loyalty to the McKinsey way and each other. McKinsey alumni who later go into business management tend to do very well—not infrequently ending up as CEOs.

McKinsey Doesn't Always Get It Right

No company would survive more than ninety years if it wasn't perceived as giving good value to its customers. Typically, these customers pay a 25 percent premium to engage McKinsey. KP paid McKinsey $16.2 million for strategic planning in 1995 alone, according to findings compiled by the California Nurses Association.

Nevertheless, no one can see the future—and McKinsey doesn't always get it right. In the early eighties, it recommended to AT&T not to invest in cell phone infrastructure because it judged that it would never be more than a niche market. McKinsey gave the go-ahead to the management of Time Warner to proceed with the disastrous $350 billion merger with AOL. While consulting for GM, McKinsey concentrated on corporate management structure rather than product quality—while GM continued to lose market share to competing Japanese companies. An article in *Business Week* in 2002 implicated McKinsey clients in the bankruptcies of Swissair, Kmart, and Global Crossing.

It's Just Business

The culture of McKinsey is strictly business. While this is not so much a problem for a company struggling to cope in a highly competitive market, it would be a problem if the advice crosses ethical lines, especially in medical care. McKinsey has been criticized for insensitivity to ethical constraints on a number of occasions. The worst of these was its involvement with Enron. Jeffrey Skilling was CEO, and twenty-one other managers were McKinsey & Company alumni. While McKinsey was never charged with a crime, it had been a long-term Enron consultant. The *Huffington Post* accused McKinsey of advising Allstate Insurance to lowball claims, and when challenged, to vigorously defend them in the courts to discourage plaintiffs lawyers from taking Allstate cases. It was a consultant to Valeant Pharmaceutics, which was best known for buying companies that manufactured single source, low priced drugs that were off patent. It then hiked the price of these drugs by hundreds of percent. The CEO for a time was a McKinsey alumnus.

Poor Match

McKinsey was a poor match for Kaiser Permanente. It was employed by Health Plan. The Medical Groups were not involved in the contract. McKinsey saw its accountability to be with Health Plan. In Kaiser Permanente, it is the responsibility of the Permanente Medical Groups to provide the medical care and to be sensitive to the ethical, quality, and service imperatives that go along with it. The role of the Health Plan is to organize the marketing and financing of KP so that there are resources for that medical care. *Medical care is the product of Kaiser Permanente—not insurance.* Without understanding the value of the partnership, McKinsey was bound to draw wrong conclusions.

Growth Is the First Priority

By recommending that KP be the lowest-cost provider of health care in its market, McKinsey saw the delivery of health care as a commodity—like sugar. Sugar (sucrose) from Russian sugar beets tastes the same as sugar from West Indian sugar cane. There is little ability to differentiate the product to justify a higher price. Thus, the primary difference that distinguishes the product is price. If one is managing a sugar company, attempting to keep the price lower than the competitors and gain economies of scale due to large size from increasing market share is a good strategy. Kaiser Permanente is not marketing a commodity.

The delivery of personalized medical care is about as far away as one can get from a commodity pricing model. There are huge differences in the quality and outcome of medical care delivered by different health care entities. Providing standardized high-quality care and service and a high ethical standard for the Kaiser Permanente product had always been the responsibility of the Medical Groups. Leaving the Medical Groups largely out of the strategic marketing decisions was a very bad omission.

The exclusive partnership with the Medical Groups was holding back growth. For something as personalized and differentiated as medical care-delivery, size does not necessarily correlate with good. The Medical Groups did in fact slow down corporate decision-making. The role of Health Plan had been to represent the business side of health care, and governance was hierarchical or top down. The role of the Permanente Medical Groups was to represent the complexities of care-delivery and ethical standards of the program. Their organization was democratic or bottom up.

In the long run, recent history teaches us that the results of democratic processes are slower but also more successful and longer lasting than dictatorial processes. KP had always been successful when Health Plan and the Permanente Medical Groups were balanced and working together. Ending this relationship is fraught with danger to both entities. *There is a big difference between a partner and a vendor relationship.* Health Plan never managed vendor relationships on a large scale, and there was little reason to believe that they could do it better than their competitors who had been doing it for decades.

The Permanente Medical Groups, in turn, benefitted from the stability of the Health Plan's facilities, financing, and marketing. Instead of wildly fluctuating economics resulting from the need to manage multiple, transient, Health Plan contracts, it was able to focus on an entirely new way of developing the rational, patient-oriented, medical care that has become the model of health care-delivery. Even though the large, often for-profit, health plans were growing at the time, they had not developed models of health care-delivery beyond existing fee-for-service models. Since health care-delivery *is* the KP product, this was a strategically important omission that was not recognized or exploited by KP or McKinsey.

Break Up the Local Medical Group and Health Plan Partnerships and Centralize Health Plan Regional Control

From the beginning, the success or failure of a region was determined by how well the Permanente Medical Group and Health Plan cooperated in that region. Each year the Kai-Perm Committee, consisting of the PMG presidents, regional Health Plan presidents, and the program executives met at a pleasant off-site location. There, program policies were developed and presented, creating a sense of program solidarity.

During these meetings, there was a cross-fertilization of ideas and important networking opportunities, often resulting in strong bonds of friendship. One such friendship, previously described and important for Hawaii, was the friendship between Bill Dung and Dan Wagster, which made the HPMG/ Health Plan relationship much smoother than it otherwise would have been between 1988 and 1991. Faced with common problems and because of the natural dependency upon each other as they solved serious regional issues together, regional loyalty by Health Plan managers was often stronger than loyalty to Central Office (Program Office) loyalty.

Following McKinsey's advice, Health Plan executive leadership acted to break down this loyalty to the region rather than to the corporation. This was done by dissolving the Kai-Perm committee and establishing divisions that combined previously independent and largely autonomous KP regions under a centralized, often distant Health Plan management. It was an impossible management structure where local managers had to report to remote managers unfamiliar with local problems. It did successfully break down interregional cooperation between Health Plan and the PMG Medical Groups. Local Health Plan managers now had to turn to Program Office for the approval of their strategic direction—as did their executive managers. They now had to report to two bosses: the regional president and the central office boss. Northern and Southern California were their own divisions. Initially, the regions outside of California (ROCs) were a third division. This division was subsequently divided into four divisions, including the Pacific Division (Northwest and Hawaii), Central Division (Colorado and Kansas City), Southern Division (Texas, Georgia, and North Carolina), and the Mid-East Division (Northeast Ohio), and Mid-Atlantic.

Retreat from Vertically Integrated Facilities

If Kaiser Permanente had not established its own hospitals during its formative years, the life would have been crushed out of it by its fee-for-service competitors working in tandem with the forces of organized medicine. It was difficult enough for the Permanente Medical Groups to evolve an entirely new way of practicing medicine without having to simultaneously counter the forces arrayed against them in hospitals dominated by enemies of the program. Prepaid hospital care itself required a whole new approach. Hospital care, like physician care, is not a commodity. The expansion regions that did not establish their own hospitals ultimately failed or were absorbed by the California PMGs.

A good example of what to expect when a KP hospital closes and hospital care must be contracted with the community was the aftermath of the closure of the Northwest Region's Bess Kaiser Hospital. The Bess Kaiser Hospital was completed during the summer of 1959, a few months before the completion of the Kaiser Medical Center in Honolulu. By 1996, at the height of McKinsey influence with Health Plan, the Bess Kaiser Hospital was aging. It would require at least $60 million for capital and seismic improvements. It was located in the inner city, an area with stagnant population growth, while metropolitan Portland growth was in the western and northern suburbs.

Health Plan, with the reluctant acquiescence of the Northwest Permanente leadership, agreed to the McKinsey-influenced recommendation to contract for patient care in local private hospitals. KP was beginning its late nineties financial freefall, so there was no reasonable expectation that capital would be available for a new hospital in any case. The storm broke immediately. Despite the problems associated with practicing in an old facility, the doctors and staff at Bess Kaiser Hospital had evolved into a very effective clinical team that had practiced together for decades. This team would now be broken up to be distributed among the various competitor hospitals and their medical staff. Based upon previous experience, they could expect that their reception into the community hospitals would not be friendly. History would show that, for the most part, their concerns were justified.

Discussions between the medical director, Dr. Allan Weiland, who had been elected to a three-year term as medical director in 1992, and the Northwest Permanente board grew so hostile that Weiland decided not to seek a second term. Fortunately, with the help of a facilitator, the board moderated its positions and asked Al to run for another term, which he did. This was fortunate because, had he not run, the transition from the Bess Kaiser Hospital to the community hospitals would have been much less likely to have been successful. Politically the Portland city government threatened to no longer offer KP as an option to city workers if the hospital and its inner-city services closed. Jesse Jackson threatened a boycott.

A costly compromise maintained urgent care services in the center city. As KP attempted to negotiate hospital contracts, it was under pressure by employers to offer hospital services in the growth areas of the city. This forced KP to make unfavorable, costly contracts with sometimes hostile competitor hospitals. One well-regarded, suburban, contracted hospital was not ready to treat higher-risk obstetrical KP patients who would be coming from Center City when Bess Kaiser closed. Ultimately, KP staff trained the contracted competitor's staff.

PMG doctors introduced efficiencies that were often welcomed by these hospitals—but not always. Medical staff relations ranged from neutral to outright toxic hostility, especially with the Southwest Washington Hospital. Medical staff leaders from this community fought KP every step of the way. At one point, they organized a regional physician monopoly and made an offer to Mike Katcher, Health Plan regional president, that they would give the Health Plan a substantial discount if the Northwest PMG doctors were excluded from the Southwest Washington Hospital. Weiland was not invited to these discussions. Accepting non-Permanente physicians as providers for Health Plan patients would have broken the exclusivity clause of the partnership.

To his credit, Katcher refused the offer, and the program accepted the consequences rather than breaking up the partnership. Harassment ratcheted up. Denial of operating room time, unfair call coverage, denial of office space, and refusal to provide specialty coverage at reasonable cost at the hospital were typical of problems that were constantly cropping up. These issues demanded disproportionate amounts of regional KP administrative attention and inefficient utilization of Northwest Permanente Medical staff.

Dr. Weiland put a positive spin on the effort by saying that by forcing KP to interact with the non-KP hospitals, it demonstrated the innovative high quality of Permanente medicine to the community. When pressed, he would also say that not having its own hospital made the hard job of delivering good care much harder. When further pressed, he would agree that what was saved in capital costs by not building a replacement KP hospital was likely more than lost in care-delivery inefficiencies and unfavorable contracts.

The difficulties of delivering care in community hospitals after the shutdown of a KP hospital were well described by Dr. Weiland's chapter 19 in Dr. Ian MacMillan's comprehensive history *Permanente in the Northwest*. The Northwest region was one of the original KP regions with a half century of experience of delivering affordable, high-quality, and innovative care when Bess Kaiser Hospital closed. At the time of the closure, the Northwest region was blessed with an optimally functioning partnership and exceptional leadership. Nevertheless, the integration into the community hospitals after the Bess Kaiser Hospital closure was extremely difficult and could have easily failed. It is not surprising that many of the newer regions, unable to establish their own hospitals, were not ultimately successful.

Al Weiland was to prove to be one of the best medical directors in Northwest PMG history. He went on to serve three more three-year terms. He deeply believed in the ideals of Kaiser Permanente. He was one of the founders of the Permanente Federation, he helped stabilize the Mid-Atlantic PMG as a live-in consultant for six months when it was faltering in the early 2000s, and he strongly promoted the electronic medical record by leading the effort to implement the Epic program in the Northwest well before the decision to implement it for the entire program. After it was decided that it would be the electronic medical record for the whole program as Health Connect, he traveled extensively to support the implementation.

Dr. Weiland was able to perform these national roles because he and the Northwest Health Plan presidents, first Mike Katcher and then Barbe West, had established a regionally cooperative relationship that was a model for the rest of the program. In 2002, Health Plan leadership terminated partner Barbe West, a respected Northwest region Health Plan veteran of twenty-five years. Despite the regional stresses and expense associated with obtaining non-KP hospital coverage as a result of the Bess Kaiser closure, Health Plan established, in the face of a capital freeze, a 2, 4, then 6 percent yearly financial regional margin (income beyond expenses) requirement. The Northwest region met the 2 percent and then the 4 percent margins, but to achieve the 6 percent margin the following year, Barbe resisted. She believed that the cuts to clinical budget required to achieve the 6 percent margin would negatively impact essential medical services. A month later, she was terminated by senior leadership and escorted from the building that day. After twenty-five years of service, it was the Medical Group, not Health Plan, that organized her retirement party. She went on to serve in an executive capacity in progressive organizations and did good things wherever she went.

The thanks of Health Plan for Weiland's interregional efforts to promote the chosen Epic based Health Connect elect and stabilize the troubled Mid-Atlantic region, was to fire Barbe West and to replace her with someone that did not believe in the partnership. She came from the fledgling Kansas City region where she ended the partnership by opening up membership to a non-KP network of outside physicians. Shortly thereafter, she was presiding over the closure of the region. When she got to Northwest KP, her theory of management was unchanged. With the blessing of senior leadership, she was to sever as many partnerships between Health Plan and Medical Groups as possible. Her theory was that these partnerships with the Medical Group were the reasons for a program's financial downfall. Dr. Weiland thought he could work with her, and he tried as did others in the NW PMG, but without success. It was a one-way relationship. The partnership was gone. In 2004, he was due to run for a fifth term. While he was willing to soldier on, this time, he would have opposition. A delegation of senior shareholders approached him and expressed their dissatisfaction with the poor relationship with Health Plan.

Mike Chaffin and Al Weiland, serving together as medical directors, were good friends. They had similar personalities. Like Mike, Al always tried to avoid confrontation while moving the region forward. After four terms as medical director—and knowing better than anyone the obstacles that he faced both from the Health Plan and the Medical Group— with some relief, he withdrew his candidacy. He felt badly that he had failed to be able to establish a partnership with the new regional president. As history would show, he should not have. While he continued his career with KP, doing many useful things, the loss of his executive leadership was a loss to the whole program. He had not underestimated the obstacles ahead. The Northwest Permanente Medical Group had four presidents over the next six years. Needless to say, isolating the Health Plan from the Medical Group failed spectacularly. The regional president who had initiated the isolationist policy was terminated in mid-2006. It took years to repair the damage to the partnership and the Northwest KP region.

Hawaii Region and McKinsey

Mike Chaffin announced at a board meeting in October 1993 that McKinsey would be coming to the Hawaii region soon to perform an analysis of our market. They didn't show up until February 1995. By then, many of the McKinsey recommendations had leaked out from the regions that had gone before. The Hawaii leadership was very concerned that a breakdown of the partnership, the loss of the hospital and ancillary services (lab and diagnostic imaging) to outside contractors, and dropping the rate to become the lowest-cost provider would result in a rapid failure of the region.

Two respected HPMG leaders, Drs. Peggy Latare and Eric Matayoshi, volunteered to represent HPMG interests by working closely with the Hawaii region McKinsey consultants. Both were excused from clinical duties by HPMG administration because of the perceived importance of a successful interaction by HPMG leadership and the long hours they would be expected to work to match the McKinsey work ethic. Between February and August, the Hawaii medical business environment was intensely analyzed. Drs. Latare and Matayoshi were indeed impressed with the work ethic of the McKinsey consultants, and they, in turn, impressed the McKinsey team. While the McKinsey team recommended an undefined partnership with the existing Queens and Kapiolani Health Plans, the Hawaii staff successfully convinced the McKinsey team that Hawaii really was different from the other regions and that the standard McKinsey recommendations would not work here. The McKinsey consultants went back to their bosses and convinced them to leave Hawaii pretty much as is.

One of the McKinsey consultants eventually married a capable KP staffer and built a successful career in Hawaii. The lesson here is that whenever consultants are invited to the Hawaii region, HPMG must be closely embedded with them.

The nineties were successful for the "McKinsey-free" Hawaii region, which amassed a $300 million surplus earmarked for the renovation of the Moanalua Hospital and the aging peripheral clinic facilities. That surplus is what eventually kept KP in the black in 1998 when it was down to three days of operating cash. The Hawaii region's reserve "disappeared" during the liquidation of the failed regions and the subsequent economic recovery of KP. This has never been forgotten within the region.

The Permanente Federation

On June 18, 1992, Ian Leverton, MD, introduced himself to the HPMG board of directors as the new director of "The Permanente Medical Groups Interregional Services" to succeed Paul Lairson, MD, upon Paul's retirement at year's end. Dr. Leverton had been chief of surgery at Redwood City in Northern California. Then he became medical director of the small Kansas City region, which was founded in 1981 and was later closed in 2001.

Paul Lairson, MD, was an important figure in Permanente Medical Group history. Paul had joined the Northwest PMG as a clinician in 1966 and remained there until 1975 when he became the medical director of the Georgetown University Community Health Plan. This early, not for-profit staff model HMO was acquired by KP in 1980, and the physicians there formed the core group of the Mid-Atlantic Permanente Medical Group. From there, in 1977, he went on to become the founding medical director of the Texas Permanente Medical Group. In 1981, he left Texas to become the first director of the Permanente Medical Groups Interregional Services—the immediate predecessor of the Permanente Federation.

Martin Bauman, MD, the Mid-Atlantic Permanente medical director, watched with concern at the McKinsey-driven, rapidly widening gulf between Health Plan and the Permanente Medical Groups. He strongly advocated for a single national organization to represent the Medical

Groups. This was an idea that had been advocated by Sidney Garfield himself. The two California regional Medical Groups were skeptical of such a plan because of fears of losing influence relative to their size. Each one of the two California regions was large than the combined Regions Outside of California (ROCs). That concern had to be accommodated. By 1996, even the California regions realized that individually they were not strong enough to resist the new direction of Health Plan. The events that pressured the PMG Medical Groups to unite included:

1. The failure of the "Change to What" committee, which sought to find a middle ground between the Medical Groups and Health Plan. Issues included the role of non-Permanente physicians, hospital closures, and the Health Plan expansion strategy.
2. The dissolution of the Kai-Perm Committee, which removed the PMG Medical Groups from program decision-making.
3. The Program Office centralization policy, which established multi-region "divisions." This model completely disrupted regional management decision-making, which normally had been done in partnership with the regional Permanente Medical Groups.
4. The purchase of the financially losing network and staff model Community Health Plan based in Albany, New York. This was a program that was more than two times the size of the existing Northeast region. It was grafted to, and dominated, the much smaller successful, but slowly growing, traditionally established Northeast region. This action was to drag the previously viable Northeast region down to failure in less than two years.
5. Health Plan expansion plans with staff and network model health plans without significant Permanente Medical Group involvement.
6. Finally, and especially alarming to the Permanente Medical Group leadership, were "leaked" McKinsey recommendations to decrease Health Plan partnership dependence upon the Permanente Medical Groups, to break up the regional partnerships in favor of corporate centralization, and to move away from integrated facilities and internalization of care in favor of purchasing outside services from the community.

A work group consisting of Drs. Ian Leverton, Jay Crosson from Northern California's TPMG, Irwin Goldstein from Southern California's SCPMG, and Allan Weiland from Northwest PMG drew up the charter of a new Permanente Federation. It was to be a legal association of all of the PMG Medical Groups. It was also located in Oakland in the same building as the Health Plan offices. Its executive director would be empowered to represent the collective interests all of the Permanente Medical Groups. It was intended to counterbalance and hopefully to partner with Health Plan to develop a national strategy. The executive director had one seat on the executive committee. To reassure the large California regions, both would have permanent seats on the executive committee. Two representatives would be elected from the regions outside of California for an executive committee total of five. No policy could be passed without the assent of one of the California regions.

Jay Crosson, an important Northern California PMG leader, was selected as the first executive director. The first executive committee also included Dr. Oliver Goldsmith, medical director of Southern California PMG, Dr. Harry Caulfield, medical director of Northern California (TPMG), Dr. Allan Weiland, medical director of Northwest PMG, and Dr. Adrian Long, the medical director of Mid-Atlantic PMG. It was a strong team. The charter was presented to all of the Permanente Medical Groups for ratification. Hawaii ratified it in October 1996. All the Permanente Medical Groups had ratified it by January 1997. Membership in the Federation required that no Permanente Medical Group could change the mutually exclusive agreement with the regional Health Plan without the approval of the Federation's executive committee.

Tahoe II: The National Partnership Agreement

By early 1997, in the face of the widening separation between Health Plan and the Permanente Medical Groups, the Federation's leadership petitioned the Kaiser Health Plan and hospital board of directors to make a presentation. By then, the Permanente Federation was up and running, and its charter had been ratified by all of the regional Permanente Medical

Groups. The Federation leaders professionally organized their presentation. The key points were:

1. The divisional structure was not working. It was extremely inefficient and was resulting in confused leadership, poor communication, and operational losses.
2. The policy of distancing the Medical Groups from Health Plan decision-making was financially risky, and it threatened the partnership.
3. Growth by acquiring money-losing staff model and network health plans to establish regions without establishing an exclusive partnership and integrated facilities would be a failed policy. Where networks were required in the early stages of new regional establishment, there were no resources in place to manage networks. Networks, in the traditional model, were under the operational control of the local Permanente Medical Group. Use of networks in parallel to the local Permanente Medical Group was even worse because it placed the local Permanente Medical Group in competition with the better-resourced community doctors for Health Plan business. Obviously, this was a serious threat to the partnership. It was failing in every region where it was being tried.

The Permanente Federation representatives warned the board that if these issues were not addressed, the future of KP was threatened. They emphasized that the Permanente Medical Groups were standing by to help. The board, appointed by Health Plan listened in stony silence. There were no comments. There were no questions. The Permanente Federation leaders got up and left. The Federation leaders felt that the presentation had been a failure. It was not – it was prophetic.

In retrospect, the Kaiser Health Plan board of directors had been given a presciently accurate view of the financial freefall that would occur before the year was out. This was the 1997 $270 million net loss—the first loss in KP history. The losses worsened in 1998 with losses totaling $1 billion. It may also have convinced David Lawrence that he was going to need the cooperation of the Permanente Medical Groups if he was going to turn around the rapidly deteriorating financial situation.

Negotiations began between Health Plan and the Permanente Federation in February 1997. An agreement was reached between Health Plan and the Permanente Federation Leadership and signed in June 1997. In that agreement, the exclusive partnership was affirmed. A Kai-Perm Program Group was established. It consisted of five Permanente Federation representatives and five Health Plan and hospital representatives. It met every month until 2014 when the Health Plan leadership abolished it. It was established to set the direction of the program—specifically all expansion region agreements. Even though it did not take place in Tahoe, it was often informally referred to by Medical Group leadership as "Tahoe II" in remembrance of the landmark Tahoe Agreements of the early 1950s that had established the foundational principles of KP for the next forty years.

The Financial Crisis

On September 19, 1997, Moody's Investor Service placed Kaiser Health Plan and Hospitals bond rating under review for downgrade. On November 13, 1997, the downgrade was announced. It also gave Kaiser a "negative" outlook classification. Moody's reported, "Kaiser management has reaffirmed its commitment to remain an integrated delivery system, utilizing the 'group model' HMO as its core product." Apparently, the national partnership agreement had its intended effect. Moody's however warned that this model would only work if the Health Plan "right sized" its facilities.

Most of the losses came from the Southern California region. In an attempt to promote growth, it had set the membership rates far too low. This resulted in record-setting membership growth. During the early nineties, there had been an overcapacity of hospital beds. McKinsey advice had been to close as many KP hospitals as possible to lower fixed costs and to buy hospital beds at below cost—available because of the then current bed overcapacity. Predictably, as the decade progressed, the weaker hospitals went out of business—and market overcapacity disappeared. KP no longer had enough hospital beds to accommodate a member growth spurt. Consequently, the cost of hospital beds and other clinical outside services skyrocketed at multiples of the internalized cost. The earlier

McKinsey-influenced decision to close facilities was now threatening the entire program. Without the facilities to serve the new membership, KP was required to make unfavorable contracts with the community hospitals and outside providers at high prices to maintain service. All this occurred in the face of a temporary nursing shortage that worsened the situation. The expansion regions, which had not been established with KP founding principles, such as vertically integrated facilities and close partnerships, were also adding to the deficit with no immediate solution in sight.

Losses continued to worsen, and a second bond downgrade was issued on June 19, 1998. The significance of a bond downgrade is that it increases the cost of borrowing money. Riskier bonds command higher interest rates to compensate for the increased risk. This is important because the non-profit Kaiser Health Plan and Hospitals is unable to generate large amounts of investment cash quickly from the stock market. It relies upon bonds to borrow large sums of money to pay for capital needs, such as new hospitals. The bonds are then gradually paid off from future planned margins derived from the yearly prepaid dues.

In June 1998, KP hired Dale Crandall as chief financial officer, chief operating officer, and senior vice president. After 2000, he was named president. In this capacity, he assumed responsibility for much of the KP financial and operational decision-making. Crandall was known for being a turnaround artist, and with his hiring, the KP turnaround began. He had little health care management experience prior to his KP hire, but he proved to be a quick study. By all accounts from the Permanente Federation leaders, led by Jay Crosson, he was much easier to work with once he understood the role of the Permanente Medical Groups in the program.

The June 1998 downgrade was the bond rating low point. Another report was issued in November 1998 that confirmed the bond rating. It noted improvements in program financial performance that were already occurring. Nevertheless, the overall outlook remained negative. By January 2, 2001, Moody's improved the outlook of KP from negative to stable. On April 11, 2002, Moody's improved the KP outlook rating from "stable" to "positive." The worst of the financial crisis was over. To achieve this, the following initiatives, some very painful, were required:

1. Poorly performing expansion regions were liquidated, including Texas, Northeast, North Carolina, and Kansas City. Some of these regions were more than twenty years old. These regions covered more than eight hundred thousand lives. Merger negotiations with Group Health Plan of Puget Sound were shut down.

2. Operational actions included opening existing hospital beds in KP hospitals to reduce contracted hospital bed utilization, reassessment of Emergency Department procedures with the goal of internalizing more care, and the employment of hospitalists by the Permanente Medical Groups to shorten hospital stays to improve the utilization of existing hospital beds.

3. Outside provider and hospital contracts were renegotiated, resulting in more favorable terms.

4. The 1997 growth spurt had been due to unrealistically low dues rates. There was a large rate increase in 1999 to compensate for this error.

5. The debt was restructured.

6. A capital freeze for the entire program was instituted for purchases above $100,000.

7. Bookkeeping was improved to better account for incurred but not reported costs (IBNR).

8. A program to require a cash margin of 2 percent during the first year, 4 percent during the second year, and 6 percent in the third year for the existing regions starting in 2000. These cash-generation requirements fell hard upon clinical services, but they did generate innovations to avoid care compromises.

9. No new expansion regions were contemplated so as to concentrate on the core program.

The program recovered quickly with the new understanding between Health Plan and the Permanent Medical Groups. Relative peace and prosperity continued for more than fifteen years.

CHAPTER 14

THE CASE FOR KP REGIONS OUTSIDE OF CALIFORNIA

Program Genetic Code Compromises That Lost Five Regions:

H enry Kaiser and the founding doctors and Health Plan administrators of Kaiser Permanente believed that the KP model could and should become the model for health care not only for the United States but for the world. Until the mid-nineties, KP actively promoted the model nationally—even helping competitors—to establish KP-modeled HMOs. Kaiser International, which promoted the model outside of the United States, was in existence until the mid-2000s. The founders believed that KP could be a "third way" where the patient's interests would come first. KP would be somewhere between government control (single-payer) where political forces would come first and an unregulated free market where corporate interests would come first. The establishment of the regions outside of California and Oregon reflected this philosophy under KP CEOs Clifford Keene and Jim Vohs. During David Lawrence's administration, the reason for expansion regions changed from modeling a new way to deliver patient-centered health care to rapid company growth.

The fate of those regions not established with genetic code principles was grim. Between 1997 and 2002, four of these regions closed. Subsequently, the management of two regions—Georgia and Mid-Atlantic (metro Washington DC)—were assumed by the California regions. In 2014, the Ohio region closed.

Does this mean that the KP model does not work outside of California? If that is so, then KP cannot aspire to be the model of medical care anywhere outside of California. Few would contend that California mirrors mainstream America even though it is often a trendsetter. Indeed, Kaiser Permanente originated in California.

The following brief analysis of the reasons for the failure of the "lost" regions may provide KP with lessons for the future. The long-term surviving regions remained largely faithful to the genetic code principles of prepayment, an exclusive partnership between Health Plan with a salaried Medical Group and integrated facilities. The regions that did not performed poorly or went out of business.

Prepayment Compromises

Kaiser Permanente has always worked best when the payment model was prepayment. This principle goes back to Sidney Garfield's first hospital in the desert. With guaranteed prepaid funding, future planning could proceed successfully. No effort or resources were wasted on coding, billing, and unpaid claims. These billing processing costs were 15 percent of the health care dollar elsewhere. Most new KP regions started out as purchases of small, usually poorly performing, health plans. Because they were too small to internalize services, these services were mostly provided by networks of private doctors and independent hospitals and pharmacies. The payment model for these networks was fee for service. Unless and until local leadership could internalize most services, and unless the region could either own or control its own hospital and pharmacy, the predominant payment model for these new KP regions was fee-for-service and not prepayment. Internalization of services requires a relentless, uncompromising commitment to an internalization of services by local KP leadership as resistance to internalization from the network providers, lab and diagnostic imaging, and hospitals can be expected. This was nearly impossible at a time when local Permanente Medical Groups and Health Plans were communicating poorly and when national Health Plan leadership was sympathetic to the idea of networks and saw the Medical Groups as holding them back. A predominantly fee-for-service payment model is not Kaiser Permanente.

Partnership Compromises

By weakening the Health Plan-Medical Group partnership, Kaiser Health Plan lost the valuable input of the doctors, the ones who actually delivered the care. As such, it also lost some of the buy-in from them. Traditionally, the Medical Groups had an overall cooperative relationship with Health Plan.

The Permanente doctors generally were proud to be an integral part of a nonprofit health care program that promised to put the patient first. During the early years, this pride was strong enough to overcome the high risk of the ever-present professional ostracism. They accepted the principle of integrating cost-effective medicine into medical decision-making so that health care would be affordable and therefore available for most patients. Furthermore, only the doctors have the extensive medical training to know how to make cost-effective medical tradeoffs without compromising care. For the medical profession at that time, this was a relatively new, professionally risky, and controversial concept. This had historically provided the cost-effectiveness advantage that allowed Kaiser Permanente to provide lower-cost care with the better coverage that had fueled its growth.

As the Lawrence administration moved away from the partnership, most of the experienced Health Plan administrators from the Vohs administration steeped in KP lore and who had managed by the genetic code were replaced. Their replacements were managers from indemnity fee-for-service health plans. They only had a passing familiarity with KP genetic code principles and had not previously managed by them. This change in leadership philosophy had not occurred in the Permanente Medical Groups who still believed in the genetic code principles of Kaiser Permanente. This contributed to the widening gap between the Medical Groups and Health Plan. Supported by the McKinsey recommendations and the new Health Plan administration, these new Health Plan managers saw the Medical Groups as an obstacle to growth. They were already experienced with, and sympathetic to, the idea of independent vendor doctor and hospital networks and had not experienced the advantages of Medical Group partnership.

The new regions that were acquired by purchase were available for purchase because they were already underperforming financially. The Medical Groups were all staff model or networks of physicians that used multiple community hospitals. The Texas (1979), Northeast (1980), Georgia (1981), North Carolina (1981), and Kansas City regions (1985) were established during the Vohs administration and grew relatively slowly but they did make a margin. Wanting to grow faster, the Lawrence administration acquired more poorly performing health plans with wide networks that were grafted onto these fledgling regions. Because KP had always been prepaid, there was no experience managing these networks of independent "outside" doctor and hospital vendors. Without the ability to financially manage these large networks, each of the new region's financial performance could be expected to be poor—and it was.

While the medical groups were supposed to be managing the networks according to the traditional model, by necessity, they were often dominated by the very network that they were supposed to be managing. Naturally, network doctors would resist internalization of services by the core program as they would lose the lucrative business. They often threatened boycotting KP or financial retaliation if their KP business was threatened by internalization. As such, for financial reasons, there was the temptation to favor network doctors over Permanente doctors by Health Plan and even by some of the Permanente Medical Groups.

The nearly unsuccessful internalization of cardiac surgery saga in Hawaii (chapter 10) is instructive. This had occurred in a well-established, strong chief Permanente Medical Group, which had a clear prerogative to manage outside services in a successful partnership with Health Plan in a financially successful region. Imagine how much more difficult internalization of services would be for a newly established Permanente Medical Group working with a Kaiser Health Plan that was following the McKinsey advice that saw the Permanente Medical Group as an obstacle to growth. Health Plan in this setting was a "partner" who would not clearly see the advantages of a partnership arrangement with the local Medical Group over a vendor relationship with network physicians. Often in these new regions, it wasn't even clear which entity—Health Plan or the Permanente Medical Group—managed the network.

Integrated Facility Compromises

During the early development of the program, internalizing medical services was a management priority. In Hawaii, the hospital, clinics, diagnostic imaging, and pharmacy facilities were built by Mr. Kaiser even before Health Plan was established. The principle of vertically integrated medical services came from an understanding that the care-delivery incentives of a nonprofit program, based upon prepayment, would be so different than those of the fee-for-service medical environment that KP could not evolve successfully without its own largely self-contained organization.

Better "Deals"

Without significant Medical Group input, the McKinsey business culture recommendations pursued by Health Plan moved away from integrated facilities in favor of, often transient, better "deals" as a result of temporary community overcapacity. Without significant Permanente Medical Group input, McKinsey was largely unaware of the significant contribution of Permanente medical practice to the program's historical cost efficiency. As stated earlier, the "big money" to be saved in medicine is not from better, transient "deals," better marketing, and better government relations, but in the way that the medical care is practiced. Indeed the doctors do control more than 80% of the costs, but their performance determines 100% of the income. While better contracting "deals," better marketing, and good government relations are important, a motivated, self-policing, high-performing Medical Group acting in partnership with Health Plan is potentially much more important. For this to occur, the Medical Groups need to evolve in a financially secure, stable, medically friendly environment with a maturing partnership relationship with Health Plan. That is the point of this book.

The low bid that would be offered would be likely offered because the hospital was having quality or financial problems to begin with. Such a hospital would also likely be the best candidate for closure in that community. Then what? With the community bed glut eventually eliminated, and with too few internal hospital beds due to downsizing, community beds could only be purchased at a significant premium over internalized costs. As community hospitals failed there would be fewer hospitals with which to bargain. It takes a long time, a lot of planning, and a lot of capital to build a hospital. During that interval, the region without a hospital will be paying a high premium for hospital beds. Thus, an immediate "good deal" on hospital beds can become a very bad deal over the long haul.

Unfortunately, that is only part of the problem. In most contracted hospitals, Permanente doctors are a minority, they are the newcomers, and they are only there because the hospital offered, a—often short-term— lowest-bid contract to Health Plan. As such, these doctors are not likely to have much leverage on their own for favorable treatment by the community hospital administration.

That same hospital administration also has to cater to the majority: competing community doctors. Usually the reception of the KP doctors by the community doctors—the competition—ranges from apathy to downright hostility. The community doctors are typically well established in that hospital, and as such, they already have the best access to the facilities such as favorable operating room time slots. There would be little incentive for the community hospital administration, for example, to move the established surgeons out of the favorable time operating room time slots to give them to KP surgeons who might be gone in a few years in any case. Unless the Kaiser Health Plan negotiators explicitly negotiated that equal services would be provided to the Permanente doctors, the KP doctors would likely be second-class citizens in that hospital. Without the strong support of Health Plan, which would be predominantly interested in price, obtaining equal access to hospital services would be up to the newly relocated Permanente doctors to negotiate these services on their own. With such weak leverage, this would be nearly impossible.

The practice environment of a non-KP hospital presents a much higher professional risk to the individual KP doctor than that of a similar practice in a KP hospital. If the economic model of the contract hospital is fee-for-service, hospital policies and procedures will reflect this bias in the hospital policies and procedures. To protect their career, there would be a powerful incentive for KP physicians to fit in. The loss or restriction of hospital privileges from a hostile hospital staff would be entered into the Physicians National Databank to follow that doctor for the rest of that doctor's career. Permanente Medicine based upon the ideals of Kaiser Permanente, would be slow to evolve if it did at all, in a contract community hospital that the regional Permanente Medical Group didn't dominate. That would be the real loss—both professionally and financially.

Ancillary Services: Pharmacy, Pathology, and Diagnostic Imaging—No Medical Effectiveness-Based Cost Controls

Using outside pharmacies exclusively would also conflict with Permanente medical practice. Within the Kaiser Permanente pharmacy infrastructure, the pharmacists work closely with Medical Group doctors to establish a formulary to eliminate useless drugs, restrict expensive "me-too" drugs that have little or no advantage over established drugs, and develop programs to rationally prescribe the remaining drugs. These actions would be disincentives for a fee-for-service, for-profit, outside pharmacy. These pharmacies have a fee-for-service incentive model—the more and higher cost drug prescriptions filled the higher the profits.

When considering the overall health care budget, the ceiling of which is set by society, the cost of drugs is the major driver of health care inflation. Pharmaceutical cost inflation is rising at three times that of physician or hospital services and is six times higher than the general rate of inflation. If KP is to be cost competitive, then pharmaceutical use needs to be scrutinized and controlled. Abdicating control of pharmaceutical utilization is likely to be vastly more costly in the long run than internalized KP pharmacy costs. Similar arguments apply to externalized diagnostic imaging and pathology and laboratory services not staffed by PMG physicians. In similar ways, the financial incentives would be driven by fee-for-service principles in conflict with those of KP. Externalized services are unlikely to cost less than internalized services unless the vendors were willing to accept capitated payments that were less than KP's internalized services—an unlikely event. Once internalized services are contracted out, it takes years to re-establish those services internally.

As stated repeatedly, within a fixed budget, inappropriate excessive utilization of resources by one entity must be compensated for by fewer resources available to the other entities. For KP to work optimally, *all* clinical services should be managed within the program. The founders were correct about the need to internalize services. A strong case can be made that violation of this principle of internalized services contributed to the demise of the failed regions.

Texas: 1979–1997

The Texas region was established as a joint venture with Prudential back when KP was trying to promote its model as the model for health care—even to potential competitors. After learning what they needed to know, Prudential left the partnership to KP. Clinics were widely spread over the huge Dallas-Fort Worth metropolitan area, which is larger than four of the fifty states. For example, even if KP had a urologist in a Dallas hospital, the distance from Dallas to Denton, Texas, in the northern suburbs, would have been forty-two miles through city traffic. As a result of this geographic dispersion, the Texas region was heavily dependent upon fee-for-service network physicians. KP was a very small player everywhere in the region. Hospitalizations were concentrated in two hospitals—one in Dallas and one in Fort Worth. In both hospitals, KP patients were never more than a small minority of admissions.

The political environment was simply hostile. During the region's existence, Texas was considered one of the best places in the country to bring a malpractice suit. Tort reform did not occur until 2003—too late for the KP Texas region. Lawsuits, in the name of the health plan rather than individual doctors as in other KP programs but not competitor plans, were misrepresented against the program by a hostile attorney general as the health plan with the most lawsuits. For example, Doctor X a non-Permanente doctor is sued for malpractice. By contract, the health plan is not sued. In contrast if a Permanente physician is sued, it is attributed to the Health Plan not the physician since the Health Plan manages medico-legal issues. This and other distortions of facts were compiled by a very hostile Texas attorney general's office to attempt to embarrass KP nationally and drive it out of Texas. The negative state report, eventually blocked in the courts by KP for its inaccuracies, had been given to the ABC network investigative news program "Prime Time Live" several days before it was even submitted to KP. That government hostility coupled with a $52 million loss from 1996 to 1997 due to an inability to internalize services quickly enough, caused Program Office to shut down the region. It was the first Kaiser Permanente region to ever fail. Ironically, it was at its membership peak of 129,000 members—a viable size if it had been centralized and followed genetic code KP principles.

Northeast: 1982–1999

Kaiser Permanente was invited by Connecticut state officials to acquire a poorly performing Hartford regional health plan. In 1992, KP operations commenced. A new sub-region in the Pioneer Valley of the Connecticut River in Western Massachusetts started in the northern suburbs of Springfield, Massachusetts, by acquiring Valley Health Plan.

By acquiring the small Westchester Community Health Plan, it expanded into Westchester County in the northern suburbs of New York and Fairfield County in Connecticut. The three small sub-regions were too far apart geographically and culturally to significantly support each other—at least initially. Even though Springfield, Massachusetts, and Hartford, Connecticut, were the two closest metropolitan medium-sized cities in the US, they were distinct societies. They were in different states with their own independent media outlets. Only in the past decade, long after the demise of the Northeast KP region did the two metro regions really begin to cooperate. As a result of this geographic and cultural dispersion, none of these sub-regions, at least starting out, was large enough to own or even dominate a hospital.

The Northeast region may have eventually made it on its own. In 1997, there were about 150,000 members with roughly one-third of the membership in each sub-region. Growth was slow but steady. The sub-regions were geographically close enough that if they continued to grow, they would have been able to coalesce using the California sub-region model. Hartford center city was only twenty-four miles from Springfield, fifty miles from Fairfield County, and seventy-five miles from Westchester County. During its existence, the Northeast region was constantly vying with Hawaii as the KP region with the best quality and service.

All this changed in 1997 when Community Health Plan and the KP Northeast region merged. Community Health Plan of Latham, New York, near Albany, was a vast 350,000-member network health plan covering the Albany metropolitan region, the entire state of Vermont, and parts of New Hampshire and Western Massachusetts. There were more network neurosurgeons in Community Health Plan than in the entire KP organization. Virtually every doctor in Vermont was a participant in the network.

Community Health Plan was losing money, and its executives thought that merging with KP would cover the losses and somehow reverse the losses. Kaiser Health Plan management, on the other hand, was obsessed with rapid growth and had few concerns about compatibility or even prospects for success when merging with a money-losing, large network model that was more than twice the size of the existing KP Northeast region. It was a very poor match. Because of its size, Community Health Plan management and physicians almost immediately took control of the region. KP had no special expertise managing networks, and any cost efficiencies from the existing KP program were overwhelmed by network losses. With the merger, losses only accelerated. In 1998, the region lost $97 million. The decision was made by Program Office to close the whole region at the end of 1998—less than two years after the merger. The Northeast Kaiser Foundation Health Plan and the Northeast Permanente Medical Group dissolved.

North Carolina: 1985–1999

At least initially, KP had cordial relationships with the North Carolina state government. Indeed, KP was recruited to set up a program within the state. Unfortunately, KP facilities were widely dispersed from the outset. Initially intended to serve the Research Triangle of Raleigh-Durham and Chapel Hill, itself a large area, it eventually expanded to Charlotte and twenty-two of the hundred counties in the state. Over this area was spread two hundred Permanente doctors but four hundred network doctors. There was no possibility of a central hospital. The large, predominantly fee-for-service network and a dispersed regional Permanente Medical Group prevented the development of a KP that could implement Permanente Medicine along with KP-first principles.

In the academic *Milbank Quarterly* 2003 article "The Rise and Fall of a Kaiser Permanente Expansion region" by David Gitterman et. al. (including HMO and KP expert Alan Enthoven), failure of the Carolina region was attributed to: (1) Marketing interference by the state government, (2) micromanagement by Program Office in Oakland that limited the ability to adapt to the new market, (3) excessive debt-service demands by Program Office, (4.) and a poor regional partnership.

In the course of writing the article, the authors interviewed both Health Plan and Medical Group executives. Each blamed the other for the demise of the region. The authors found the arguments inconclusive. As in any partnership, working with the partner instead of blaming them is the better course of action. Shortly before the closure of the region, Health Plan experimented with private physician networks in competition with the Carolina Permanente Medical Group. This is a terminal event for any KP partnership, and it would be a terminal event for any KP region that tries it. It was the terminal event for the Carolina region.

Between 1985 and 1992, the Carolina region had a net loss of $113 million, including startup costs.

The region was profitable between 1992 and 1995 with a total profitability during those years of $17 million, but then losses accelerated until its closure in 1999. The total loss to the program by the Carolina venture was $280 million. At the time of its closure, the membership had peaked at 134,000. In a traditional KP region, this would have been large enough to internalize most services, but that would not have been possible with the dispersed North Carolina model. KP sold the Carolina health plan to health plans in Charlotte and the Research Triangle. The medical group continued on for a time as an IPA, the "Carolina Premier Medical Group," but it filed for bankruptcy in 2000.

Kansas City: 1985–2001

Kansas City Healthcare was incorporated in 1981 and was acquired by Kaiser Permanente in 1985. Kansas City had a metropolitan population of approximately two million spread over fifteen counties in two states. Such a large area combined with a relatively low population density required a large network to service patients locally. The membership never exceeded sixty thousand. Such a small membership scattered over such a large area meant there was little prospect of a Kaiser Permanente-based Permanente Medical practice of internalized services ever taking hold. The Kansas City region was incorporated into the Colorado Division in 1997, which proceeded to liquidate the Kansas City region. It was purchased by Coventry Health Care.

Ohio: 1969–2015

Kaiser Permanente was established in Ohio at the invitation of labor unions. It grew to a membership of 210,000 with the traditional KP structure and identity. In 1994, with both of its hospitals needing replacement and the national program at the peak of its McKinsey influence, it was decided to obtain hospital beds from the Cleveland Clinic rather than rebuild its own hospitals. The Cleveland Clinic is a world-renowned medical institution, and at the time, it was building a local network to decrease its reliance upon out-of-area and international business. The relationship with the Cleveland Clinic was excellent as long as Health Plan and Cleveland Clinic administrators were willing to tend to the relationship.

Changes in leadership at the Cleveland Clinic and a simultaneous rapid turnover of Ohio Regional Health Plan presidents caused the relationship to break down. As long as KP was identified as an affiliate of the Cleveland Clinic, it maintained a lower but sustainable membership. By the time that the relationship broke down, a separate KP Ohio regional identity was long gone, having been subsumed into the Cleveland Clinic identity, and with the breakup, membership steadily decreased. Unsuccessful efforts to reestablish the relationship with the Cleveland Clinic continued until the Cincinnati-based Catholic Health Partners acquired the Ohio region in

2013 when the negotiations ceased. Catholic Health Partners was more interested in working out a relationship with the University (Case Western) Hospital System, which was the Cleveland Clinic competitor in Cleveland.

By 2013, the Ohio region had shrunk to eighty thousand members and fifteen clinics. In its last year as a KP region, Ohio lost $30 million. The plan was sold to Cincinnati-based Catholic Health Partners, the largest health plan in Ohio in 2013. Catholic Health Partners, a hospital-based corporation, was establishing a venture known as Health Partners, which it hoped could provide comprehensive Health Plan services. The former Ohio KP was to be the core Medical Group, and it was a mandatory part of the sales agreement with Kaiser Health Plan. The Ohio Permanente Medical Group remained intact to serve this new entity.

The attempt by Catholic Health Partners to duplicate the KP delivery of services was unsuccessful. Losses persisted and then accelerated. Catholic Health Partners closed its money-losing Health Partners Division at the end of 2015. The medical group then dissolved, having survived less than two years after its dissociation from the Kaiser Health Plan.

Group Health

Group Health Cooperative of Puget Sound, based in Seattle, was a large member-driven, nonprofit, staff model health plan founded in 1945. In the early days of HMOs, it was often mentioned in the same breath as Kaiser Permanente as an HMO model. During the mid-1990s, it began movement toward a merger with the Northwest KP region with a change to a group rather than staff model.

In 1997, the Health Plan leadership of both regions canceled the merger progress. The Medical Group however pursued an affiliate association with the Permanente Medical Group Federation as the Group Health Medical Group. Upon the acquisition of Group Health by KP in 2017, the Medical Group changed its name to the Washington Permanente Medical Group, and it has fully integrated into the Permanente Federation.

Paralleling KP, in the mid-1990s, Group Health downsized its hospital presence. It partnered with the Virginia Mason Hospital, and Virginia Mason used the Group Health ambulatory surgical facilities. There was also a large Group Health network outside of the core plan. Even with this model, Group Health continued to sustain losses, which resulted in its acquisition by KP. The region's leadership is now seriously considering decreasing its dependence upon networks by strengthening its specialty capabilities and building out its own hospital infrastructure. With an established 700,000 membership base, if it is able to successfully accomplish this, its future is bright. The official turnover to KP occurred on February 1, 2017, so only time will tell.

What Have We Learned?

History's greatest value is it that it can guide us away from what has previously failed and toward policies that have been successful in the past. Much of this predictive value is rooted in human nature, which hasn't changed much in thousands of years. The genetic code guided Kaiser Permanente successfully from about 1945 until 1992. It was a period of financial success, increasing membership, steady quality, and service improvement as well as geographic expansion. Starting in 1992, experiments with the "KP Genetic code" throughout the decade resulted in near bankruptcy, geographic contraction with consequent loss of membership, and near dissolution of the partnership. By largely returning to first principles after Tahoe II, the program was restored to health. That was to last for another 15 years when Health Plan decided to repudiate the agreement.

These failures, from which KP recovered, were not the result of a conspiracy of evil minds in Health Plan. Dr. Jay Crosson, leader of the Permanente Federation during the recovery, and an important participant in it, probably had more contact with high-level Health Plan leadership than anyone. He would be the first to say that the Health Plan leaders were well-meaning people who obtained their own health care and that of their families from Kaiser Permanente. They were honestly worried—nearly panicked—about the rapid changes occurring in health care that threatened to relegate KP to the dustbin of history.

With the transfer of power from Jim Vohs to David Lawrence, there was also a change in Health Plan leadership at lower levels. Most of these leaders came from indemnity medicine. While often excellent managers, their management models came from fee-for-service networks. Coming from a model that often saw care providers as financial adversaries, they had not experienced the advantages of prepayment, partnership with the medical staff, and integrated facilities. Their knowledge of KP heritage was scant. Program efforts to educate them were minimal. It is understandable that they were open to lowering fixed costs by closing hospitals and other KP facilities, embracing fee-for-service networks at the expense of the regional Permanente Medical Groups, and compromising with prepayment. After all, that is what one of the most prominent business consultant groups (McKinsey) was telling them to do to achieve rapid expansion.

There were legitimate issues of concern within KP in the early nineties. There were whole regions and sub-regions (now called Service Areas-For example the San Diego Service Area was part of the Southern California Permanente Medical Group)where Health Plan and the Permanente Medical Groups were locked in conflict, bringing true partnership and progress to a standstill. As occurs periodically in all large organizations, complacency, "bureausclerosis," and "not invented here" resistance to improvement slowed program progress. These maladaptive behaviors are an expected product of human nature and can be overcome with good management. It was only when the short-term tactical solutions compromised the strategic genetic code principles that KP was nearly finished off.

Establishing New Regions: Lessons Learned

There have been no new Kaiser Regions established in more than thirty years. The last region established was in 1985. The last new region to survive independently was founded in 1969— half a century ago. Of the two regions that were established in 1969—Ohio and Colorado—only Colorado survives. The executive management of the Mid-Atlantic region (Metro Washington-Baltimore) comes from Northern California (TPMG) and for the Georgia region (Metro Atlanta) from Southern California (SCPMG). It should be recalled that both California regions have preserved the original genetic code. The new Washington region (2017) is the acquisition of the Seattle-based former Group Health Cooperative, which has been flirting with various KP associations for more than twenty years. If the executive management implements core KP principles, then its future is very bright.

Does this mean that Kaiser Permanente expansion was a historical accident possible only during the fifties through the eighties. Has the market evolved better competitive models? Not necessarily. The difference between the older successful regions and the newer regions is that the older regions were established and maintained using the classic genetic code principles. The relatively unsuccessful newer regions were established with compromised genetic code principles. These included:

1. Partnership Compromises: These were characterized by isolating Health Plan decision-making from the Permanente Medical Groups. These were decisions that compromised financial performance of the core program of the new regions. Widely dispersed clinics staffed by small numbers of Permanente Medicine doctors in a region where much of the care, especially specialty care, is delivered by network physicians strongly inhibits or even prevents the establishment of Permanente Medicine.

2. Integrated Facility Compromises: No region established without its own hospital has survived independently. The exception is the Colorado region. While Colorado didn't own its own hospital, Colorado Permanente Medical Group (CPMG) physicians so dominated St. Joseph's Hospital, almost from the beginning, that for CPMG physicians, there was no impediment to Permanente practice. Ohio initially had two hospitals, but both were closed in 1994 and were not replaced as part of the Health Plan early nineties' policy of closing KP hospitals in favor of using contract hospitals. The region went into steady gradual decline after. The Ohio Permanente Medical Group physicians were not major players in the community hospitals in which they practiced. As noted, the program was closed in 2013. In the Northwest Region the consequences of not replacing the Bess Kaiser Hospital but relying on community hospitals is another cautionary tale.

3. Prepayment Compromises: Large networks require the ability to manage fee-for-service practices. KP went into these extensive network contracts with little or no experience negotiating extensive

fee-for-service network contracts. This new, large administrative expense, 10–15 percent of the budget of most indemnity health plans, diverted resources from the care-delivery of the core plan. This was Sidney Garfield's first lesson—prepayment saved his hospital. Few network physicians are interested in capitated payment models. The regions with large networks failed or were annexed by the California regions. As long as most care, especially specialty care, is network care, Permanente Medicine can't really evolve.

Why Establish New Regions?

It was Jim Vohs policy to ease out long term Kaiser Heath Plan manager with special retirement projects. His reasoning was that it would wasteful not to avail the organization of their long experience while making room for younger leadership. There was a project building devoted to just this humane policy. It ended with his retirement as CEO.

As a retirement project, Dr. Bruce Sams, the former long-term TPMG medical director, and Daniel Wagster, former regional president of Southern California, then Northwest, then Hawaii, were tasked with summarizing the successes and failures of the expansion regions. It was ninety-one pages long and entitled "The Kaiser Permanente Expansion Study." It was issued in February 1993 and based upon data up to the end of 1992. That was the year David Lawrence became KP CEO, succeeding Jim Vohs. For anyone interested in rejuvenating the idea of expansion regions, this monograph, which is in the KP and Hawaii archives, should be required reading.

The two authors had been militant representatives of their own entities—Dr. Bruce Sams for the Medical Group and Dan Wagster for the Health Plan. Nevertheless, they both believed in the traditional principles of Kaiser Permanente. Their belief in the value of partnership is evident in this important document. Unfortunately, the timing was bad. In the document, both authors reasoned within KP "Genetic Code" principles. The new, McKinsey-influenced Lawrence administration saw the KP genetic code principles as obsolete and a "constraint" to growth and financial success. As noted, the "genetic code" principle compromises led to near bankruptcy by the end of the decade and the closure of five regions. So why reconsider the policy of expansion regions? This remains an important strategic question for the future leaders of Kaiser Permanente. What is the case for Kaiser Permanente semi-autonomous regions?

KP as a Model of Health Care

The Kaiser Permanente founders deeply believed that the KP model was the answer to the problem of health care-delivery, and they acted accordingly. Between 1960 and 1985, nine new regions were established in addition to the original three. The intention was to establish a national network of KP regions, and through the KP International Department, to promote the model internationally. KP was widely seen in academic circles as a viable solution to health care-delivery. Things changed with KP's poor financial performance of the late 1990s and the subsequent failure of five expansion regions. The apparent failure of the expansion regions outside of those established before 1970 has given comfort to KP critics who maintain that the KP model is not viable outside of California and a few regional "historical accidents." It is too soon to tell if the new Washington region will embrace the KP genetic code principles or even if it will remain as an independent region.

Geographic Diversification

KP is heavily concentrated in the California regions, which alone cares for 70 percent of the entire membership. Executive Permanente Medical Group management of the one million member Mid-Atlantic and Georgia Regions—another 8.3 percent—is also controlled out of the California regions. This parallels the long-standing Program Office trend to steadily weaken all regional management and to substitute it with Program Office control.

Could the program survive if something really bad happened in California as it did in 1997? The two big risks that come to mind are natural and political earthquakes. The urban areas where most KP members reside and where most of the facilities are located are on or near active fault lines. Program Corporate offices in Oakland are within sight of the very active Hayward Fault. It is not a question of whether the "big one" is going to happen in California—but when. Fortunately, in the early 2000s, having learned the folly of outsourcing to competitor hospitals, KP went on a massive hospital- and clinic-building program to replace its old hospitals using the latest earthquake-resistant technology. One can only hope that "earthquake resistant" will be enough.

The political earthquake that comes to mind is the institution of a single-payer payment program managed by the state of California. The present governor of California ran on such a platform. How would Health Plan fare with a California single-payer government payment program? A single-payer program would pay providers directly. Why would alienated Permanente Medical Groups need Kaiser Health Plan. Having dispersed, successful, autonomous, well-populated regions could hold the program together in such an event. In addition, it would be in a position to provide rapid financial or other support California in a financial or other disaster as Hawaii did in 1997.

Financial Diversification

Recall that during the financial crisis of 1998, at its low point, KP was financially reduced to cash for only three days of operations. This amount approximated the cash available from little Hawaii's cash surplus, which plugged the hole in the dike just long enough for the program to turn itself around. That financial catastrophe was largely due single-year rate-setting error in the Southern California region. At the time, Hawaii represented only about 2.2 percent of the program membership. Despite McKinsey recommendations, Hawaii did not close its hospital. It did not lower its rates to become the lowest-cost health plan in Hawaii, and it continued to internalize services as quickly as possible. As a result, the nineties were a good decade for Hawaii, and by the end of the nineties, it had a $200–300 million surplus.

That was a very close call, and small Hawaii would not have been able help the program for very long if a rapid KP financial turnaround had not occurred. Indeed, it probably would have been dragged down into bankruptcy with the rest of the program. There is a saying in business that a business is either growing—or it is dying. A principle of successful investing is diversification. Both of these principles, financial and geographic diversification, would support a return to regional autonomy and expansion defined as a centralized strategy based on the KP genetic code principles at the national level and regional tactics in compliance with these principles but with enough tactical agility to accommodate local challenges.

Innovation

Different regions provide different financial environments and different challenges. It is often easier to design and implement solutions to these challenges in medium sized regions. They are small enough so that everyone knows everyone yet these regions are large enough to be able to resource an innovation. Throughout KP's history, the smaller regions out of proportion to their size, have pioneered many innovations adopted by the whole program. By having multiple regions in many different financial environments following the KP "Genetic Code", myriad adaptations would be available to the financially dominant California regions should the need arrive. The dinosaurs perfectly adapted to the earth's environment, dominated the earth for more than 140 milllion years – then about 65 million years ago the asteroid struck-the ultimate black swan. Fortunately there were other animal designs available for the recovery. We live in the "age of mammals. The dinosaurs never came back.

Learning from Our Mistakes

The value for an organization to understand its history is to guide it away from repeating past errors. What doesn't kill an organization can make it stronger if organizational memory is retained-if heeded. Many lessons were learned from the failed regions, and many were foreseen in the Sams-Wagster expansion monograph. Unfortunately, the monograph was apparently ignored as KP turned away from its traditional organizational principles.

By the time of the February 1993 monograph, all the expansion regions had reached a positive cash flow—and their collective debt to the program was decreasing. A good case could be made for their long-term survival had the program maintained its genetic code principles. For various reasons, they didn't and were gone within nine years. Reading this book, it should be clear that the Hawaii region had at least four near misses during its history that were as serious as anything faced by the failed regions. The author, who personally experienced three out of four of them, would maintain that when everything seemed lost, it was the aspirational ideal of the traditional Kaiser Permanente promise in the minds of the leadership and the line staff that held it together.

So, half a century after the establishment of the last independent, successful region, let's say leadership was going to try again. Many of these concepts were prophetically presented in the 1993 expansion monograph but not implemented. What lessons did KP learn about establishing new regions?

Finance Adequately

As noted earlier, the Hawaii region, with integrated facilities in place even before the program was marketed, a strong Permanente Medical Group, and both local and national Health Plan support, didn't break even for four years. It wasn't self-sustaining, having the ability to sustain rate-setting cycles and having adequate capital reserves for facility expansion and replacement, for three years after that. As noted in the 1993 expansion study, this sort of time line was generally true for all of the expansion regions. In the business case study analyzing the failure of the North Carolina region, the demand to generate cash to pay off its loans before it was securely established contributed to its premature downfall.

When establishing a new region, it needs to be seen as an investment. A large amount of capital needs to be set aside prior to making the attempt. A long cash burn, five years to the break-even point and up to ten years to self-sustainability should be anticipated. Serious deviation from the KP "genetic code" principles will likely lengthen these time frames or more likely result in long-term regional failure. In the long run it is a good investment for the program as a whole.

Establishment and Support by the Permanente Federation and Health Plan: Support Not Control

The strategic direction to invest in new regions for reasons of geographic diversification, financial diversification, and innovation should be a joint program decision by Health Plan and the Permanente Federation. Otherwise, only the California regions would be large enough to sponsor and rescue failed regions. Having new regions only as subsidiaries of the California regions would further decrease financial and geographic diversification. Consideration should be given to not expecting the loan to be paid back but as an investment in the future of all of KP. Once a region is declared autonomous, it would then be expected to contribute its share for future regional investments and common program expenses. If program leadership really believes that the KP ideals should be spread because it is the right way to deliver medical care, investing in new regions would be KP putting its money where its mouth is. If the mission of KP is about generating money rather than offering an ethical, practical model for delivering healthcare, then all of these founding KP "genetic code" principle are simply quaint.

Compact—Not Diffuse Market Areas

All the expansion regions established after 1979 were established in geographically large metropolitan regions thinly served by KP in predominantly primary care clinics. The designers of this model thought that patients would want small, nearby clinics. Hawaii patient surveys have consistently demonstrated that when ranked in order of importance, nearby facilities ranked between sixth and eighth—well below doctor quality and service, proper billing, and comprehensive care. The KP promise is very difficult, if not impossible, to fulfill with a model of widely spread out clinics served by small numbers of Permanente doctors, contracted non-Permanente fee-for-service specialists, and hospitalized in contracted hospital beds in multiple hospitals. *A building with a Kaiser Permanente logo on it is not Kaiser Permanente.* The Kaiser Permanente promise is a promise of high-quality, preventive, well-coordinated, scientifically based medical care that is as comprehensive as possible to be affordable to the largest population possible. Again, none of these decentralized expansion regions survived independently.

In the 1993 KP expansion study, thirteen reasons were given for reversing the clinically decentralized model of regional care delivery back to the traditionally centralized regional model of care. One of the most important reasons was loss of the KP identity. With a decentralized model, it is hard to differentiate KP health care-delivery from coexisting independent practice associations (IPAs). The decentralized model pits KP in competition with the strengths of the IPAs: localized care without the advantages of the KP identity characterized by the "genetic code" principles; partnership, well-integrated (hospital, pharmacy, diagnostic imaging, pathology and other services), comprehensive, prepaid, high-quality care with an emphasis on prevention.

Other reasons included the high cost of inefficient small clinics. In the KP expansion study, the regional cost of clinics went down as the size of the clinic went up. A four-doctor clinic was up to 40 percent more costly to maintain than a twenty-four-to-forty-eight-doctor clinic. Also noted were much higher startup costs until most of the care was internalized, very difficult to accomplish if a region consists of small scattered predominantly primary care clinics. Also noted was difficult leadership communication, and high travel costs. Doctors can either be serving patients or driving from clinic to clinic to hospital in congested urban traffic at a cost to the program-and therefore the members-of $250 to $400 per hour.

The best demographic for a new KP region would be a compact, medium-sized metropolitan region with a population of 500,000 to 1,000,000. As a second option, if KP were to attempt to set up a new region in a large metropolitan region, it should concentrate its facilities to a single suburb that could financially support the plan during its establishment phase and then expand from there.

Let us imagine an alternative history for the Northeast region. The metropolitan population of Springfield, Massachusetts, is ~700,000, for Fairfield County, Connecticut, and Westchester County, New York ~1,000,000 each, and for Hartford, Connecticut, and Albany, New York ~1,200,000 each for a total population of five million. Each of these five metropolitan regions is a compact and self-sufficient urban entity. For each of these sub-regions, early internalization of services out of central hospital-based facilities would greatly lower costs and insulate each region from competitor price gouging.

With good management combined with adherence to the KP genetic code, history suggests that a realistic potential market share of 15 percent within ten to fifteen years could be attained. That would result in a KP region of 750,000 members, which would make this imaginary Northeast region the third largest region of KP. With such a region already established in the northern suburbs (Westchester County) of New York's twenty-four million-person megalopolis, there would be tremendous potential for even further growth.

Integrate Facilities and Internalize Care

A Kaiser-owned hospital, within easy walking distance of a Kaiser-owned building for clinic, ancillary, and administrative services, with space for parking and expansion would be ideal. This building could contain primary care physicians to cover the local population but also hospitalists, centralized regional specialty departments to allow for sub-specialization and the associated specialty procedure suites, outpatient surgical suites, and ancillary departments, including diagnostic imaging, pathology, and pharmacy. As important, it should be the center of regional governance with offices of Permanente Medical Group and Health Plan executive leadership in close proximity to promote coordinated leadership. Finally, to support leadership and clinical innovation activities, there should be adequate meeting room space and an auditorium with the latest AV and remote capabilities to act as a nerve center for the rest of the regional clinics.

Obviously, a newly established region would not have the capital to do all of this from the start, but it should be considered as a master facilities plan. It which would promote coordinated leadership, easy communication, efficient care-delivery, and a template for rapid internalization of care. It would serve as the "mother ship" of a growing region on a rapid path to autonomy, at which point, it would provide mutual support to all the other KP regions.

Restore the Partnership

The program evolved such that the Health Plan and Permanente Medical Groups are in MAD status if the partnership fails. MAD was a Cold War term that stands for "mutually assured destruction." Attempts at establishing Independent Physician Association (IPA) clinics in subregion expansion areas without a Permanente physician core has consistently failed wherever it has been tried. Examples include Northern California (Modesto), Southern California (Palm Springs and Ventura), Colorado (Colorado Springs), and Hawaii (Kauai). These examples either needed to be converted to a traditional Kaiser Permanente model or closed.

Point-of-service programs, if they covered their expenses, were too expensive to be popular and never amounted to much. If they didn't cover their expenses, they were diverting resources from the core program and decreasing the entire regional program to compete. On the other hand, no Permanente Medical Group has persisted more than two years after ending its partnership with Health Plan. Most Permanente Medical Groups simply dissolved at the time of the regional closure. Anything that increases the cooperation between the Health Plan and the Permanente Medical Group leadership is good for the Health Plan, good for the Permanente Medical Group, and ultimately good for the local community.

Community Rating—Sort Of

Community rating meant that the cost of providing care to everyone in the community would be estimated—and then everyone would pay that rate up-front with few or no additional costs. The sick and the well pay the same rates. Community rating is the basic premise of all insurance.

In 1991, the concept in its pure form had to be abandoned by KP if the program were to survive. The HMO Act of 1973 had nothing in it about health plans being nonprofit—nor was community rating required. By the late eighties, an increasing number of health plans were for-profit. This causes a potential disconnect between the actual cost of care and rate setting. In the for-profit setting, if the cost of care is lowered, and the rate is not lowered but maintained, profits—and therefore stock prices and dividends—increase. There was now a third partner in the rate-setting equation—the stockholder. In contrast, the incentives of nonprofit health plans were efficient delivery of health care thus conserving health care resources that could be devoted to improved service, lower costs, and wider benefits. This model is well aligned with patient interests. There are no investors' interests that must be served.

The incentives of patients and stockholders were not so well aligned in the for-profit models. The best way to increase profits and therefore increase stock value was for the for-profit health plans to lower the cost of care but not necessarily to lower monthly rates. This initially led to some control of waste, which was admittedly not always well managed in nonprofits, but it quickly progressed to the denial of appropriate care and marketing only to the profitable well patients.

One of the best ways to lower health care costs is cherry-picking: signing up patients who don't need any care and driving away patients who do. One of the best ways to do this was to design "skinny" plans that set very low monthly rates but very high deductibles. The low cost would be attractive to those who didn't think they needed health care and especially to the employers that usually paid for employee health insurance. These same plans were unattractive to patients who actually need care because of the very high deductibles. This is where we are today. Without a level playing field, this trend will continue. At some point, it isn't going to be insurance any more but fee-for-service medicine—unless the playing field is leveled. There will need to be equal community rating for both for-profit and nonprofit with standardized and enforced categories of coverage—platinum, gold, silver, bronze—and hopefully not sand, dirt, or worse categories.

KP held on to community rating for as long as it could, but by the early 1990s, it was being priced out of the market by companies offering low monthly rates and high deductibles. In 1991, its leadership reluctantly threw in the towel and began a form of "experience rating"—sicker patients paid more—called "adjusted community rating." KP deductibles prior to this change had always been minimal. To remain competitive, KP had to increase the deductibles to make up for the lost up-front prepaid monthly dues revenue. For the first time in KP history, deductibles were a looming threat over the KP-covered family budget if someone got sick. This was a serious blow to the comprehensive-coverage, low-cost identity of KP. Furthermore, the administration of a high-deductible program requires a costly infrastructure that KP had never needed previously. At least initially, KP didn't do it well. Eventually, KP got it mostly right at a cost to its budget and reputation.

None of this means that community rating is a bad idea. KP should be doing what it can to encourage patients to elect comprehensive coverage with the low out-of-pocket cost. It was a good idea during the first forty years of the program's existence, and it still is. This could be accomplished by:

- Promote comprehensive care aggressively in advertising and marketing.
- Discount comprehensive care plans. Take into account the cost of managing deductibles. Explicitly return the savings as a discount to patients electing comprehensive care. Insurance companies do it all the time.
- The Marketing Department should structure higher commissions for the more comprehensive plans. This should not be restricted to on-the-ground salespeople but implemented into the incentive pay structure all the way to the top of Kaiser Health Plan Management as an ethical stand of Kaiser Permanente.

Exploit the Partnership: Use the Medical Expertise of the Permanente Medical Group to Design Plans

If KP really believes in preventive care, the medical expertise of the Medical Group should be employed to help structure plans. These plans would front-load into the least comprehensive plans scientifically validated preventive care medical benefits at low, or better yet, no cost. Examples that come immediately to mind include antihypertensive medications, prenatal checks, screening mammography, immunizations, and exercise programs for seniors. There are many more. Not only is it better medicine, if KP really believes that preventive care is cost effective, the KP promise of preventive care would be kept for even those who can't afford the richer plans. At the same time, this population, being healthier because of the preventive care, would consume fewer health care resources later on. This use of Permanente Medical Group's expertise would be partnership at its best. Comprehensive care was one of the most highly regarded and distinguishing features of KP. It could be again.

It Is All about Leadership: Recruit It and Prepare It

In the KP expansion study, the authors noted that the program had underestimated the importance of leadership in the new regions. Leaders were selected somewhat haphazardly and then thrown ill prepared into administrative shark-infested waters and left to sink, swim, or be eaten. One of the authors of the KP expansion region monograph compared the survival of an expansion region executive leader to that of a junior officer in an active battle zone. When examining the history of the expansion groups, that longevity estimate was not far off. These were the recommendations. They apply as much now as they did then.

New Regions Require Major League Leadership—Not Little League Leadership

Managers should be experienced, successful KP managers who understand the KP heritage and promise.

Requirements: Energy, Entrepreneurial Spirit, and a Willingness to Take Risks

These leaders are going to have to be able to bend the will of the region to reflect the KP promise.

Training

The Kaiser Permanente Executive Training Program (KPEP) from the eighties spent about half its time training together promising Health Plan managers and Permanente physician leaders about the heritage and desired culture of Kaiser Permanente. The rest of the training was more technical: basic economics, management theory, accounting, and marketing. While it is useful for Permanente medical directors to understand what double-entry bookkeeping is, they and the regional presidents are not going to be doing it—nor should they be. Their job is to drive together, as partners, the strategic direction of the KP region. Ideally, they would attend a resurrected KPEP program, preferably together, before being dumped into the administratively risky fray of an expansion region.

Communicate Openings

The Sams-Wagster monograph noted that executive management openings were poorly communicated. One possible reason is that regions did not want to lose their best managers. If KP is to be one program, this obstacle will have to be overcome. Expansion regions will need the best and brightest managers and not the failed, inexperienced, or talentless ambitious ones.

Mentoring

To quote from the KP expansion study: "Expansion region managers should have ongoing relationships with other knowledgeable people in the Program for continuing help with problem solving and education. This should be a serious relationship with expectations on both sides." This sounds a lot like what the Kaiser Permanente (Kai-Perm) committee was supposed to do. Is it time to bring it back for this and a number of other reasons, especially partnership restoration? Without such mentoring early in its history, it is unlikely that the Hawaii region would have survived.

Retention

Promising and experienced managers, whether Health Plan or Permanente, placed into the executive leadership of an expansion region is placing them

ALBERT J. MARIANI, M.D.

into a very high-risk position. The historical, metastatic cancer-like job-survival rates are eloquent testimony to this. Besides recruiting, training, and mentoring such individuals, there should be adequate compensation and security to offset the increased risk and responsibility. It is harder to manage a startup expansion region than a larger but established region.

Good managers are hard to find and shouldn't be wasted. If they fail, as long as the failure isn't due to criminal or unethical behavior, they should understand that efforts would be made to find a home for them somewhere in the program. Not every manager performing excellently at midlevel responsibility has skills that are transferrable to executive responsibility, especially in the Wild West environment of a startup region. Usually, they can still return "home" to positions of productive responsibility, chastened and wiser for the executive experience. With any luck, they won't come back with posttraumatic stress disorder.

Clear Path to Autonomy: If Failing, End It Mercifully

In the end, regions must be able to support themselves long term. Expansion regions are a long-term investment. As earlier stated, they can take an average of four or five years to break even, and seven to ten years to generate enough margin to be self-sustaining and contribute to the program as a whole. At that point, a region should be awarded full autonomy.

If, after ten years, a region is still on financial life support, it should be closed so that the resources can be better utilized elsewhere in the program. The program should be slow to close a region that has already achieved autonomy because economic cycles can cause good and bad years. Every region has gone through these cycles. These cycles often occur in some regions and not at the same time in others, proving the value of geographical diversification.

For the regions that fail, KP should accept at least some responsibility for the failure and learn what lessons there are to be learned. As such, closure should be done mercifully for the patients who will lose their coverage and the doctors and staff who will lose their jobs.

Final Thoughts

There have been no expansion regions established since 1985. There has also been little interest in establishing new KP regions from scratch since then. This is likely due to the failure of most of them. Every one of those failed expansion regions sacrificed major components of the KP genetic code principles.

While it would be a major undertaking to start expanding again, history would suggest doing so by resurrecting the genetic code principles next time. A quote from G. K. Chesterton comes to mind: "Christianity has not been tried and found wanting; it has been found difficult and not tried." Actually, expansion regions *were* successfully established, but that was a long time ago, and the KP genetic code was used to establish them. We should relearn this lesson from our history.

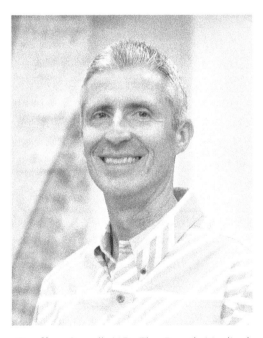

Geoffrey Sewell, MD: The Fourth Medical
Director of HPMG (2007–present).

CHAPTER 15

GEOFFREY SEWELL, MD: THE FOURTH PRESIDENT OF HPMG

The Perfect Storm

I n late 2006, because of accelerating membership and financial losses, a high-level Program Office team led by Gregory Adams, later chief operating officer of National Kaiser Health Plan and Hospitals, journeyed to Hawaii to make preliminary arrangements for a Program Office takeover of the region. Historically, after such takeovers occurred in other regions, they were shut down within two years.

Among the ideas surfaced in the proposed recovery plan were a capital budget freeze, canceling the Moanalua Medical Center expansion, renting community beds, lowering rates enough to become the preferred Medicaid provider, outsourcing the capital-intensive but high-performing cardiac program, laboratory, and pathology services, and Health Plan taking back control of clinic nursing services from HPMG. If these policies had come to pass, the forty-six-year-old Hawaii region would have almost certainly shared the fate of the other closed regions. This was serious HPMG leadership led the defense of the region. It was pointed out that:

1. The Hawaii region still had the lowest cost of care delivery in the program despite the very high cost of doing business in Hawaii.

2. Membership and financial losses were largely due to major problems with rate structure relative to HMSA, inaccurate patient billing, and a poor co-payment collection rate—not patient service and quality of care. These had been rapidly improving since 2205. Soon, even patient service and quality of care would suffer if the capital budget and therefore care-delivery resources were frozen.

3. Doubling down on Medicaid by lowering rates, already a losing line of business, would only worsen the financial crisis. St. Francis West hospital, serving a predominantly Medicaid population, was financially failing for this reason. Eventually, it did fail.

4. In Hawaii, community hospital beds cost more than three times more than internalized beds. This loss did not even include the major additional operational costs of physician travel time or the loss of quality and cost control in these outside hospitals. If there were such an excess of community hospital bed why was the region being charged so much for renting beds in the community.

5. In a carefully prepared analysis, the high performing Heart Program would be three to four times more costly if outsourced—again with far less control over quality and cost. Similarly, outsourcing pathology and laboratory services, one of the best services from the earliest days of the program, would also result in loss of control over quality and cost.

6. HPMG simply was not going to give up the operational control of clinic nursing. It would have been a partnership breakup issue.

7. As for leadership issues, the Medical Group was about to elect the young, energetic, and visionary Dr. Geoff Sewell its new HPMG president. He had an administrative team of young, similarly energetic doctors ready to go. The issue of ineffective Health Plan leadership was on Program Office—not HPMG. Mike Chaffin interceded with his substantial contacts in Program Office to send a promising candidate to Hawaii as the next Health Plan president. This was taken to heart by Program Office leaders and soon remedied. The candidate was Janet Liang. Janet was recruited to KP from Group Health in Seattle where she had been a rising

star. She was young, ambitious, and energetic. She was appointed Health Plan president of the Hawaii region in March 2007. She was to prove to be a good match for Geoff Sewell. In January 2007, a follow-up analyst team was sent from Program Office. To their credit, the Program Office team decided to defer the takeover and give the region a reprieve; it was a reprieve but not a dispensation.

Hitting the Ground Running

At the January 4, 2007, board meeting, it was announced that there would be no 2006 divisible surplus because of the Hawaii region's poor financial performance. An exception was made for the top 10 percent of the peer-to-peer (PtoP) and patient-satisfaction (PSat) physicians who received a $1,000 bonus. This, plus a scattering of hundred-dollar recognition chits from the chiefs for performance, helped cement the importance of the peer-to-peer and patient-satisfaction results in the mind of the individual HPMG doctors.

On February 1, it was announced to the board that Sewell would assume all executive functions on July 1, 2007. On March 1, a delegation from the Emergency Department made a presentation to the board to reconsider financial penalties for poor peer-to-peer and patient-satisfaction performance. Furthermore, they proposed that the Emergency Department be held to a lower standard. The board listened politely, but no action was taken.

On March 15, as scheduled, the penalty structure for five physicians ranging between 7.5 and 20 percent of salary went into effect. During the previous year, of the twelve physicians at risk for a penalty, three physicians had improved markedly, avoiding the penalty, and nine had resigned. On March 15, Janet Liang made her first presentation to the board.

On April 5, it was announced to the board that Ohio was now declared a turnaround region. Five years later, it was sold. It was not lost on the board that it could happen here. At the April 19 board meeting, Mike Chaffin announced that this would be the last board meeting over which he would preside. From May 17 on, Geoff Sewell presided. His HPMG organizational structure was announced. He requested the pro forma resignation of all vice presidents and chiefs and noted that he was in the process of appointing the members of his administration. He also announced that HPMG would be in conformity with standardization of Permanente titles. There would be no physician vice presidents but instead associate medical directors (AMDs). The vice president title would be reserved for non-physician administrators. His title would be president and executive medical director (EMD).

On that date, Gladys Ching, RN, the effective and long-serving vice president in charge of clinic nursing, announced her retirement. With no obvious successor in place, and to keep clinic nursing under HPMG control, clinic nursing was added to the responsibilities of Leighton Hasegawa, the stalwart and multitalented HPMG chief financial officer (CFO).

In 2014, Leighton relinquished the clinic nursing title to Sally Lee, RN, MSN, who had consistently distinguished herself by her administrative skill and tact. She became the obvious choice to succeed Gladys as vice president of clinic operations. At the time of this writing, she was the supervisor of more than 1,300 clinic staff.

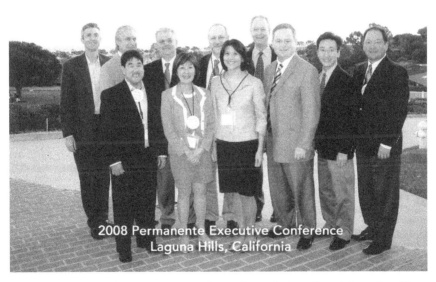

2008 Permanente Executive Conference
Laguna Hills, California

The First Sewell executive team (2008). Back Row (l to r) Drs. Geoff Sewell, Karl Pregitzer, Al Mariani, Jim Griffith, Geoff Galbraith. Front Row (l to r) Leighton Hasegawa, Dr. Chris Fukui, Janet Liang, Drs. Mike Caps, Grant Okawa, and Daryl Kurozawa.

During the next six weeks, Dr. Sewell proceeded to appoint and then obtain the board ratification of his appointees. They included the beloved Ben Tamura, MD, the current chief of medicine who would be the AMD of primary care. Reporting to him would be the AAMD, chiefs of internal medicine (Vernon Ansdell), family practice (Peggy Latare), behavioral health (John Drager), and obstetrics and gynecology (Keith Ogasawara).

Ben would be succeeded a year prior to his planned retirement in 2017 by board acclamation by Dr. Samir Patel. The author was to be AMD of specialty and hospital care. This included surgical specialties and anesthesia led by AAMDs (Dr. Mark Santi), medical specialties (Dr. Tarquin Collis), hospital specialties (Dr. Kelly Yim), and ancillary services, including pathology, laboratory and diagnostic imaging (Dr. Stacey Honda, the capable chief of pathology).

As planned, upon the author's retirement near the end of 2009, each of these four individuals was appointed an associate medical director in their own right. Dr. Daryl Kurozawa, a well-liked surgeon practicing in Kona and former physician in charge of the Big Island of Hawaii, was appointed AMD of the neighbor islands. Dr. David Ulin physician in charge of Maui would later succeed him when Dr. Kurozawa was appointed AMD of sales and marketing, service delivery planning, and community benefit. Dr. Ulin would capably represent HPMG during the difficult transition from state of Hawaii to Kaiser Hospital management of the Maui Memorial Hospital.

Dr. Christine Fukui moved from chief of medical specialties to AMD of quality care. Upon her retirement near the end of 2009, after twenty-nine years of service, she was succeeded by Dr. Karen Ching. Dr. Dave Bell was appointed AMD of professional development and service. He had the tremendous responsibility of maintaining the quality of care, quality of service, and peer-to-peer teamwork initiative within HPMG, thus making concrete the HPMG values statement. He presided over the PPRO upon the retirement of the author.

Dr. Bell didn't stop there. He expanded the quality initiatives to department and population quality of care as well as patient access. Dr. Karl Pregitzer continued in his role as managing physician business services, network management, and occupational medicine—with his title changing from vice president to associate medical director. He was also placed in charge of coding and the associated compliance. He would become a nationally recognized coding expert. In 2014, after thirty-nine years of HPMG service—the longest in the history of HPMG—he would retire.

In 2013, Geoff Sewell asked him to recommend his successor. That was to be Dr. Michael Caps. He had been an elected board member and was a widely respected and exceptionally capable vascular surgeon. He was appointed associate medical director of occupational health, network management, and physician business services. He subsequently managed outside services, which represented 7 percent of the HPMG budget and helped manage the Health Plan outside services, which represented an additional 15 percent of the regional budget.

Dr. Anthea Wang was appointed AMD of government programs and population health solutions. Finally, Dr. Grant Okawa was appointed AMD of knowledge management. The author who was chief of staff of the Moanalua Medical Center upon retirement was replaced by the very capable pediatric pulmonologist and intensivist Dr. James Griffith who served until his own retirement. He was succeeded, in turn, by the proven and experienced Dr. Keith Ogasawara, chief of obstetrics and gynecology.

Historically, both HPMG and Health Plan and Hospitals had shared a corporate attorney. As interests diverged, HPMG felt the need to hire its own corporate attorney. George Apter, Esq., was made an HPMG vice president and ably represented HPMG interests during subsequent crises.

As the scope of HPMG expanded, later additions to the executive committee included Richele Thornburg, MS, who continued her role directing strategy, leadership development and communications as a vice president. Jill Shinno, APRN, was appointed vice president of quality and care delivery integration. The remarkable quality of all of these individuals is borne out by the fact that these choices were the executive structure of HPMG for the subsequent thirteen years and continued at the time of the writing of this book. There had been no for cause removals from office. The only changes were due to retirements, splitting of expanding department responsibilities, or promotions. With this group of capable and experienced medical administrators, on July 1, 2007, Dr. Sewell and his team were ready to hit the ground running—and they did.

Building HPMG Morale

Richele Thornburg deserves special mention. Richele joined the Human Resources (HR) Department of KP early in her career. There she was mentored by Carolyn ("Kaki") Jennings, the experienced and successful HR director who had mentored many, including the author. Kaki had done much to break down the medical versus business cultural differences between the Medical Group and Health Plan. Eventually, both entities felt the need to develop their own Human Resources (HR) Department. To Kaki's credit, there had been little interest in this while Kaki was at the helm of HR.

Richele had rare sense of empathy, loyalty, and total dedication to the HPMG mission. She truly embraced HPMG as her life's work. Without shortchanging family responsibilities, church, and outside social responsibilities, she was hardworking to the point that friends, including the author, worried about her health. Emails or messages sent from her at three o'clock in the morning were not unknown. No member of her team could say that they worked harder than she did—and work hard they did. Her department was not for employees with a nine-to-five mind-set, free spirits, or those who favored high levels of independence. Direction was specific, detailed, and perfectionistic. She gradually built up an extremely loyal, hardworking, disciplined, efficient, and capable team. The mission of her department was to successfully bring about Geoff Sewell's vision to durably unify HPMG and build the morale of the group. This was accomplished to never-before-seen levels through a multitude of HPMG events produced at highly professional levels of organization and production. Social events intended to unify the group included:

The HPMG Annual Anniversary Dinner

This is an evening of fun, food, and fellowship highlighted by service awards and accomplishments and awards by individuals, HPMG, and the program as a whole. For the first time, neighbor islands HPMG professional staff were transported and housed in Oahu at HPMG expense. This finally ended the neighbor island/Oahu disunity that had plagued HPMG since it opened the first neighbor island clinic in 1967.

HPMG Annual Community Day of Service

This widely praised event is held yearly on Martin Luther King Day. HPMG participating staff are given the day off to participate in HPMG-organized activities supporting local nonprofit organizations at multiple sites on Oahu and the neighbor islands. This would be in addition to the activities of the more than two thousand HPMG staff and clinic operations personnel who were already participating in community volunteerism on their own.

Family Day

This event is meant to recognize the sacrifices that families make to support the demands of medicine made by the professional staff. This biannual event is held during the summer school vacation. It is held at a local water park, and families are encouraged to attend. neighbor island staff are also transported and housed for this event.

Professional Development Days

At least once a year, professional development days are held to present a variety of medical profession topics designed to inform the professional staff of policy and medical practice trends that better enable them to adapt to these changes.

Research and Innovation Symposium

Every other year, a day is devoted to presentations of original clinical research, population management, and awards for distinguished research, innovative practices. The many contributions of the HPMG professional staff to state-of-the-art medical advancements, formerly sporadically publicized, were now on display to the entire Medical Group in an organized fashion.

Communication efforts were not limited to event coordination. Richele's department was also responsible for issuing periodic written publications. They included:

Making Waves

This quarterly color publication presents Hawaii region news in addition to news of the program, announcements, awards, and heritage articles. It replaced Bill Dung and Mike Chaffin's presidential newsletter, which went back to 1970.

Kina'ole

This is a monthly newsletter highlighting regional continuous quality-improvement initiatives.

O KP Kakou

The overarching theme of this book is that a well-functioning partnership is the key to the success of the program. Upon the arrival of David Underriner in 2018, as the new regional president, he and Geoff Sewell agreed to issue a regional newsletter highlighting the progress of the Hawaii program. That ended with Mr. Underriner's resignation.

Grand Rounds

The pride of being in an elite organization rouses a contagious effort by everyone in that organization to constantly strive to do better. Psychologic studies show that in low-skilled jobs, the difference between best performance and being terminated is relatively small. For the professional, the difference between the best performance and bare minimum performance is nearly unlimited. A culture of excellence that drives pride of performance taps this vast reserve of performance that is almost independent from fair compensation once such fair compensation is achieved. It is a powerful antidote to complacency. It is something that money just can't buy.

For the first two decades of its existence, the quality of the medical care delivered by KP and specifically HPMG was disparaged by the competing medical community and by those who listened to them. This was not objectively justified. Before the end of the first decade of HPMG's existence, the 1969 University of Michigan study sponsored by the Hawaii Medical Association (HMA) compared Hawaii KP care to fee-for-service care. KP medical care was found to be superior to fee-for-service care in almost all categories. It was attributed to better coordination of care. This was not the expected outcome. Needless to say, no further such studies were commissioned by HMA. Nevertheless, the continued semiofficial stance of KP public relations was one of quiet humility—not a vigorous response to accusations of mediocre care. It got to the point where in social situations HPMG physicians were reluctant to reveal where they were employed.

Strenuous HPMG efforts to improve the quality of medical care were detailed in earlier chapters. They included sub-specialization (1960), early recognition of the importance of board certification (1960), multiphasic screening for early disease detection (1968), disproportionate amounts of published, internationally peer reviewed clinical research compared to the rest of the community, residency sponsorships for the University of Hawaii, and the prestigious Stanford and University of California San Francisco residency programs and the HPMG Research Symposium (1963), which required community physician review. Organized by the education committee was Saturday-morning Grand Rounds in the old Waikiki hospital auditorium. At these Grand Rounds, most of the Medical Group would gather for a one-hour presentation by one of the staff on a topic of medical interest. This program provided a framework which evolved into a coordinated, scientific medical practice.

As long as most of HPMG was on Oahu, this worked out well. With the proliferation of peripheral clinics on Oahu with Saturday-morning clinics in the 1960s, neighbor island clinics first on Maui in the late sixties, and then the Big Island in the 1980s, a significant portion of HPMG could not participate in Grand Rounds. Because of the technological limitations and expense of remote video, there was no practical way to transmit Grand Rounds to multiple sites on three islands.

In 1985, when the Kaiser Moanalua Medical Center opened, Grand Rounds faded away. There were individual efforts by departments to give educational talks to other departments, but they were sporadic, unfocused, and often sparsely attended. Presentations by physicians from pharmaceutical company speaker bureaus occasionally snuck in. In time, there were fewer and fewer educational efforts as HPMG struggled with the establishment of the electronic medical record, the dispersion of the Medical Group to multiple sites, and other administrative and clinical challenges. These required physician adaptation at an ever-accelerating pace. The joy of practicing state-of-the-art clinical medicine was being sucked out of HPMG practice by new, necessary, ever-growing administrative and documentation requirements.

In 2005, the concept of Grand Rounds was resurrected. Several developments made this possible:

1. By the mid-1990s, evidence-based medicine was actively being promoted by academic medicine. Evidence-based medicine establishes rigorously defined, statistically valid standards of evidence. In descending order of validity, these standards were 1. meta-analyses of multiple prospective, 2. statistically valid, randomized double-blind studies, single such studies, 3. case-controlled randomized prospective studies, 4. retrospective studies, 5. case series, and 7. anecdotal case reports. Collective expert opinion and individual opinion were the lowest standards of evidence. This was a positive development. The KP promise demanded a practice grounded in scientifically valid evidence-based medicine.

2. With the successful implementation of Health Connect, the electronic medical record, in the clinics (2005) and Hospital (2009), a medium for simultaneous dissemination of clinical information to all of HPMG was now feasible through a common medical record.

3. Remote audio-visual (AV) technology was now cost-effective, and the program had a mature, skilled Hawaii region AV Department, ably led by Vernon Hiroe. HPMG's hardworking and talented

Kwok Wut, assigned by Richele Thornburg, worked closely with Vernon.

4. The Moanalua Hospital auditorium was equipped with a state-of-the-art AV capability. Every clinic had real-time, interregional AV capability in at least one of their conference rooms. If not already in place, it was installed.

5. The specialty departments were now successfully subspecialized and eager to give clinical presentations to a region-wide audience. The primary care doctors, especially on the neighbor islands, were just as eager to receive them. The primary care departments had their own areas of expertise to share with the rest of HPMG through Grand Rounds.

6. There was a new, energetic HPMG administration. Richele Thornburg mobilized her department to organize the new HPMG Grand Rounds.

For Grand Rounds presentations, the following rules apply:

1. The presentation must be a topic of general interest to all of HPMG. It should represent the department's message to the rest of HPMG. For example, urology could present its recommended prostate-specific antigen (PSA) regional screening policy for prostate cancer. A presentation about the research history of PSA and the clinical significance of PSA subunits might be appropriate for an internal Urology Department meeting—but not for the rest of HPMG.

2. The presentation represents the consensus—not necessarily unanimous—of the department's recommended approach to a disease process. If following the recommended protocol, referring doctors would not expect to be reproached by a member of that specialty department.

3. The presentations are to be the responsibility of the specialties, including primary care. Guest lecturers are discouraged because they would not necessarily be representing the consensus of the specialty department. Guest lecturers sponsored by pharmaceutical or medical equipment manufacturers are banned.

4. Presentations are to be held one hour prior to clinic start times on the first Friday of the month. They would be pre-announced in a broadcast email well ahead of time. Presentations are to be available in real time at all clinics in their audiovisual room. There should be local clinic personnel assigned to correct any audiovisual problems in real time. There would be a ten minute question-and-answer period during which questions from all clinics sent though messaging could be entertained. All presentations would be confined to a total of sixty minutes.

5. All presenters are expected to write a brief summary that could be read within two minutes. It was to be placed into the reference side bar in the Health Connect electronic medical record and be available at all times with a few clicks of a mouse. Presenters were instructed to review the summaries every three years to ensure that the recommendations were current.

6. Considerable background administrative work was done to ensure that Continuing Medical Education Level 1 credits were awarded to all attendees for each presentation. As part of the CME affirmation form, a survey is added. Points were awarded for the value to all of HPMG of the information presented, the technical quality of the presentation, the use of evidence-based medicine, and an exposition of the clinical capability of the presenting department, which was often unknown outside of that department. After almost every presentation, viewers should come away with increased appreciation of that department's clinical capability. Presentations should attract reward chits. More important would be the recognition by colleagues that the individual was going above and beyond to give back to the total HPMG knowledge base. Contribution to HPMG is one of the four criteria of the peer-to-peer survey. During the research symposia, the results of all the surveys should be the basis of the department and individual rewards.

While the benefits of Grand Rounds were clear—the standardization of scientifically valid medical practice, best practice utilization of resources, and repeated demonstrations of HPMG's state-of-the-art clinical capabilities—it would take an enormous amount of administrative work to make it happen. This was one of first demonstrations of the new administration's energy and efficiency. It was spearheaded by Richele's department. While there was widespread physician support, the project was enormously complex and required a considerable resource outlay. Audiovisual rooms had to be coordinated at all eighteen clinical sites on three islands with real-time staffing to fix transmission glitches. Specific announcements had to be broadcast for scheduling purposes. Timing of the presentations had to be precisely fifty minutes, starting on time and ending on time. Presenters were instructed in presentation skills. The submitted questions from all eighteen sites needed to be submitted and collated on the fly prior to the precisely timed ten-minute question-and-answer period that followed the main presentation. Summaries needed to be incorporated into Health Connect. Videos of the presentations required archiving. Continuing Medical Education credits need to be credited for all attending physicians. It was a lot of work, but if all of this wasn't carried out with near perfection, the whole initiative would fail. The team knew this and spared no effort.

Preparations were started in early 2009. The first trial presentation was made by Dr. Phil Bruno in October: a timely and compelling case for flu immunization. It went off flawlessly. The first official presentation was in February 2010 by the author on the topic of the evaluation of hematuria (blood in the urine). The program settled into ten presentations per year at eight o'clock on the first Friday of the month. The attendance remained at more than half of HPMG. Grand Rounds was especially popular on the neighbor islands.

As time went on, the presentations became more and more refined. The production and presentation professionalism was at the levels of the best national and international academic and medical meeting standards that physicians attended. The goals of Grand Rounds—clinical cooperation, standardization of scientific medical care, efficient utilizations of resources, and the satisfaction of being part of HPMG—were more than met. Thus, in February 2019, Grand Rounds celebrated its tenth anniversary and has become an integral part of the HPMG culture of excellence.

In the original plan, there would have been weekly Grand Rounds on a three-year cycle with each department given a set number of slots. One of the responsibilities of the chief would have been the responsibility to organize a department education program. The department would use those slots to present a coordinated clinical message to the rest of HPMG. Unfortunately, in 2009, that would have been a bridge too far. It would have required at least four times the resources that were available to Grand Rounds and would have floundered under its own weight—prematurely ending the entire initiative. It was wisely decided to prioritize quality over quantity. As for expansion of Grand Rounds? Maybe in the future.

Accelerating Momentum

By 2010, HPMG had resolved most of the internal conflicts that had diverted the collective energy of the Medical Group away from its primary mission. From a historical perspective, things were pretty good. The compensation package was competitive and defensible because it was based upon national average physician compensation. There was little physician turnover. That same national average salary formula had virtually eliminated all the conflicts surrounding specialty compensation differences. Endorsing the salary scales was now a pro forma, routine, year-end board action. Bringing neighbor islands doctors to Hawaii for major HPMG events had healed the long-standing neighbor island-Oahu schism. Engaging all of HPMG in well-organized yearly events further healed medical center versus clinic differences. Well-thought-out policies and procedures developed carefully during the previous half century were available to process the day-to-day operational problems in a consistent and rational way. Peer-to-peer and patient-satisfaction survey outcome enforcement, combined with robust counseling and assistance, largely eliminated performance issues. A culture of excellence was well established.

Historically, such success often led to periods of peaceful complacency. Complacency is one of the greatest threats to any organization because it encourages resistance to change, and change is always occurring, especially in business. This was not to be. The young, energetic, idealistic, activist leadership led by Geoff Sewell further accelerated the drive toward excellence. For the first time in HPMG history, HPMG with most internal conflicts resolved, was able to turn its full considerable talent and energy toward external threats. This was to bear abundant fruit.

Threat to the Hawaii Partnership

In 2011, Hawaii Pacific Healthcare (HPH) was the umbrella organization managing the Kapiolani Medical Center for Women and Children, the Straub Clinic and Hospitals, the Pali Momi Hospital on Oahu, and Wilcox Hospital, the only hospital on Kauai. HPH was closely affiliated with Hawaii Pacific Health Partners. These were doctors either employed by these hospitals or admitting to them. It was the second largest hospital system in the state and moving toward a vertically integrated system.

Dr. Mark Santi, AMD of surgical services, had a return flight canceled after a Permanente Executive Leadership conference in Los Angeles. In the hotel, he ran into Ray Vara, the chief executive officer of HPH. They spoke for a while, and he asked Mark how Bernard Tyson, the soon-to-be CEO of Kaiser Health Plan and Hospitals, was doing. He noted that he and Tyson were old friends and that Tyson would soon be flying to Hawaii and having dinner with him. At the time, HPH was in a public dispute with HMSA over hospital reimbursements. In their view, HMSA had an effective monopoly in Hawaii and was making the most of it by lowering hospital reimbursements. This had been the motivation for the predecessor of HPH, the Kapiolani Health Systems, to attempt to establish its own health plan in the mid-1990s as a counterweight to HMSA. That and a similar effort by the Queens Hospital system had failed after an existence for a few years. As a result, HPH was looking for another Hawaii partner, and KP was the second largest health plan in Hawaii.

A partnership with HPH would have necessarily included the doctors of the Hawaii Pacific Health Partners. Program Office, Health Plan, and Hospitals had in recent years demonstrated openness to the idea of violating the exclusivity arrangements between the Permanente Medical Groups and Kaiser Health Plan and Hospital. Examples had been the attempted marketing expansion of the point-of-service offerings and the establishment of clinics outside of the areas of Permanente staffing. The only thing that kept the exclusivity of Kaiser Health Plan and Permanente Medical Group contracts intact was that the Permanente Medical Groups had management authority over all community doctor staffing. HPMG was now on alert for any Kaiser Health Plan-Hawaii Pacific Health "partnership" ideas, especially those that might "partner" doctors from HPH with Health Plan.

As anticipated, shortly thereafter, the idea of a partnership was raised in a strategic work group (SWG, pronounced "swig"). The SWG meeting was a monthly regional summit meeting of four principal leaders of HPMG and four principal leaders from KP Health Plan and Hospitals. When the issue was presented in the SWG meeting, the HPMG members were clearly and completely opposed.

Dr. Santi, representing the HPMG position in his usual amiable way, stated that while we might remain friends for a while for historical reasons, enactment of any policy compromising the exclusivity clause of the medical services agreement would result in the end of the partnership. There was some enthusiasm for exploring the idea in some local Health Plan circles, but Janet Liang, president of the Hawaii Regional Health Plan, to her credit, even though she was under pressure from her superiors, realized that a breakup of the partnership would threaten the very existence of the Hawaii program. When the issue came up at the next SWG meeting, Janet shut down the idea from the Regional Health Plan side. Here was another example of a local Health Plan president supporting the interests of the region in alliance with a PMG president against an ill-considered Program Office initiative. Unfortunately, the Program Office concentration of authority at the expense of regional leadership has continued. It is a threat to the entire program. Without local support, the idea of a Kaiser and Hawaii Pacific Healthcare partnership faded away. A serious local crisis with program-wide implications was averted.

An Era of Good Feeling

The election of Dr. Sewell as HPMG executive medical director in late 2006 and the replacement of Jan Head with Janet Liang in 2007 was another turning point in the KP Hawaii Regional history. Dr. Sewell and his exceptionally talented team made the most of the stability of HPMG. This all bore fruit with regional membership growth from 205,000 to 255,000 and increased local and national recognition for quality and service. The

HPMG doctors now recognized as never before the importance of good leadership. Physician leadership was no longer seen as something to be done in spare time or on a rotating basis. It was now recognized that leadership was its own "specialty," needing training and experience, and that good leaders should be judged more by results than affability. Good leaders were no longer seen as disposable, "anyone can do it" colleagues. As a result, Dr. Sewell and his team achieved unprecedented levels of respect and popularity. By 2017, the "Climate Survey" of physician satisfaction, which had been run since 1971, and typically had run in the low- to mid-eighties in earlier years, now stood at 96 percent "happy with being a part of HPMG." That was about as good as it could get.

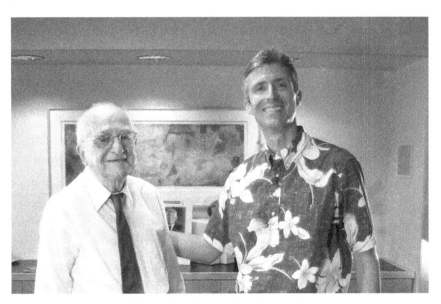

Morrie Collen, MD, (l) and Geoff Sewell, MD, (r): A rich past and future Permanente heritage.

In KP, at the national level, Geoff Sewell was increasingly recognized as a fresh face with clearly articulated, principled, and visionary goals for Kaiser Permanente. By 2012, there was local concern that he would be recruited away from Hawaii. In August 2012, almost eleven months prior to the end of his first term, he was effortlessly reaffirmed for a second term, which would continue his leadership to 2019.

In 2006, the bylaws had been changed to establish a two-term limit for HPMG presidents. If Sewell was to lead Hawaii beyond 2019, this had to be changed. Upon his appointment to chair of the National Permanente Executive Committee (NPEC) and CEO of the Regions Outside of California (ROCs), HPMG concern increased. A motion to reverse the two-term limit was passed by the board and then the associates on November 2015. In an unprecedented board action, he was authorized to run for a third term, which, if completed would extend his HPMG leadership to 2025. His election to the third term was ratified with essentially no opposition on December 6, 2016. Also in October, it was announced that for the first time since the peer-to-peer and patient-satisfaction survey started, no HPMG doctor was below the mandatory action plan of 80 percent highly satisfied on the Art of Medicine patient-satisfaction survey and less than 3.0 (above average) on the peer-to-peer survey. The overall performance was a record-setting 96 percent highly satisfied on the patient-satisfaction survey and 3.6 on the peer-to-peer survey.

The Mouse That Roared

Remembering the fate of Al Weiland and the Northwest region maybe it shouldn't have. The Hawaii region had never been more than 2.5 percent of Kaiser Permanente. As long as the national leadership of KP saw itself as a socially valuable "middle way" alternative to single-payer, government-controlled health care versus a purely market-driven commercial enterprise, the little Hawaii region was safe as a small, successful outpost of a spreading national Kaiser Permanente.

Extraordinary attention from the highest levels of KP had been devoted to the success of the Hawaii region, especially during the politically unstable early years. That effort bore fruit as the region matured into a high-performing entity generating more than its fair share of care-delivery innovations. These innovations were often applicable to the whole program.

In the early 1990s, things changed with the retirement of Jim Vohs as CEO. The administration of David Lawrence placed a new emphasis on corporate interests in the face of rapid, threatening, medical market changes. In retrospect, ill-advised experiments with the genetic code principles in the 1990s resulted in the loss of several regions and a weakening of the others that eventually resulted in the program-threatening financial crisis of 1998. They had included compromising the Health Plan Permanente Medical Group partnership, de-emphasis of regional autonomy, and inadequate support of the newer regions that had been established without implementing important genetic code principles, such as integrated facilities.

With the new KP corporate focus and de-emphasis on the importance of the ROCs (Regions Outside of California), the Hawaii region now faced more risk of closure by Program Office from short-term financial setbacks. If the Hawaii region couldn't be a "milk cow," consistently providing funds to Program Office for other regions with more growth potential, in the mind of Program Office executives, there was little reason to keep it open. The region indeed faced challenges not found in other regions.

1. It was the smallest region in the program with limited growth potential. As of 2018, the population of the state of Hawaii was only 1.4 million with a total KP membership of 255,000. Many service areas of KP California were larger.
2. Hawaii is the most geographically isolated state.
3. Politically, Hawaii possesses one of the least friendly business climates in the country.
4. Its competitor is HMSA. For decades, HMSA has held a near-monopoly statewide health care presence that allowed it to enforce some of the lowest provider reimbursement rates in the country. These, in turn, allowed it to offer some of the lowest dues rates in the country. KP Hawaii had to match these low rates.
5. HMSA does not have to pay a burdensome out-of-state Program Office tax for mandatory services from its operating funds.
6. Hawaii is one of the most expensive states to live and do business. Combined with constrained rates, this high cost of doing business leaves limited margin for expansion and depreciation.

A good case can be made that all of these challenges made KP Hawaii leaner, more aggressive, more innovative, and more flexible. It wasn't easy, but sixty years after a difficult founding, it is still here and stronger than ever. Nevertheless, there have always been revenue cycles of good years and bad years. Support from Program Office during the bad years was now far less assured.

In 2009, Geoff Sewell had been in office for two years, and his leadership in partnership with Health Plan had already turned the region around. It was now going from success to success. The other Permanente Medical Group presidents were either approaching retirement or newly elected. Geoff was offered a position on the select KP steering committee. It was a tough decision.

On one hand, membership on this committee would allow networking with top KP executives. This could protect the Hawaii region from short-term, ill-considered Program Office initiatives that could harm or even shut down the region.

On the other hand, the lesson of Dr. Al Weiland's experience in the Northwest was instructive. To recapitulate, Dr. Weiland, the successful Northwest PMG president for twelve years (four terms), had become heavily involved with the National KP Electronic Medical Record initiative, and had provided six months of on-site management guidance to the troubled Mid-Atlantic region. Things were going well in his own region. He had left management of the Northwest to a capable and trusted team working with an excellent regional Health Plan partner. Shortly after his return, Program Office fired the long-standing Northwest Regional Health Plan partner and appointed an adversarial replacement who was intent on destroying the partnership. Having served for twelve years and realizing the difficulty continuing his position with an uncooperative Health Plan, he decided not to fight off an internal challenge. This ushered in an extended period of political instability for the Northwest Permanente Medical Group and financial failure for Northwest Regional Health Plan.

This was a critical time for Hawaii and the program. The Program Office drive toward centralization was continuing. Sewell agreed to serve on the KP steering committee. He had both the energy and youth to make it a success, and he did. Geoff was eventually appointed to chairman of the Permanente executive committee, and in April 2013, he announced Jack Cochran's election to another six-year term.

In 2015, Jack Cochran, president of the Permanente Federation since 2007, suddenly and unexpectedly stepped down. In August 2015 the

Permanente Federation leadership was reorganized into the National Permanente executive committee (NPEC) with the Northern and Southern California medical directors as co-chief executive officers (CEOs) and Geoff Sewell as Chair of the NPEC and CEO of the Regions Outside of California. He brought Richele Thornburg and Dr. Dave Bell to the NPEC, and they were appointed as co-executive vice presidents of people and leadership strategy. Both were distinguished for their work on the Medicine and Management training program developed for promising PMG leaders.

Dr. Bell had been designated to succeed Dr. Sewell in the event of his incapacitation in October 2015 by the HPMG board of directors. Also brought on board of the NPEC as executive vice president of products/sales and marketing was Dr. Daryl Kurozawa. He had held the similar AMD position in HPMG. Thus, three out of nine members of the NPEC were now from the Hawaii region. Thus, while smaller than the other regions, it was still large enough to provide outsized leadership to the Permanente Federation. While the involvement in the Federation was a disproportionate drain on HPMG's talent and resources, it also gave the Hawaii region a disproportionate share of national KP influence. Strategically, this was seen as protective against temporary local financial downturns that could threaten the region. Ultimately it wasn't.

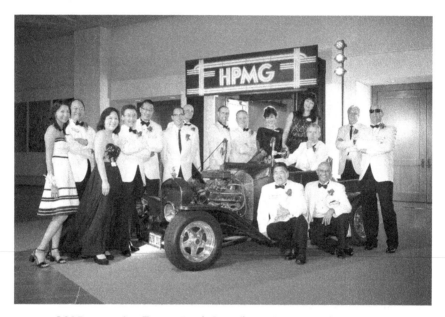

2015 executive Team: Back Row (l. to r.) Drs. Anthea Wang, Daryl Kurozawa, Karen Ching, Grant Ozawa, Keith Ogasawara, Tarquin Collis, Dave Bell, Mark Santi, Mike Caps, vice presidents Richele Thornburg and Sally Lee, Dr. Karl Pregitzer, and George Apter, JD. In the driver's seat: Geoff Sewell. Bottom Row (l. to r.) Leighton Hasegawa and Dr. Samir Patel.

Maui Memorial Hospital

Hawaii has a long tradition of paternalistically caring for the common people. It goes back to the royalty of the kingdoms of Hawaii, carried forward during the plantation era, and finally to the policies of the Hawaii state government. Of the six major islands of Hawaii, Oahu has had 70–80 percent of the population since statehood.

While Oahu had several modern, well-equipped, self-supporting hospitals, including the Kaiser Moanalua Hospital, the small remaining population, scattered among the five main populated islands outside of Oahu, could not individually financially support modern, comprehensive, free-standing hospitals. This was a serious health care problem for the residents of the neighbor islands.

Unlike the other sparely populated areas on the mainland, which were usually well served by land-based ambulance services, the islands were separated by rough ocean. Practical water passenger service between the islands does not exist. There are frequent interisland flights, but they are appropriate only for noncritical ambulatory cases. For critical cases, the only alternative is an air ambulance service, which is prohibitively expensive for routine use. The state government solution was to establish and operate state hospitals on each of the islands. These hospitals were managed by Hawaii Health Systems, an arm of the Hawaii State Department of Health. This worked fairly well for basic and emergency hospital services. The problem was that state government was not well adapted to manage the operational complexities of hospital administration. Much of the hospital workforce was represented by the politically powerful Hawaii Government Employee Association (HGEA). This was the state government workers' union. Labor negotiations were conducted at the state government level—not at the hospital level. As such, negotiated compensation and benefits were much more generous than those of the other hospitals in the state. Labor costs typically make up 60 percent of hospital operating costs. Finally, the cost of providing highly technical medical services, such as cardiac surgery, or neurosurgery to small populations is prohibitively expensive. The neighbor island hospitals were destined to get further and further clinically behind even as state government subsidies were getting higher and higher.

The resulting chronic and accelerating state hospital budget deficits were covered by state tax revenues. By 2016, the state hospital subsidy had reached $121 million a year—15 percent of the entire state government budget—and it was steadily rising. The cost of a day of hospitalization at these hospitals was often greater than that of major medical centers on the mainland.

For the state government, the solution to the accelerating deficits was privatization to an organization with experience managing hospitals. The plan was for the state to continue to own the hospitals with long-term (thirty-year) hospital management contracts to be put out to bid. The first test case would be the Maui Health System, which included Maui Memorial Medical Center, the main hospital on Maui, Maui Memorial Outpatient Clinic, Kula Hospital, Kula Clinic in "upcountry Maui," the small communities on the flanks of the massive Haleakala volcano, and Lanai Community hospital and it's associated clinics. This plan was approved by the state legislature in April 2015. Initially, KP was uninterested in bidding because of political and financial uncertainties. As the situation clarified in 2015, KP decided to make a strong bid for the management of the Maui Memorial Hospital health system. There were good reasons to do so. KP had sustained continuous losses on Kauai because Hawaii Pacific Healthcare—a direct competitor—owned the only hospital on the island. This removed any leverage KP might have on pricing. Worse yet, there was no HPMG physician presence on Kauai to coordinate the day-to-day care. This was a pattern seen everywhere in the program where sub-regions were established without Permanente Medical Group direct-patient management over hospitalization, laboratory, pharmacy, and diagnostic imaging facilities. The KP Kauai subsidy did not threaten the program because the member numbers were small—about four thousand—less than 10 percent of the Kauai population—and it did give KP a presence on all of the major islands. This was a requirement necessary to fulfill the contracts of some of the largest accounts.

Maui was different. With a population of approximately 152,000, more than one-third were KP members. It had the highest KP market share of any island, including Oahu. It represented one-fifth of the entire regional membership. The only other bidder for the Maui Health Systems contract was Hawaii Pacific Healthcare (HPH). If HPH managed the

Maui Memorial Hospital system, a repeat of the Kauai experience could be expected. Kaiser Permanente would lose control of the hospitalization, lab, diagnostic imaging, and hospital pharmacy costs on Maui as well as the quality assurance and credentialing mechanisms. The only quality and cost control alternative would be to duplicate as many hospital services as possible and send the rest to Oahu. While operationally difficult, it was definitely possible, and there was a well-oiled transfer procedure that had been in place for decades. KP was popular with the Maui members who often preferred to have major procedures done at the Kaiser Moanalua Medical Center in any case.

Hawaii Pacific Health (HPH) was a formidable competitor for the contract. The Kapiolani Women and Children's Specialty Hospital was very well regarded for pediatrics and obstetrics and gynecology. The Straub Clinic had a legacy reputation for specialty services, while the Pali Momi Hospital was a modern, single-bed-per-room hospital known for good patient service. HPH could also claim neighbor island hospital management experience, having managed the only hospital on Kauai. HPH presented itself as a nonprofit, experienced, local organization fully capable of managing Maui Health System.

Kaiser had its own advantages. It had long ago overcome quality-of-care and service concerns and was regarded as at least the equal of the other health care systems in Hawaii. For most residents of Maui and the Big Island of Hawaii, KP set the standard for on-island health care with the best care coordination for advanced care on Oahu. Unlike the other health plans, KP paid for round-trip patient transportation to Oahu as well as lodging. This care coordination was well regarded, well established, and had been in place for decades.

Unlike KP, the Health Plan partners of the other hospital systems (mostly HMSA) saw their function as limited to paying for health care provider services, but they took little or no responsibility for assuring local island physician staffing. That was left to market mechanisms that were, in turn, dependent upon the size of the populations that would financially support them—inadequate for the small neighbor island populations.

Finally, there was the KP resource base. By 2015, the Kaiser Foundation Health Plan and Hospitals of Hawaii partnered with Hawaii Permanente Medical Group had been an integral part of Hawaii health care for more than half a century. It cared for almost one-fifth of the state population and had a presence on all of the main islands. Even that was dwarfed by the resources of national Kaiser Permanente, which managed thirty-nine hospitals and 680 medical clinics on the mainland. Kaiser Permanente hospitals were among the highest rated in the country for quality outcomes and patient satisfaction. As such, an enormous amount of clinical and administrative talent, expertise, and experience could be brought to bear by KP from both local and national sources. This resource base could not be matched by Hawaii Pacific Health.

The campaign was tightly coordinated by Health Plan and HPMG working together to effectively make the KP case in a number of presentations. The already existing, long-standing, arguably dominant clinical KP presence on Maui and the overwhelming resources that KP could bring to bear on the management of Maui Memorial Hospital prevailed. Consequently, on September 23, 2015, it was publicly announced that the long-term Maui Memorial Hospital contract was awarded to Kaiser Permanente.

Political and labor issues needed to be overcome first. KP didn't officially assume Maui Health Systems Management until July 1, 2017, after these issues were resolved. Maui Health Systems was now a wholly owned subsidiary of Kaiser Foundation Hospitals. There was an enormous amount of reorganization that needed to take place. Large numbers of doctors and skilled medical staff positions needed to be filled, and they were. Almost all employees were rehired under employment contracts that were negotiated directly by the hospital management. Almost all employees accepted the new contracts. Volumes of policies and procedures needed to be established. The regional electronic medical record needed to be implemented, but now non-HPMG staff needed to be accommodated in addition to the HPMG staff. Kaiser Permanente had to invent a new billing system to replace the antiquated and ineffective existing system. This new billing system had to accommodate non-KP care providers and other health plans in addition to KP.

The greatest hurdle was going to be redefining the Permanente Medical Group-Kaiser Health Plan and Hospitals relationship. For the previous fifty-eight years, the Hawaii KP relationship between the two partners had been like a marriage. There was a level of trust that prevented many disputes and pressured both entities to compromise when disputes did occur. Now, for the first time, there was another partner in the marriage: community non-HPMG doctors and other health care providers. In real marriages, this usually doesn't turn out well.

On one hand, Health Plan and Hospitals could see this as a new line of business—hospital management without Permanente Medical Group involvement. This would decrease its dependence upon the Permanente Medical Groups. On the other hand, the Permanente Medical Group could respond by noting that if Health Plan wanted to hire and/or partner with the community providers—HPMG's competitors—the obvious solution would be for HPMG to partner with the competitors of Kaiser Health Plan. This would mean independent contracts with other health plans including HMSA- Kaiser Health Plan's main competitor in Hawaii. Maui would be a nicely isolated testing ground for this "new" idea. Of course, it could also be a model for "divorce" as the loyalties of both entities would now be divided as each followed their own separate economic interests. The likely lethal consequences to both Health Plan and the Permanente Medical Groups of a KP partnership breakup have already been discussed at length. This was one potential path—the bad one.

The problem to be solved was that there was no model for Kaiser Hospital management of a hospital that had a community monopoly on hospitalization services. As such, Kaiser Health Plan and Hospitals would be required to give equal access to all non-HPMG providers and health plans as it had promised to do. Historically, when KP went into a new area, the regional Permanente Medical Group controlled all the contracting of physicians and the professional staff caring for KP members while Health Plan managed KP hospital contracts and the other Health Plan and Hospital contracts. These hospitals were independent entities with their own administrations. Their relationship with KP was that of a vendor to a customer.

This was an entirely new relationship. Whose interests were going to get precedence: Maui Health Systems, Program Office Health Plan and Hospitals, or the KP Hawaii region partnership? The only answer must be that all had to benefit; otherwise, it would not work. This was going to be a difficult needle to thread.

The first issue to arise was the management of the medical staff of the hospital. On Maui, as always, the HPMG physicians would continue to care for the KP members by capitation, according to the medical services agreement. The issue of who would manage the doctors caring for the remaining non-KP Maui patients was unclear. Health Plan maintained that they should control the hiring, firing, quality assurance, quality of service, hospital staff governance, and payment of physicians employed by the hospital. HPMG maintained that they should administer non-KP physician issues through an independent management contract as they had traditionally done in the partnership. To manage this, HPMG had established the Hawaii Pacific Permanente Group (HPPG). HPPG was separate but wholly owned subsidiary of HPMG. It was modified to accommodate the requirements of providing staff to a community hospital with fair treatment of all providers to maintain quality and service.

An understanding could not be reached between Kaiser Health Plan and Hospitals and HPMG. The hiring of hospital physicians commenced under the HPPG contract but also independently by Kaiser Health Plan and Hospitals. Conflicts arose almost immediately. For example, the hospital made a direct contract with a local specialist against the advice of HPMG/HPPG because of the specialist's known limited practice capabilities. Soon, a high-risk, complicated case presented itself that the physician specialist in question could not manage. As it had done in the past, under that standard medical services agreement, Kaiser Health Plan and Hospitals turned to HPMG to manage the case with its own staff or contracted staff. HPMG declined following the principle of "with responsibility must go authority."

If the hospital was going to make independent contracts with physicians outside of HPMG, they would have to accept and manage the consequences of those hires, including referrals to community physicians outside of HPPG and HPMG. Arranging for the management of this case turned out to be very difficult for Kaiser Health Plan and Hospitals. They learned that they would independently need to develop an extensive and expensive suite of physician-management systems if they were going to bypass HPMG/HPPG. These issues had for decades been well handled within the partnership as a "no-charge" partnership obligation of HPMG. There was nothing to prevent Health Plan from setting up separate policies for their (not HPMG) Maui M.D. hires. This would require policies for hospital governance, physician hiring and firing, clinic staff hiring and firing, hospital quality assurance, outside referrals, physician cost-effective input for planning and marketing, and all the other things that HPMG did for Kaiser Health Plan and Hospitals in the partnership. Nevertheless, to do all of this just for Maui would be costly, operationally confusing, and duplicative, especially since HPMG had managed such responsibilities well since the founding of the Hawaii region and would continue to manage these responsibilities for the KP members. Demonstrating the value of such HPMG/HPPG services would highlight the value of the partnership and why there was a partnership in the first place. At the time of this writing, that restatement of the partnership was yet to be resolved.

Many other complex and potentially contentious issues emerged. One example of the decision-making complexity was the establishment of high-tech specialties, such as cardiac surgery and neurosurgery, on Maui. One of the aspirational goals of the previous hospital administration had been to make Maui Memorial Hospital (MMH) a full-service medical center. This superficially laudable goal was to offer as many of the medical services that were otherwise only available on Oahu for the convenience of Maui patients who would now be able to obtain these services locally. When Kaiser Health Plan and Hospitals took over the hospital contract, the MMH administration expected that this policy would be continued.

Theoretically, any level of medical care, no matter how advanced, can be delivered locally if resources are unlimited. Ferdinand Marcos, dictator of an impoverished Philippines, established the state-of-the art-National Kidney and Transplant Institute in Manila by presidential decree in 1981. Conveniently, in 1983 and again in 1984, Marcos secretly underwent kidney transplants there to treat his renal failure.

With the assumption of the hospital management contract, Kaiser Health Plan and Hospitals was responsible for working through the complex financial and clinical realities of maintaining safe and fiscally responsible Maui neurosurgery and cardiac surgery services. After all, it was these concerns that prompted the state to offer the long-term management contract for Maui Health Systems to begin with. To help illustrate the complexity and difficulty of just one of these issues—cardiac surgery— some time will be spent drilling down into the continuance of the Maui cardiac surgery program decision. Even within this magnified view, each point has multiple ramifications of its own.

1. The incidence of open-heart surgery is roughly one per thousand. Due to advances in minimally invasive coronary artery procedures performed by interventional cardiologists, even that incidence has been dropping. For the Maui population, minus the KP members who are treated at the KP Moanalua Hospital, that would be fewer than one hundred cases per year.

2. To maintain surgeon and operative team competence and full-time availability, cardiac specialty societies have recommended a minimum program caseload of 150–200 cases per year.

3. HPMG learned over the decades that the internalization of a high-intensity specialty like cardiac surgery or neurosurgery requires a minimum of two surgeons to provide twenty-four-hour call coverage and assistance with difficult cases. On Oahu, after HPMG hired the first surgeon to anchor a new internalized department, coverage and other requirements could be covered by contract with willing community surgeons of good reputation until the program grew large enough to hire a second surgeon. It remains doubtful that the Maui population could financially or clinically support even one cardiac surgeon never mind two. There is no Maui pool of willing cardiac surgeons to partner with—nor would there be in the foreseeable future. The use of temporary or part-time, unknown contract cardiac surgeons is fraught with potential lack of availability, quality, and cost problems. These would have to be borne by the patients—both financially via plan dues but especially in clinical outcomes.

4. Because of the expensive baseline program infrastructure required to maintain a cardiac surgery program, the cost per cardiac surgery case program drops for every case up to about 250–300 cases as the fixed costs are distributed among more cases. Thus, the cost per case for a small program is high compared to a "right-sized" program. Any transfer of KP member cases to the Maui cardiac surgery program would hurt the core program in two ways. Each case would cost more than doing the case at the Kaiser Moanalua

program. Since there would be fewer cases performed at the KP Moanalua program, the cost per case would go up there as well because there would be fewer cases bearing the fixed high costs of the Moanalua cardiac surgery program. Who would be willing to step up to fund the substantial subsidies required to maintain a local Maui program and make up for the extra overhead costs of the Moanalua program? Would that be the Kaiser Hawaii Health Plan and Hospitals? Such a diversion of funds would weaken the core program. If an extra HPMG cardiac surgeon is expected to be a second surgeon on Maui, who would pay for that position? Not HPMG. That point is moot because there wouldn't be enough cases to maintain the surgical and clinical skills of two surgeons in any case. Would Program Office cover the subsidy? Even if they would, there would still be the serious clinical concerns.

5. The KP Moanalua cardiac surgery program has been in place for more than twenty years and has a very good reputation with very good risk-corrected clinical outcome scores. For comparison, any Maui cardiac surgery outcome numbers would be small and, as such, statistically it would be very difficult to make any valid quality comparison between the two programs. Would KP members even choose to be operated on in the Maui program versus the Kaiser Moanalua program if offered the choice? They should be offered that choice.

The previous description just begins to outline the complexity of issues surrounding KP management support of the Maui cardiac surgery program. The Maui Hospital, to support its own fledgling cardiac surgery program, would like the Hawaii region to refer its Maui patients to the Maui Memorial Hospital cardiac surgery program instead of its own program at Moanalua. Should the Maui cardiac surgery program exist at all? This brief analysis just scratches the surface. What about the need to improve the capability of other required support services at Maui Memorial Hospital? What about the need to back up minimally invasive interventional cardiac procedures such as coronary stents? At the time of this writing, these issues remain unresolved.

Principles of True KP Partnership for Community Hospital Management

It is fortunate that this community hospital management experiment is being conducted in the Hawaii region. Hawaii has a long tradition of innovation and cooperative partnership between HPMG and the Regional Kaiser Health Plan and Hospitals if not always with Program Office. If the issues are worked out, it will be because of the trust that a strong partnership engenders. The underlying idealism of the KP promise, the talent and experience and resources of the program should be able to skillfully resolve each of these thorny issues and the others that will arise. Barring short-sighted external interventions from political special interests or Program Office initiatives to operate hospital management as a new line of business without Permanente Medical Group involvement, all these issues can be satisfactorily solved. If successfully resolved, the new idea of KP managing community hospital contracts will have been another Hawaii-originated innovation well out of proportion to its size. As such, it would be a model that could be applied across the entire program.

Kaiser Permanente has survived seventy-five years largely intact and growing because it has a mission that most persons of goodwill would support. It accomplished that mission by adhering to its founding principles—the most important of which was the Medical Group-Health Plan partnership.

The founding principles provided a framework for innovation based upon the ideal of patient service. KP has survived because it has proven again and again that it had the flexibility, resources, and talent to meet the inevitable challenges of a rapidly changing political and market environment. It has been seventy-five years since its founding and sixty years in Hawaii—and KP is still here. The proof of its formula has been its persistent success.

Professional Dreams Surpassed

On the evening of October 27, 2018, the fifty-eighth anniversary dinner of the Hawaii Permanente Medical Group was held in the huge Coral

Ballroom at the Hilton Hawaiian Village Hotel—formerly the Kaiser Hawaiian Village Hotel during Henry's days. It was a festive affair with a homecoming theme attended by eight hundred HPMG physicians and family members, including retirees. It was organized, as usual, by Richele Thornburg's department with class and military precision. The theme of the meeting was HPMG's mission of excellence, service, and inclusiveness in partnership with Health Plan. The highlight of the meeting was a presentation showing that year's program accomplishments. A partial list included:

- HPMG: 172 HPMG doctors were included on one or both national peer-nominated Best Doctors in America and America's Top Doctors.
- KP Moanalua Hospital: An "A" rating was received from the Leapfrog Group for hospital safety for the seventh straight ratings period.
- The American Heart Association awarded the Heart Failure Gold-Plus Quality Achievement Award for the seventh consecutive year.
- Healthgrade's 2018 Outstanding Patient Experience Award placed the Moanalua Medical Center in the top 15 percent of all hospitals in the nation.
- *US News and World Report*'s Best Hospitals rated the hospital as high performing in colon cancer surgery, heart failure, and chronic obstructive pulmonary disease (COPD).
- The Joint Commission on the Accreditation of Healthcare Organizations (JCAHO) Hospitals award the hospital with the highest score of any hospital in the national KP program.
- The 2018 Women's Choice Award of America's Best Hospitals for Obstetrics, Cancer Care, and Bariatric Surgery.

Hawaii KP Program

The National Committee for Quality Assurance (NCQA) rated the program as best in the state for its Medicare, Medicaid, and commercial plans. Its Medicare plan was in the top eight nationally with the highest possible rating of 5.0.

The Triple Crown on workplace safety was awarded for the third year in a row. The Human Rights Campaign foundation awarded the Hawaii program another "Leader in LGBTQ Healthcare Equality" award. There were many more detailed in Dr. Sewell's four-page, small-print, year-end presidential newsletter.

Those of us, now long retired, who went through periods of crisis decades ago, left that celebration with a tremendous sense of professional satisfaction. For those who were in leadership positions, we ask ourselves if we were good leadership "ancestors." Whatever we left HPMG, the current generation has certainly made the most of it. It is not often in life when the professional dreams of forty years ago are exceeded beyond one's imagination.

WILL KAISER PERMANENTE SURVIVE?

Will the Kaiser Permanente model survive? At least in California, it has existed largely in its current form for approaching eighty years despite predictions that the model was too complex and idealistic to succeed. Not only has it succeeded, it has delivered almost constant growth and quality improvement. While an eighty-year existence suggests that there is something about the model that underlies its success, large, old, established companies fail all the time. Consider Kodak, Pan Am and Polaroid—and Kaiser Industries. Henry Kaiser was correct when he said he would be remembered mostly for his hospitals. These companies failed because they lost their sense of mission. Human nature will bring on complacency, self-centered careerism, resistance to change, and the loss of a commitment to excellence. These behaviors also harm a medical organization's ability to compete, serve its patients, and adapt to changing markets. This could happen to Kaiser Permanente at any time, especially if it loses that idealistic culture derived from its founding principles.

The theme of this book has been that Kaiser Permanente was founded as an idealistic culture of health care-delivery—not simply another health care business. Indeed, KP history teaches us that when it did compromise its founding principles, when it became so bureaucratic that it lost sight of its mission, or when it attempted to adapt to short-term market changes by abandoning founding principles, it did falter. When it did recover, it was because there was a recommitment to the Kaiser Permanente mission and its founding principles: its culture. The CEO of Kaiser Permanente's closest competitor in California once said that you could copy just about everything Kaiser did and still fail because KP's strategic competitive advantage is its culture.

The founding principles are still relevant because they align with the better angels of human nature. Consider the longevity of the Ten Commandments and "do unto others as you would have them do unto you" as guides for optimal as well as good human behavior, even apart from their religious connotation. Briefly restated, the foundational principles of Kaiser Permanente are:

Exclusive Partnership

The exclusive partnership between the Kaiser Health Plan and Hospitals and the Permanente Medical Groups has been key to its success. Health Plan represents the business realities—"no margin no mission"—of health care while the Permanente Medical Groups protect the ethical imperatives of health care-delivery. This exclusive relationship requires an explicit conversation between the two entities to solve the paradox of infinite demand and finite resources. Removing exclusivity removes the requirement to have this essential conversation—for both entities.

One health plan cannot manage hundreds or even thousands of independent physicians. Similarly, individual physicians cannot simultaneously team up with dozens of health plans—all of which have differing objectives—when all that binds them together is money. KP history demonstrates clearly that where the partnership thrives, the program thrives. From the Kaiser Health Plan side, there are no instances where non-Permanente networks have been successful. From the Permanente Medical Group side, there have been no Permanente Medical Groups that have survived more than two years without partnership with Kaiser Health Plan. The breakup of the partnership would almost certainly result in program-wide "MAD" (mutually assured destruction). Despite dreams of divorce by the leaders of both entities who have tired of the perpetual but necessary negotiation, loss of the partnership would be the greatest risk to the continued existence of Kaiser Permanente.

Integrated Facilities

Without clinical control of its own care providers, hospital, pharmacy, lab, and diagnostic imaging, no region has survived independently. The KP philosophy of practice is so integrated that if these essential services are not under its direct management, large chunks of costly care, such as pharmacy, diagnostic services, or the largest one of all—hospital costs—are not within its control. Most of the cost of health care (~85 percent of the health care budget) is controlled by how the care is delivered.

Prepayment, Comprehensive Care, and Community Rating

Prepayment explicitly demands a real-time, on-the-ground solution to the paradox of unlimited demand for medical services and limited resources to provide those services. It provides strong incentives to prioritize preventive care, which, in turn, is better care. At the same time, preventive care conserves resources. Dr. Sidney Garfield's original vision was correct. The program saves big money by keeping people well. Also incentivized is efficient care and the explicit recognition of the importance of scientifically driven, cost-benefit decision-making to eliminate waste. Cost-benefit decisions also conserve resources. In a nonprofit setting, these conserved resources are put back into the organization to fund more comprehensive care at lower cost.

Sadly, market realities, supported by laissez faire laws, have weakened the advantages of prepayment for KP as fewer health care costs are covered with prepayment and more are covered by fee-for-service like co-payments by the patient. At some point, health care-delivery by this model will simply revert to fee-for-service with all of its problems.

The original idea of a set prepayment for necessary comprehensive medical care for everyone in the community was a good one because it spread out the cost of medical care across the sick and the well, large populations, and time. This is how insurance is supposed to work. It made comprehensive health insurance affordable for most of the working population. At least in the Hawaii region, the program proved that it could adapt to a government-financed safety net for the rest. This model worked well for KP until the early 1990s.

By the early nineties, for-profit health plans realized that that caring only for the healthy could result in huge profit margins. This gave rise to business models that denied care through limited benefits, benefit structures designed to cherry-pick low-risk patients, and the "hassle factor" denial of needed care. To survive, KP had to abandon full community-rated comprehensive care or be priced out of the market. In the absence of a level playing field, the risk to society was that health insurance would only be affordable to those who mostly didn't need it and unaffordable to those who did.

It was a difficult transition for KP. It could not pay for the care of the sick with a rapidly declining pool of well patients. Within KP, there was no existing infrastructure to price out or collect the new large volume of co-payments. This had been unnecessary during the previous three decades since the vast majority of its funding was through prepaid dues. After some initial missteps, it did successfully adapt to the new market realities by setting coverage levels with fewer and lower co-payments for patients who select more comprehensive coverage plans. It distinguished itself by providing low-cost or free preventive care for even the most basic coverage plans. It can extend this "brand value" by explicitly encouraging comprehensive care and by establishing internal incentives from the top to the bottom to incentivize comprehensive care. This would be nearly impossible for plans without partnering medical groups. KP can—but only if Health Plan takes advantage of its partnering Permanente Medical Groups. Doing this, KP would be well positioned to flexibly adapt to whatever future changes occur in the political and health care market climate. The stark business reality is this: "You don't have to run faster than the bear—you only have to run faster than the other guy."

Regional Autonomy

Regional autonomy from the National Health Plan ("Central Office") was KP policy almost from the beginning. It demonstrated that the KP vision of health care was not a historical accident; it could be a model for health care-delivery anywhere and adaptable to diverse medical market conditions. Each geographic region succeeded by having the local managers of the Health Plan insurance arm and hospitals partnering with the local Permanente Medical Group doctors. By this diversification, the regions outside of California decrease the dependence of the organization's survival upon events in California. The crisis of 1998 demonstrated this nicely.

Historically, because the leaders in those programs outside of California had to adapt to challenges different from those in California, they became innovation incubators out of proportion to their size. Barring "not invented here" resistance, these innovations instructed the entire program. Unfortunately, since the early 1990s, the KP trend toward central control has inhibited the dynamism of those regions outside of California (the ROCs) through burdensome mandatory Program Office "taxes" and management confusion as a result of simultaneous dual-reporting relationships to Program Office as well as the local management team. This is not a healthy trend.

High Program Office taxes imposed upon the regions for mandatory Program Office-controlled services put a tremendous financial drag on the competitiveness of regions whose competitors do not have similar external financial burdens. By making the services mandatory, the growth of an unaccountable, constantly growing Program Office bureaucracy is almost inevitable. With no possibility of critical pushback, this will progressively increase the KP Program Office's region-killing tax burden. Making these services elective, rather than mandatory, would force fiscal and performance discipline upon these Program Office programs.

The long-term Program Office trend of centralizing authority at the expense of regional autonomy will weaken the organization. The advantages of regional diversification have been already discussed: KP as a model for health care outside of California, less dependence on California for KP survival, innovation incubation, and a source for new talent. As Cora Tellez, an emeritus, successful president of the Hawaii region wrote to the author: "Regional autonomy recognizes that all medical care is local. Decision-making devolved to the lowest level fosters patient loyalty, employer and community commitment to KP as local providers of care, more efficient decision-making and of course, engenders a system of upward mobility for employees. Not everyone wants to move to Oakland." The author certainly didn't. She continued: "Regional autonomy also attracts the kind of talent that Kaiser Health Plan will need as markets become more complex and competitive. Those leaders are entrepreneurial and willing to take strategic risks in the interest of their respective regions. They have a strong incentive to work with their Medical Group leaders as coequal leaders. Such leaders don't thrive under central control." It could not have been better expressed.

At its height in 1993, all twelve independent regions of Kaiser Permanente were in the black. KP was well on its way to becoming a national health plan. After that, when KP changed direction, abandoning several founding principles, the number of independent regions has dropped from twelve to six with the additional Washington state program recently added in 2017. Once Program Office declared a region a "turnaround region" and brought in its own leadership, the prognosis was guarded: five dead (Texas, Northeast, North Carolina, Kansas City, and Ohio), two wounded (Northwest, Colorado), and Hawaii, and two that lost their independence to California control (Mid-Atlantic and Georgia). Of the three that survived independently, Hawaii, Colorado, and Northwest had been established and operated under the founding principles of Kaiser Permanente.

Dual Option

This was KP policy from the earliest days of the program. The idea was that no patient should be forced into KP and that every patient would have the option to choose a different health plan. This was a powerful argument against KP enemies who maintained that KP patients were forced to join the "socialist-industrialized medicine" of Kaiser Industries against their will. It also provided an escape for those who were, for various reasons, unhappy with the program.

In the late 1980s, with the rise of Health Plan brokers, KP competitors offered "one-stop shops" with standard fee-for-service to individual physicians, discounted independent physician associations (IPAs), and HMO options while KP only offered its standard HMO plan. This placed KP at a major disadvantage.

The solution was for KP to offer brokers a non-HMO option called the point-of-service program. The idea was that patients would see Permanente Medical Group doctors, but they had the option to go outside. This solved the broker problem, but it introduced problems that threatened the entire program. A recurring theme of this book is that major cost efficiencies do result from delivering health care with the KP HMO model. These savings are lost when patients go outside the program; therefore, the actual cost of point-of-service coverage would be expected to be considerably higher than the core HMO product. Of course, the point-of-service would be most attractive to brokers and the KP sales force if priced similarly to the HMO product. The Permanente Medical Groups noted in response that if the point-of-service program was priced the same as the HMO product, the point-of-service program would be diverting financial resources and members away from the core product. Such a point-of-service product would be subsidizing the competition while at the same time weakening the KP core product. When priced correctly, the higher price of a point-of-service product limits the popularity of this option, but more important, it limits damage to the core product. In all fairness, indemnity plans do the same thing. They charge more for unrestricted fee-for-service versus restricted care options. Point-of-service can remain a useful tool to market a one-stop shop for brokers and to introduce new members to KP. Many point-of-service patients, after trying KP, eventually do switch to the core HMO product. That was the original intention: but point of service is not the answer.

Lesson of the Principles

The theme of this book is that the founding principles have defined Kaiser Permanente Health Care. For more than seventy years, the program has prospered when they were observed, and when they were not, the program failed. *Kaiser Permanente is a prepaid, nonprofit, affordable, comprehensive medical care program spreading risk by community rating, controlling quality and cost through the vertical integration of facilities delivering quality health care by scientifically and ethically informed program principles. This is made possible by the regionally autonomous but united exclusive partnership of the Kaiser Health Plan and the Permanente Medical Groups.* A Kaiser

Permanente building with a Kaiser Permanente logo on it is not necessarily Kaiser Permanente Health Care.

Historically, the principles of Kaiser Permanente Health Care prompted more than three generations of health care and management professionals to take professionally dangerous personal risks and make the necessary self-sacrifices to promote this visionary culture of health care. This was especially true in the early years. The author witnessed it again and again during his almost thirty-year career with KP. It has been an essential component of KP's long-term survivability. If Kaiser Permanente loses its commitment to these principles, it may survive for a time as a name, but its identity will be lost. Few physicians would care to make a personal and professional commitment to a health care company that is indistinguishable from all of the others—or worse, a for-profit company the main mission of which is to increase shareholder value—potentially at the expense of patient care.

It was this commitment to the idealistic foundational principles of Kaiser Permanente that motivated generations of Permanente Medical Group and Health Plan leaders to successfully combat the foibles of human nature that cause internal complacency and bureaucratic, self-interested careerism. This commitment enabled the program to steadily improve quality and service as well as to adapt to the massive economic and political changes in the delivery of American health care. As this book demonstrates, the continuing march toward a medical culture of excellence in the Hawaii Permanente Medical Group did not occur suddenly or spontaneously. It developed gradually by the persistent efforts of idealistic leaders who were inspired by the Kaiser Permanente promise. Lose these first principles, and the program will likely lose that idealism and all that comes of it, including survival. That would be a societal tragedy.

In the arena of health care population-management policy, Kaiser Permanente has already won. Were Kaiser Permanente ever to fail, it will go down in history as a program that transformed the delivery of health care in America and elsewhere. To name a few of the innovations:

1. The efficient management of health care for large populations.
2. The value of preventive care.

3. The value of prepaid, nonprofit, comprehensive scientific care to control cost.
4. The ability of salaried doctors and Health Plan managers—despite their cultural differences—to work together to provide efficient, scientific, affordable, high-quality medical care.
5. The value of applying computer technology to medical care to provide better preventive and acute care-delivery coordinated through an electronic medical record and the medical decision support that it provides.

These concepts were all pioneered and successfully demonstrated for large populations by Kaiser Permanente.

ABBREVIATIONS AND CONCEPTS

alignment of Interests: Any human endeavor that aligns the interests of the parties involved is likely to be successful. This may explain the success of Kaiser Permanente, which, when functioning properly, aligns the interests of the patients, the doctors, the workers, and the community. It is not that easy, which happens to be the theme of this book.

cherry-picking: This is a policy of structuring a health plan so that only low-risk patients are attracted—and high-risk patients are excluded. Techniques include very low premiums but very high co-payments, exclusion of preexisting conditions, and offering benefits that would attract only young, healthy patients (health spa memberships, etc.). It can be very profitable because only a small proportion of the population uses a disproportionate amount of the medical resources, which is, of course, the reason for medical insurance to begin with. Those health plans that do not follow suit are driven into a death spiral. The logical end point would be a society in which medical insurance is only affordable for those who don't need it while being unaffordable and therefore unavailable to those who do need it.

CIS (clinical information system): An ill-fated attempt by KP to partner with IBM to develop a proprietary electronic medical record.

When George Halvorson became the fourth CEO of Kaiser Permanente, it was shut down and the Epic Company derived Health Connect was implemented program-wide.

Colorado River Aqueduct: A 242-mile aqueduct bringing Colorado River water from Lake Havasu on the California-Arizona border. It is an important source of water for Southern California. The aqueduct was built between 1933 and 1939. About halfway across the Mohave Desert was located Dr. Sidney Garfield's twelve-bed Contractors General Hospital, which was built to provide health care to the workforce.

community rating: It is a form of dues setting whereby all patients in a given geographic area pay the same premiums. It spreads risk across that geographic area. It has the potential to provide care to the sick and healthy at affordable rates for all because the medical risk is spread across time and the whole population. It was the way that KP delivered its care during its first forty years. As experience rating (you pay for what you individually use) became more sophisticated in the late 1980s, KP was forced to follow suit or face a death spiral. It did so with "adjusted community rating," which is another form of experience rating.

CON (certificate of need): This is a program run at the state level to prevent expensive duplication of medical services for the purpose of lowering overall health care costs. Unintended consequences include the establishment of bureaucratic barriers subject to political pressures, which can establish government protected monopolies. These, in turn, can raise health care costs rather than lower them.

death spiral: In a community where experience rating is extensively employed to structure insurance premiums designed to attract young and healthy patients, the health plans that do not do so go into a death spiral. They are left with the old and sick patients who use up disproportionate medical resources. These health plans must raise rates to stay in business. With higher rates, they are even less attractive to low-utilizing patients, and only sick patients stay with the plan until they too are priced out of the market. As these health plans go out of business, the old and sick patients have no insurance. It is good for the experience-rated health care companies' bottom lines—but not so good for old and sick patients or society.

experience: What you gain if you learn from your mistakes. It usually takes time.

experience rating: A method of setting health care insurance premiums in which rates are set based upon claims made. In other words, patients in a high-risk group pay higher premiums. Fee for service care-delivery is the logical end point of experience rating.

fee-for-service payment model: Payment is for services rendered after the fact. More care is incentivized whether effective or not. Preventive care could be a dis-incentivized as it could reduce the need for future care.

Fleur de Lac: Henry Kaiser's estate on Lake Tahoe. It was one of the sites of the "Tahoe Conferences" that settled fundamental issues between Kaiser Health Plan and the Permanente Medical Groups. It can be seen as the Godfather's house in *The Godfather II*.

gag order: These were inserted into contracts between physicians and health plans. They prohibited a physician advising a patient that appropriate care would require an intervention not covered by the health plan.

genetic code of Kaiser Permanente: The genetic code espoused the principles of (1.) prepayment for comprehensive medical care, which would provide predictable and stable financing to incentivize preventive care and the early treatment of disease (2.) cost-effective care through broad community rating so that the care is affordable by as much of the population as possible (3.) vertical integration of facilities to control costs and to provide a cultural environment in which preventive and cost-effective scientifically based care can be safely delivered by the medical staff (4.) dual option to avoid forcing patients into the KP program, which by necessity, had a closed panel of doctors and finally and most important (5.) the exclusive health plan—salaried Medical Group partnership to balance of interests of economics and medical care.

Grand Coulee Dam: One of the largest dams in the United States, it was built between 1934–1942 in a semiarid remote region of eastern Washington state to provide irrigation and hydroelectric power for the region. Edgar Kaiser managed the project for Kaiser Industries and contracted with Sidney Garfield, MD, to organize comprehensive medical care for the thousands of industrial workers and their families. It was during this experience that the power of integrated facilities and a subspecialized Medical Group was demonstrated.

Grand Rounds: A medical presentation for all of the HPMG doctors, which started shortly after the establishment of the Medical Group in 1960 and ran until 1985. It was reestablished in 2009 as a monthly one-hour presentation aired in all clinics simultaneously intended to inform and standardize HPMG's state-of-the-art care.

hassle factor: Unnecessary bureaucratic hurdles used by insurance companies to deny patient services or payments for services provided.

Health Connect: The electronic medical record adopted by the Kaiser Permanente Program based upon the Epic electronic medical record record (EMR).

HPMG (Hawaii Permanente Medical Group): The independent medical group founded in 1960, which provides on an exclusive, contractual basis the clinical care of the members of the Kaiser Foundation Health Plan and Hospitals of Hawaii.

HPPG (Hawaii Pacific Permanente Medical Group): A wholly owned subsidiary of the Hawaii Permanente Medical Group (HPMG), organized to provide staffing management for Maui Health Systems physician staffing.

Industrial Insurance Exchange: The insurance company insuring the Colorado aqueduct partly owned by Kaiser Industries. The actuary Harold Hatch recommended to A. B. Ordway that prepayment be considered to support Dr. Sidney Garfield's twelve-bed Contractors General Hospital, which was in danger of closing because of difficulty collecting fees for medical services rendered. The plan was a tremendous success, and prepayment allowed Garfield's medical services to expand until the end of the project.

Kai-Perm Meeting: This was an annual meeting of all of the Health Plan regional presidents and the Permanente medical directors to set the general direction of the program and ratify policies. It promoted cooperation between the medical directors and regional presidents.

As part of the Program Office centralization, these meetings were canceled in 1996. This action stimulated the organization of the Permanente Federation.

Kaiser Industries: An agglomeration of more than one hundred industries under the Kaiser name, including construction, concrete, mining, and entertainment. It broke up into individual companies by the late 1960s. Henry Kaiser retired from Kaiser Industries in 1955.

KP (Kaiser Permanente): A prepaid, nonprofit, affordable, comprehensive medical care program spreading risk by community rating, controlling quality and cost through vertical integration of facilities, and delivering quality health care by scientifically and ethically informed principles. This is made possible by the regionally autonomous, but united, exclusive partnership of the Kaiser Health Plan and the Permanente Medical Groups.

MGMA (Medical Group Management Association): This company was judged by HPMG as having the most accurate compensation and resource support information for a large, urban, multispecialty medical group such as HPMG. It has been in use by HPMG since 1991.

M&M (Medicine and Management): A middle management medical group training program organized and sponsored by the Hawaii, Northwest, and Colorado Permanente Medical Groups.

MMA (Medical Management Analysis): A prospective quality assurance program based upon research done at Dartmouth Medical School. That research demonstrated that screening for twenty-three adverse events could detect 80 percent of adverse hospital occurrences. This was the name of a proprietary program marketed by Dr. Joyce Craddick in the early 1980s that was based upon the Dartmouth research. It replaced retrospective disease audits in the Hawaii region and became the basis of hospital and later the clinic quality assurance program.

HPMG Operations versus Policy: This was a governance policy established by Dr. Dung, the second president of HPMG. Consistent with the concept of "with responsibility must go authority," Dr. Dung established a "strong chief" program continuing the policy of Dr. Chu and his mentor, Dr. Saward, the Northwest Permanente

Medical Group president. According to this policy, the elected board of directors would make HPMG general policy: ratifying the hiring and firing of HPMG physicians as proposed by chiefs, compensations issues, ratification of the president, associate medical directors, and major chiefs. The chiefs would be responsible for recruiting, scheduling services, department organization, the appointment of subsection chiefs, and day-to-day operational issues.

Pacific Medical Associates: A group of five prominent Honolulu doctors recruited personally be Henry Kaiser to provide medical care for the Kaiser Health Plan that he was to establish. Because it was unable to reconcile traditional fee-for-service practice with prepaid practice, it was unable to maintain cost and service competitiveness and was dissolved. It was immediately succeeded by the Hawaii Permanente Medical Group, which was organized along established Permanente principles of prepayment and an exclusivity contract with the Kaiser Health Plan.

Permanente Medical Groups Interregional Services: A position established in 1981 by the by the Permanente Medical Group medical directors to have a full-time representation in the Health Plan Program Office. It was the precursor of the Permanente Federation.

PMG (Permanente Medical Group): Salaried medical groups organized on a regional basis with their own governance. They provide services to the Regional Kaiser Health Plan and Hospitals on an exclusive basis through yearly negotiated medical service contracts.

POS (point-of-service plan): A program designed to preserve the dual option so that patients are not forced to get their care exclusively within the traditional KP program. While it can introduce patients to KP, if not priced appropriately (higher than the core program) it can have the unintended consequences of subsidizing the infrastructure of the community medical competition while at the same time cannibalizing the core KP membership.

PPRO (physician performance review and oversight committee): Committee of chiefs founded in 1998 for the purpose of carrying out the HPMG Values Statement by defining the standards of HPMG physician performance. It incorporates the findings of the quality assurance committee, patient-satisfaction survey, peer-to-peer survey, and malpractice data. These standards are then recommended to the HPMG executive committee and HPMG board of directors for ratification after which they become HPMG policy.

Pre-paid medical care model: Payment for medical care is prepaid in the form of monthly dues. With a known, fixed budget, preventive care, efficient care, and cost-effective care are incentivized.

quality assurance (QA): In the Hawaii region, a hospital committee reports directly to the hospital executive committee. It prospectively measures hospital and clinic medical care and sets standards of performance. It recommends these standards to the Hawaii region hospital executive committee for hospital care and hospital privileges—and to the HPMG board of directors for enforcement.

ROC Regions (regions outside of California): They include the Hawaii, Northwest (centered on greater Portland, Oregon), Washington (centered on Seattle) and Colorado (centered on Denver). Former ROCs included the Northeast, North Carolina, Ohio, Texas, and Kansas City regions. The Mid-Atlantic region is administered from the Northern California region, and the Georgia region is administered from the Southern California region.

strong chief program: This is the management policy of the Hawaii region. This policy states: With responsibility for favorable outcomes must come the authority to achieve these outcomes. Operational policy is distinguished from Medical Group policy and is under purview of the chiefs. The chiefs are not elected or rotated; they are appointed by the president or associate medical directors appointed by the president with a ratification by the elected board of directors. Subsection chiefs are appointed by the chiefs without ratification. With the clear lines of authority, the responsibility for outcomes is clear.

SWG (Strategic Work Group): A monthly meeting of four senior executives of Health Plan and four senior executives of HPMG to set regional program direction. It started in 2006 and ended with the resignation by David Underriners resignation as President of the Region in 2019.

Tahoe Agreement: This was the foundational agreement between Health Plan and the Permanente Medical Groups. Some of the meetings were held at Henry Kaiser's compound, hence the nickname the Tahoe Agreement. There were a series of meetings that were often contentious. In the end, it was agreed that Health Plan would control the facilities, including the hospitals, and the Permanente Medical Groups would control the medical care, including outside medical services. The Health Plan and Permanente Medical Groups would negotiate an exclusive yearly medical services agreement.

Tahoe II: An agreement reached between the Health Plan and the Permanente Federation Leadership and signed in June 1997 to help reverse the disastrous financial performance of the program. In that agreement, the exclusive partnership between Health Plan and Hospitals and the Permanente Medical Groups was affirmed. A Kai-Perm Program Group was established to replace the Kai-Perm Committee. It consisted of five Permanente Federation representatives and five Health Plan and Hospital representatives. It was to set the direction of the program—specifically regarding all expansion region agreements. Even though it did not take place in Tahoe, it was often informally referred to by Medical Group leadership as "Tahoe II" in remembrance of the landmark Tahoe Agreements of the early 1950s. It was ended by Kaiser Health Plan in 2014.

TPMG (The Permanente Medical Group): The Northern California Permanente Medical Group that served the Northern California Kaiser Health Plan and Hospital Patients. It was the first Permanente Medical Group, hence named "the" Permanente Medical Group (TPMG).

PEOPLE

This history was written by the actions of literally thousands of people. This is but a short listing. To those who are not in the glossary and should be, my sincere apologies.

Alfred Apaka: The best-known Hawaii vocalist from the late 1940s to his sudden unexpected death at the age of forty in 1960 at the height of his fame. He was the headliner at the Kaiser Hawaii Village (now Hilton Hawaiian Village) Hotel. When Henry Kaiser built the hotel, he specifically created the Tapa Showroom for Apaka. The Tapa Tower now stands on that site.

Mary Ann Barnes: She began her forty-three-year career with Kaiser Permanente as an intensive care nurse. In 2014, she was appointed regional president of the Hawaii region and was instrumental in the successful bid for the Maui Health System management contract. She ensured that regional Health Plan worked cooperatively with HPMG and retired in September 2017.

David D. Bell, MD: He joined HPMG in 2002 as a family practice doctor. He was popularly elected by the associates to serve on the 2006 presidential search committee and also appointed chief of hospital specialties. Under Dr. Sewell, he was appointed associate medical director (AMD) of professional development and service. In this position, he was responsible for HPMG physician performance.

In 2016, he was appointed executive vice president of people and leadership strategy of the Permanente Federation.

Bruce Behnke: With hospital administrative experience at the Mayo Clinic and the Southern California region, he was appointed by D. J. Mailer as her successor as hospital administrator of the Kaiser Moanalua Medical Center in 1984. He followed her as regional president in 2000 and resigned in 2003. He went on to a career as a published art photographer.

Conrad Bohuslav: He was the Hawaii regional president from 1968 until 1975. He had a difficult working relationship with Dr. Dung.

Tom Brown, MD: He joined HPMG as a radiologist, and after the death of Dr. Chu, he led one of the two major HPMG factions. He accepted the election of Dr. Dung, and as such, he served as Dr. Dung's vice president of operations from 1971–1975. After Dr. Dung's 1975 administrative reorganization, he left HPMG but did return at the end of his career to lead the Diagnostic Imaging Department during a period of crisis. He then retired from HPMG.

Gladys Ching: Dr. William Dung managed to acquire management supervision of clinic nursing for HPMG from Kaiser Health Plan and Hospitals. This is the nursing staff for the clinics and is separate from hospital nursing, which is supervised by Kaiser Hospital. Gladys Ching, RN, was appointed to supervise clinic nursing in 1975 and served until 2007. Her soft-spoken but clear management style established a tradition of accountability for clinic staff to the doctors of HPMG.

Yi Ching, MD: Joined HPMG in 1967 as a pediatrician straight from training. An excellent clinician, he was a strong supporter of quality and education. He early on recognized the potential of computers in medicine. He became chief of pediatrics in 1976, succeeding Dr. Alex Roth. He built the department into one of the strongest in HPMG. One year prior to retirement in 1997, he resigned as chief of pediatrics in favor of Dr. Marsha Marumoto who succeeded him and carried on the legacy.

Michael Chaffin, MD: He was the third medical director of HPMG (1992–2007). He initially joined HPMG in 1977. He was chief of medicine in 1984–1985 and the physician in charge of the windward

Oahu Koolau Clinic (1985–1989). During his fifteen-year term as medical director, the Hawaii program grew by forty-three thousand members and became a statewide program. Peace, prosperity, and cooperation characterized his administration. A rational and stable policy of market-based physician compensation vastly improved the ability to recruit outstanding physicians to HPMG. That, along with the development of a standardized and objectively measured and enforced physician-performance program, accelerated the establishment of the culture of excellence. The successful governance structure established during Dr. Dung's administration was further strengthened and employed to establish operational policies and procedures that provided a rational approach for most day-to-day operational issues. He also presided over the difficult establishment of the Hawaii region-wide electronic medical record—the first in Hawaii.

Philip Chu, MD: He was the first medical director of HPMG (1960–1970). A strong leader, during his administration, HPMG the program was established on a firm financial and clinical footing. It was a period of stability and growth. The first neighbor islands clinics were established on Maui, and HPMG was established as a Hawaii professional corporation, providing the legal basis for the subsequent establishment of the excellent benefit and retirement program.

Jack Cochran, MD: In 1990, he joined the Colorado Permanente Medical Group as chief of plastic surgery. An eloquent speaker, he subsequently served as medical director of CPMG. In 2007, he succeeded Dr. Jay Crosson as the president of the Permanente Federation until 2015.

Morris Collen, MD: First chief of medicine in the Kaiser shipyard worker's hospitals and clinics of Northern California during World War II. He organized the initial research effort that demonstrated that these hospitals and clinics, by emphasizing prepayment, managed care, and preventive care, delivered superior outcomes. He was a militant defender of the physician's role in the Kaiser Permanente program and an important TPMG leader. He went on to establish the computerized multiphasic preventive medicine screening clinics that were established in many KP regions, including Hawaii. Clinical research derived from the data generated from these clinics further validated the value of preventive care. He remained an active promoter of KP medicine until his death at the age of one hundred in 2014.

Tarquin Collis, MD: He joined HPMG as an infectious disease specialist in 2001. He was appointed section chief of that department in 2005. One of the most popular doctors in HPMG history, he was elected to the board of directors and represented the board members on the 2006 presidential search committee. He has served as associate medical director of medical specialty services since 2007.

Jay Crosson, MD: He joined the Northern California Permanente Medical Group (TPMG) in 1977 as a staff specialist in pediatric infectious disease. An important administrator in TPMG, he was unanimously chosen by the medical directors to become the first executive medical director of the Permanente Federation. In this capacity, between 1997 and 2007, when he retired, he ably represented Permanente Medical Group interests in partnership with the CEO of Kaiser Health Plan and Hospitals.

Cecil Cutting, MD: One of the founding "fathers" of Kaiser Permanente, he was the first medical director of the Permanente Medical Group (TPMG) in Northern California.

William Dung, MD: He was the second president of HPMG (1970–1992). During his administration, HPMG acquired management control of clinic nursing. Also during his administration, the largely intact governance structure was established in which chiefs had operational authority while the elected board of directors ratified the chiefs appointed by the president and determined HPMG associateship and financial policies.

Scott Fleming: He was an important Kaiser Industries corporate attorney who was influential in the establishment of Kaiser Permanente policy. He played a particularly helpful role in the establishment of the Hawaii region and HPMG during its difficult birth.

Pauline Fox: She served as chief counsel for the Medical Legal Department, then was vice president, and eventually became assistant general counsel of the Northern California region from 1994–1999. From

1999 to 2012 (retirement), she served as the Permanente general counsel. She returned to the Permanente Federation in 2016 and served as the executive vice president and chief legal officer of the Permanente Federation until 2019. She was an important source for this book.

Christine Fukui, MD: Joined HPMG as a pulmonologist and section chief of pulmonology until her retirement in 2009. An able and popular clinician, she was elected to the HPMG board of directors twice. From 2005 to 2007, she was chief of medical specialties, and from 2007 to 2009, she was associate medical director of quality.

Sidney R. Garfield, MD: A visionary, he is credited with bringing together the concepts of prepayment, capitation, an exclusive partnership between Health Plan and Medical Group, integrated facilities, and a partner, salaried, multispecialty medical group that became Kaiser Permanente. In 1955, his responsibilities shifted from direct administration to planning. During the remainder of his career, he envisioned and promoted new hospital designs, the electronic medical record, team models of health care-delivery, and preventive care. Right up to his death in 1984, he remained a respected, often revered, advisor to the Medical Groups.

James Griffith, MD: He was a well-respected pediatric pulmonologist who served as the Kaiser Moanalua Medical Center chief of staff until his retirement.

Leighton Hasegawa: He joined HPMG in 2000 as chief financial officer. A capable "franchise player," he served in other roles as needed. His leadership could be characterized as sensitive, dedicated, and self-effacing, but the job always got done and done well. Many long conversations with Leighton about the fundamental nature of HPMG and KP contributed mightily to this book.

Jan Head: She was the regional president of the Hawaii region from 2003 until 2007.

Vernon Hiroe: The director of AV Services joined the Hawaii program in 1990 and organized and managed the highly regarded audiovisual program for the Hawaii region.

Stacey Honda, MD: She joined HPMG as a staff pathologist in 1997 and was appointed chief of pathology in 1999, which she has capably led. In 2009, she was appointed associate medical director of ancillary services, which includes the pathology laboratory and diagnostic imaging services.

Lee Jacobs, MD: He was the Hawaii chief of medicine from 1980 until 1984. He established a formal personal care provider program in the region in which each patient had their own primary care physician to coordinate their care, greatly improving accountability and patient satisfaction.

Carolyn ("Kaki") Jennings: She joined the Hawaii region in May 1978 as department supervisor of human resources. By May 1981, she was appointed director of human resources for the Kaiser Permanente Program in Hawaii. She served in this capacity until her retirement in 2006. During her tenure, a unified Human Resources Department served both HPMG and Kaiser Health Plan and Hospitals well. She mentored many, including the author, from both Health Plan and HPMG in the principles of human resource management.

Alyce Chester Kaiser: She was mentored personally by Sidney Garfield while on his administrative team. Recognizing her as one of the best nurses in the program, he recommended her to Henry Kaiser to provide private duty nursing care for Bess Kaiser during Bess's long decline due to renal failure. Henry shortly after married Alyce despite their age difference reportedly with Bess Kaiser's blessing. Henry Kaiser established the Walnut Creek Hospital with Alyce effectively as administrator. It sparked a Health Plan Medical Group crisis that was seen by the Permanente doctors as an attempt to break up the Permanente Medical Group. It was ultimately unsuccessful, but it was one of the conflicts that led to the Tahoe Agreement.

Bess Kaiser: Beloved by all, she was the first wife of Henry Kaiser. Bess Kaiser Hospital in the Northwest region was named after her.

Edgar Kaiser: A son of Henry J. Kaiser was an important executive of Kaiser Industries. He was tasked with the management of the construction of the Grand Coulee Dam. He hired Sidney Garfield to provide medical care for the project. Dr. Garfield's management demonstrated the value of integrated facilities and a subspecialized salaried physician group.

Henry J. Kaiser: An entrepreneur extraordinaire, he was one of the greatest American industrialists of the twentieth century. His shipyards built a quarter of the US shipping during World War II. At its height, Kaiser Industries encompassed more than one hundred businesses, including broadcasting, aluminum, steel, cement, banking, real estate, and large-scale construction projects. He partnered with Dr. Sidney Garfield to establish what would become Kaiser Permanente.

Clifford Keene, MD: The first CEO of Kaiser Permanente, he took a personal interest in the establishment of the Hawaii region during the crises of 1960 and 1970. He was the effective CEO of KP from 1960 until 1970. During his administration, the program grew from 800,000 to 2.2 million members. It also grew from three to six regions.

Paul Lairson, MD: He joined the Northwest PMG as a staff physician in 1966 and remained on staff until 1975. In 1975, he became the medical director of the Georgetown University Community Health Plan, which eventually became the core group of the Mid-Atlantic Permanente Medical Group in 1980. In 1977, he became the founding medical director of the Texas Permanente Medical Group. Between 1983 and his retirement in 1992, he served as the first director of Permanente Medical Groups Interregional Services, the predecessor of the Permanente Federation.

David Lawrence, MD: He served as the third CEO of Kaiser Permanente from 1992 until 2002. At a time of rapid change in the health care industry, experiments with elements of the genetic code, the Kaiser principles of exclusive partnership, integrated facilities, and prepayment proved to be dramatically unsuccessful.

Peggy Latare, MD: She joined HPMG as a family practice physician. She served terms on the elected board of directors and was a popularly elected member of the search committee. She promoted and led "Thriving in a Busy Practice," an effective physician-performance program and was lead physician on the regional implementation of the Health Connect electronic medical record. As of 2019 she is the director of the obesity program, which integrates lifestyle programs with the medical and surgical treatment of obesity.

Martin Leftik, MD: He was chief of medicine from 1985 until 1997. After that, he was one of the team leaders who implemented the electronic medical record.

Ian Leverton, MD: He joined TPMG as a staff general surgeon. He served as medical director of the Kansas City Permanente Medical Group and then as Dr. Paul Lairson's successor of the Permanente Medical Groups Interregional Services from 1993 until 1997.

Janet Liang: She was appointed to succeed Jan Head as regional president in 2007. She had an energetic and successful administration in Hawaii. In 2014, she went on to become chief operating officer then regional president of the Northern California region and was appointed COO of Kaiser Health Plan.

T. K Lin, MD: He was a respected cardiologist and the first chief of medicine of HPMG. He was considered as successor to Dr. Chu. He declined the offer to concentrate upon clinical medicine. He left HPMG during the leadership/salary crisis of 1975.

Michael Linderman: He served as the first business manager of HPMG from 1975 until 2000. He was responsible for putting HPMG business operations on a firm financial footing.

D. J Mailer: She was appointed hospital administrator of the Kaiser Moanalua Medical Center by Cora Tellez. She followed Cora as regional president of the Hawaii region in 1994 and served in that capacity until 1999. She was an excellent partner to HPMG. She went on to a successful career capped off as the successful CEO of the Kamehameha Schools.

Albert J. Mariani, MD: The author joined HPMG in 1980 as a staff urologic surgeon. In 1983, he was appointed chief of surgical services. In addition, from 1998 until 2005 he was chief of the heart program. From 2005 until 2007, he served as chief of specialty services and then from 2007 to 2009 (retirement), he served as associate medical director of specialty and hospital services. As chair of the Physician Performance Review and Oversight Committee (PPRO) of the chiefs from 1997 to 2009, he guided the development of the quality assurance, quality of service, and peer-to-peer programs that set the HPMG standards of physician performance. From 1984 until 1986, he served as Moanalua Hospital chief of staff and again from 2007 to 2009 (retirement).

Marsha Marumoto, MD: She joined HPMG as a pediatrician in 1987 and was soon the pediatrician of choice for the children of the medical staff. An elected board of directors member, she was appointed chief of pediatrics in 1996 to succeed Yi Ching, MD, on January 1, 1997. In this capacity, she has continued his legacy of departmental excellence for twenty-two years and counting. She is a classic example of an elected board member who, once familiar with the complexities of Medical Group management, went on to become a successful chief.

Paul McCallin, MD: He was the longstanding chief of obstetrics and gynecology and served as interim president of HPMG from July to September 1970 during which time the Articles of Association were passed, allowing HPMG to become a Hawaii corporation. This, in turn, provided a framework for the generous HPMG benefit program.

Donna McCleary, MD: She joined HPMG as a pediatrician serving on Maui. From 1981 to 1998, she was the physician in chief of the neighbor islands, and as such, she presided over the expansion of the program on Maui and the establishment of the program in Kona and Hilo. In 1998, she was appointed vice president in charge of Medicare and Medicaid for HPMG.

Lorrain McVety, RN: She served the Hawaii region of KP for her entire career. As a preretirement project, she was assigned to hospital quality assurance. She identified a prospective quality assurance program based upon research at Dartmouth Medical School and marketed by Joyce Craddick, MD, in 1984 called Medical Management Analysis. Working with the author, she completely redesigned the Hospital Quality Assurance Department to implement the program. The program was later expanded to include the clinics and has remained largely unchanged at the time of the writing of this book (2020).

Stephen D. Miller, MD: He joined HPMG in 1979 as a staff ophthalmologist and retinal surgery subspecialist and section chief of ophthalmology. Shortly after, he was appointed chief of surgical services. In 1983, he was appointed vice president of finance under Drs. Dung and Chaffin. He retired in 2002 to assume a leadership role and eventually chairmanship of the SEVA Eye Foundation. He served as a part-time consultant to HPMG from 2002 until 2007. SEVA provides eye care and establishes self-sustaining eye care infrastructure internationally for impoverished populations.

A. B. Ordway: An important Kaiser Industries executive, he worked with Harold Hatch, an underwriter for Industrial Insurance Exchange. Together, they worked out a prepayment reimbursement program that financially saved Sidney Garfield's twelve-bed Contractors General Hospital. Later, he recommended to Edgar Kaiser that he meet Dr. Garfield to organize the industrial health care for the Grand Coulee Dam. The largest building in Oakland, the twenty-eight story Ordway building, is named after him.

Fred Pellegrin, MD: He was the chief of medicine of the new Walnut Creek Hospital and was Henry Kaiser's personal physician. He was invited by Henry Kaiser to reside at his Honolulu estate for six months to study the feasibility of a Kaiser-type medical program in Hawaii. He advised against it. This was not what Henry wanted to hear as he was already working with architects on the Kaiser Hospital. Dr. Pellegrin was sent back to California and never heard from Mr. Kaiser again.

Karl Pregitzer, MD: The longest-serving HPMG doctor (1977–2015), he was recruited to be chief of the Emergency Department. He professionalized the department by requiring board certification. He was instrumental in the establishment of the Industrial Medicine Department. Dr. Chaffin appointed him vice president of special projects and outside services where he brought under control outside services expenses. His service to HPMG continued under Dr. Sewell as associate medical director of business services. In this capacity, he organized the coding and compliance programs. This service became essential when political and economic change brought on an increased dependence upon accurate coding for program reimbursement.

Alex Roth, MD: An allergist, he was recruited from the faculty of the University of Kansas by Dr. T. K. Lin. He was Dr. Dung's first pick for executive vice president in 1971. That attempt failed. He was reappointed in 1975 and served in that capacity until 1984. He preceded Dr. Yi Ching as chief of pediatrics.

Mark Santi, MD: He joined HPMG in 1994 and was appointed section chief of orthopedics in 1997, chief of surgical services in 2005, and then associate medical director of surgical services in 2009. He was appointed a member of the Regional Strategic Work Group in 2009. He is an able administrator and strategic thinker with an exceptional sense of humor.

Earnest Saward, MD: He was the founding medical director of the Northwest region in 1945 and successfully led the region for twenty-five years. Working with Dr. Clifford Keene, he was instrumental in successfully helping the Hawaii region work through the HPMG founding crisis in 1960 and the Dr. Phil Chu succession crisis of 1970.

Alfred Scottolini, MD: The longstanding chief of pathology was a strong supporter of Dr. Dung during the 1975 leadership crisis.

Geoffrey Sewell, MD: He was the fourth and current executive medical director (president) of HPMG. His administration successfully implemented and improved upon previous established standards of Medical Group governance, quality, and service. This resulted in robust program growth and unprecedented levels of high physician morale and performance. This was recognized by the HPMG associates by ratifying him for a third term shortly after his second ratification. Barring unforeseen events, his term of office won't end until 2025.

Clifford Straehley, MD: He joined HPMG as a thoracic and vascular surgeon. He was one of the three founders of the University of Hawaii surgical training program. He established a surgery residency affiliation with the Stanford program. He was chief of surgical services and a strong supporter of quality assurance. He supported Dr. Dung during the 1975 leadership crisis.

Ben Tamura, MD: He was an excellent internal medicine physician and was very well-liked by all. He served as chief of medicine from

1997 until 2007 and then associate medical director of primary care from 2007 until 2017.

Cora Tellez: She was a protégé of James Vohs KP CEO (1970–1992). He appointed her associate regional president of the Hawaii region, reporting to Dan Wagster, and then succeeded Wagster in 1991. She successfully teamed up with Dr. Michael Chaffin to establish what began a decade-long period of cooperation between Health Plan and HPMG. This, in turn, led the program into a sustained period of success during the 1990s. She resigned in 1994 over philosophic conflicts with the direction the national KP leadership was taking as it was moving away from the traditional KP model. She went on to a successful executive career in health care.

Richele Thornburg: She was the Permanente Federation's executive vice president of leadership strategy and HPMG vice president of strategy, leadership, and communications. She is a dedicated, hardworking, and skilled HPMG and Permanente Federation events organizer. Her team's high level of professionalism is demonstrated organizing the Permanente Federation biannual Permanente Executive Leadership Meeting, and for HPMG anniversary dinners, region-wide Martin Luther King Day charitable events, Grand Rounds, and publications such as *Making Waves,* and much more. She and her team have been key to the high morale and unity of HPMG-characteristic of Geoff Sewell's administration. This history would not have been possible without her support.

Eugene Trefethen: One of the most important managers in Kaiser Industries, he had a practical, moderating effect on Mr. Kaiser and a special interest in the establishment of the Kaiser Permanente program. He recommended diversifying Henry Kaiser's physician choices for the first medical group to serve the members of his new Hawaii health plan. The Trefethen Winery was founded by his son and his daughter-in-law.

David Underriner: He was appointed president of the Hawaii region in 2018 to succeed Mary Ann Barnes. A believer in the partnership, under his leadership, Health Plan in Hawaii worked cooperatively with HPMG. He resigned approximately one year later as a result of a policy decision by Program Office, which he felt would be injurious to the region.

James Vohs: He was the second CEO of Kaiser Permanente from 1970 until 2002. A gentleman's gentleman, he believed deeply in the principles of Kaiser Permanente and managed according to those principles. His administration was a golden age for KP. During his administration, the program grew from 2.2 million members to 6.6 million members and grew from six to twelve regions. KP came as close as it ever would to becoming a national health care program.

A little known Voh's policy was that of Executive salaries. He felt that the manager of a non-profit organization should be limited. Even though KP was the largest corporation of its kind at the time, he limited his salary to $1 million dollars ($1.845 million in 2019), thus preventing other Kaiser Executives from having salaries that were higher than his CEO salary.

Hau Vu, MD: He joined HPMG as an obstetrician gynecologist in 1965. Energetic and with a flair for administration, he ran for medical director in a closely contested election after the death of Dr. Chu. He never really accepted the election of Dr. Dung and was the leader of one of the two main factions in HPMG. Nevertheless, he served as vice president of finance but left HPMG in 1975 when Dr. Dung reorganized the leadership of HPMG. He went on to an active clinical and administrative career in Southern California.

Dan Wagster: He was one of the most experienced administrators in the KP program. He had previously served as regional president of the Southern California and Northwest regions. The Hawaii appointment as regional president was to be his last operational appointment. His confrontational style did not work well in Hawaii, but he did work well with Dr. Dung, and he supported Cora Tellez as his associate regional manager and designated successor. He went on to coauthor the regional studies monograph with Dr. Bruce Sams, emeritus long-term medical director of Northern California. This excellent monograph was finished in 1993 but was tabled as the national program was embarking on a policy that was to de-emphasize the importance of the partnership and the regions.

Ron Wyatt: A former hospital administrator in the Ohio region, he was appointed Health Plan regional president for Hawaii in 1976. With his courtly style, he worked well with his HPMG partner, Dr. Dung, and HPMG itself. In 1986, he was replaced by Dan Wagster.

CREDITS

The author would like to thank the HPMG administration, especially Geoff Sewell, Leighton Hasegawa, and Richele Thornburg who provided steadfast encouragement, support, and cooperation. Vernon Hiroe, director of AV services of HPMG, gave invaluable assistance locating and preparing the illustrations and historical photographs. Lincoln Cushing, archivist for Kaiser Health Plan, provided valuable insights into the principles of preserving and archiving program historical documents.

Special appreciation is due to those who carefully read and made recommendations as to the content of the book, especially Steve Miller, MD—who also served as an editor— Cora Tellez, Leighton Hasegawa, Katrena Kennedy, Mark Santi, and Karl Pregitzer. Special thanks to Vernon Hiroe, Vorawat "Wally" Chaiprakorb, and Lincoln Cushing for their invaluable assistance in obtaining and processing the images. "Gully-Boy" Wilson, noted Hawaiian waterman, provided the insights related to the Kaiser Bowls surf spot.

Without the careful documentation of the early history of the program that was carefully preserved, especially by Sumi Croydon (forty-four years) and her successor Shelly Young (twenty years), the valuable primary source historical documents would not have been available. Thanks is also given to the family of William Dung, MD, the second and longest-serving (twenty-one years) medical director who presented to the author his private administrative diary for the critical years of 1975 to 1977 and for the many hours that Dr. Dung himself spent telling the author stories about the early history of the group. Further thanks are extended to those in KP who took the time to be interviewed for this book and then to review their interviews for accuracy. Many of the above also provided unvarnished but invaluable editing advice, especially my wife, partner, best friend, and companion, Aurora. Any errors in this book are unintentional, but they are my responsibility.

This story comes from the actions of all those within Kaiser Permanente who strived to advance the ideals of the program—often against long odds. It was a privilege to serve beside you. Finally, thanks go to my family, including my dedicated nephew/caregiver John Belizon, whose steadfast support and patience made this book possible.

A NOTE ON SOURCES

The core source of this book is the author's own memory of significant events in the history of HPMG between 1980 and 2009. From 1983 to retirement in late 2009, the author participated at the executive level in the governance of the Medical Group. Fully aware of the limitations of personal memory, especially for events that occurred decades ago, these memories were checked against the testimony of others and primary sources wherever possible.

Chief among the primary resources were the original archives of HPMG. The author archived, read, and created a HPMG timeline from the more than eight thousand pages of general staff meetings, board notes, presidential newsletters, and historically significant general circulation memos. Letters from Phil Chu to his Health Plan counterpart and Bill Dung's aforementioned private administrative diary, which were located and transcribed into the archive, gave important insights into the visionary thinking of these two key HPMG founders.

Three books were valuable secondary sources: *Can Physicians Manage the Quality and Costs of Health Care? The Story of the Permanente Medical Group* by John A. Smillie, MD, *The Story of Dr. Sidney R. Garfield: The Visionary Who Turned Sick Care into Health Care* by Tom Debley, and *Permanente in the Northwest* by Ian C. MacMillan, MD.

In the mid-1980s, Kaiser Permanente embarked upon a serious oral history program while most of the founders were still alive. Transcriptions of these comprehensive interviews are made available to the public by the Bancroft Library Regional Oral History Office of the University of California Berkeley. The oral histories of Robert J. Erickson, Scott Fleming, James Vohs, Drs. Cecil Cutting, Clifford Keene, and Ernest

Saward regarding the Hawaii region as additional primary sources were especially valuable.

Other primary sources included the *Honolulu Advertiser* and *Honolulu Star Bulletin* articles from late August to September 1960, which provided day-by-day reporting of the conflict between the Pacific Medical Associates and Henry Kaiser, which led to the founding of HPMG. The two newspapers combined to become the *Honolulu Star Advertiser* in 2010. These sources were supplemented by discussions and interviews with the founders of HPMG. Other cited newspaper and magazine accounts were also of value describing Henry Kaiser's impact on Hawaii, America, and the regional closures of the Texas, Northeast, North Carolina, Kansas City, and Ohio regions. The internet, if used properly, can be a valuable aid to historical research. In the case of this book, it guided the author to additional primary sources, such as the KP bond rating history from the late 1990s to early 2000s. Because of the widely variable reliability of internet information, every attempt was made to back up internet sources with a second independent source.

Among the most valuable primary sources resulted from the generosity of those who consented to interviews from their time in KP. They included Cora Tellez, Bruce Behnke, and Kaki Jennings. A 2011 interview with Drs. Morris Collin and Fred Pellegrin provided eyewitness accounts into the early days of the Permanente Medical Group, Tahoe I, and Henry Kaiser's thinking about his new health care program in Hawaii. That interview was recorded for the national Kaiser Permanente archives in 2011. An interview with Jim Vohs in 2013, twenty-one years after he retired as KP CEO and arranged by Cora Tellez, filled in many blanks. Interviews, formal and informal, were granted by HPMG founders: Drs. William Dung, Marciano Aquino, Argyl Bacon, and Yi Ching. They provided insights into the early days of HPMG. Contributors from the middle generation included Gladys Ching, Mike Linderman, Drs. Michael Chaffin, Steven Miller, Karl Pregitzer, Christine Fukui, Peggy Latare, and Peter Clapp, and many others. Interviews with the current generation included Janet Liang, Mary Anne Barnes from Health Plan, Leighton Hasegawa, Richele Thornburg, Sally Lee from HPMG administration, and HPMG Drs. Geoffrey Sewell, Mark Santi, David D. Bell, Michael Caps, James Griffith, and Keith

Ogasawara brought the history up to date. For those whose names I must have missed please accept my sincere apologies.

Permission to use the images was given by the kind cooperation of the Kaiser Permanente National Archives, the Hawaii Permanente Medical Group Archives, and the *Honolulu Star Advertiser*:

Kaiser Permanente Archives: Images 1–7, 12–14, 18, 25, 28. Hawaii Permanente Medical Group Archives: Images 15–17, 19–24, 25–35. *Honolulu Star Advertiser*: Images 8–11.

Proceeds from the sale of this book will be contributed to the Hawaii Permanente Medical Group Charitable Foundation.

INDEX

K

L

M

CPSIA information can be obtained
at www.ICGtesting.com
Printed in the USA
LVHW112304261120
672805LV00028B/102